Fourth Edition

INTRODUCTION TO
NURSING
RESEARCH

Incorporating Evidence-Based Practice

The Pedagogy

Introduction to Nursing Research: Incorporating Evidence-Based Practice, Fourth Edition drives comprehension through various strategies that meet the learning needs of students, while also generating enthusiasm about the topic. This interactive approach addresses different learning styles, making this the ideal text to ensure mastery of key concepts. The pedagogical aids that appear in most chapters include the following:

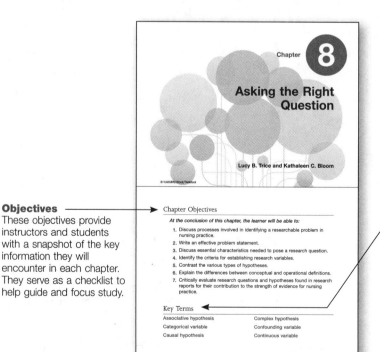

Chapter **8**

Asking the Right Question

Lucy B. Trice and Kathaleen C. Bloom

© VLADGRIN/iStock/Thinkstock

Chapter Objectives

At the conclusion of this chapter, the learner will be able to:

1. Discuss processes involved in identifying a researchable problem in nursing practice.
2. Write an effective problem statement.
3. Discuss essential characteristics needed to pose a research question.
4. Identify the criteria for establishing research variables.
5. Contrast the various types of hypotheses.
6. Explain the differences between conceptual and operational definitions.
7. Critically evaluate research questions and hypotheses found in research reports for their contribution to the strength of evidence for nursing practice.

Key Terms

Associative hypothesis
Categorical variable
Causal hypothesis

Complex hypothesis
Confounding variable
Continuous variable

Objectives
These objectives provide instructors and students with a snapshot of the key information they will encounter in each chapter. They serve as a checklist to help guide and focus study.

Key Terms
Found in a list at the beginning of each chapter, these terms will create an expanded vocabulary.

Table 8-1

Problem Statements

Declarative Statement Format	Question Format
Music therapy decreases the level of maternal anxiety during cesarean section.	Does music therapy decrease the level of maternal anxiety during cesarean section?
Nursing home residents who participate in regular exercise have fewer falls than those who do not.	Do nursing home residents who participate in regular exercise have fewer falls than those who do not?
Participation in a support group improves morale in family caregivers of Alzheimer's patients.	Does participation in a support group improve morale in family caregivers of Alzheimer's patients?
Diabetic patients who perceive themselves as obese will participate in a weight management program.	Will diabetic patients who perceive themselves as obese participate in a weight management program?
The number of medication errors made by nurses increases when the number of medications per patient is greater than three (3).	Does the number of medication errors made by nurses increase when the number of medications per patient is greater than three (3)?

❓ **THINK OUTSIDE THE BOX**

Identify the elements of the PICOT format for each of the problem statements in Table 8-1.

Think Outside the Box
Students can work on these critical thinking assignments individually or in a group while reading through the text.

■ **Hypotheses**

A research question asks whether a relationship exists between variables in a particular population. In contrast, a **hypothesis** stipulates or predicts the relationship that exists. For example, if the research question is "Does the presence of a parent in the room affect the anxiety level in children ages 3–5 years undergoing initiation of intravenous therapy?", then we might develop several hypotheses:

1. The presence of a parent in the room affects the anxiety level in children ages 3–5 years who undergo initiation of intravenous therapy.
2. The presence of a parent in the room reduces the anxiety level in children ages 3–5 years who undergo initiation of intravenous therapy.
3. The presence of a parent in the room has no effect on the anxiety level in children ages 3–5 years who undergo initiation of intravenous therapy.
4. The presence of a parent in the room increases the anxiety level in children ages 3–5 years who undergo initiation of intravenous therapy.

⚠️ **RED FLAGS**

- Quantitative studies address research problems, research questions, and/or hypotheses.
- Qualitative studies do not use hypotheses, but rather explore research problems and research questions. If a qualitative study discusses a hypothesis, thought should be given to its focus and validity.
- A hypothesis must have at least one independent variable and one dependent variable; it is usually stated in a declarative statement format rather than as a question.
- Key variables within a study should have at least the operational definition provided for consideration.

Red Flags
At the end of every chapter, these bullet points alert students to areas in research that may raise concern.

Multiple-Choice Questions

1. Developing a research study to investigate the availability of health care for minority children whose families are on welfare is an example of a research problem generated primarily from:

    A. Practice.
    B. Social issues.
    C. Healthcare trends in society.
    D. Theory.

2. Problems involving moral or ethical issues are not researchable because:

    A. They are too costly to perform.
    B. Most researchers are not interested in these studies.
    C. They are based on individual values.
    D. Data collection is problematic.

3. Determining if studying the problem will lead to results that are applicable to nursing practice is essential when analyzing the _____ of the problem.

    A. Feasibility
    B. Profitability
    C. Cost
    D. Significance

4. Which of the following topics would be inappropriate for a researchable problem?

    A. The morality of abortion as a form of birth control
    B. The relationship between cigarette smoking and weight loss
    C. The effect of severe dietary restrictions on wellbeing
    D. The relationship between religious beliefs and pain perception

5. Which of the following is the best example of a problem statement containing all parts of the PICOT format?

    A. Children whose parents stay with them experience less pain.
    B. Hospitalized patients who have a relative with them experience less pain than those who do not.
    C. Hospitalized children ages 3–5 years whose parents stay with them during painful procedures experience less pain than those who do not.
    D. Patients who have a relative with them during a transfusion will experience less anxiety than those who do not.

6. Which of the following best represents a well-constructed problem statement?

    A. What affects pain perception?
    B. Obesity negatively impacts self-image in first graders.
    C. This study will compare the effectiveness of antacids.
    D. Does time of day affect appetite?

Multiple-Choice Questions
Review key concepts with these questions at the end of each chapter.

Discussion Questions
Students can use these assignments to apply information in the text to everyday practice.

Discussion Questions

1. You work in a cardiology clinic that treats patients who have coronary artery disease and are recovering from a myocardial infarction. Many of these patients have hypertension and are overweight, and you have noticed that some of them have more difficulty following their medical regimens than others. You want to develop a research study to investigate this problem. How would you go about doing so? What would be a possible problem statement?

2. You are a BSN student enrolled in a research course. The instructor has given you the following problem statement: "Does completion of a mandatory health promotion course affect the incidence of smoking cessation among college students who smoke?" Develop four hypotheses that might be drawn from this problem statement: a null hypothesis, a directional hypothesis, a nondirectional hypothesis, and an associative hypothesis. Can all of these hypotheses be developed? If any of them cannot be developed, why not?

3. Read the abstract and then provide the following information:

    a. Identify the population of interest.
    b. Identify the variables.
    c. Construct a research question that could have guided this study.
    d. Construct a null hypothesis.
    e. Construct a directional hypothesis.

Abstract: A major goal in the care of patients with neurological problems is to prevent or minimize episodes of increased intracranial pressure (ICP). Elevations in ICP in response to nursing interventions have been acknowledged since the 1960s when ICP monitoring was first introduced in the clinical setting. Until recently, few studies have specifically examined the effect of oral care on ICP, and oral care and other hygiene measures were combined or not specified, prohibiting a direct interpretation of the influence of oral care alone on ICP. The purpose of this study was to describe the relationship between routine oral care interventions and the changes in ICP, specifically focusing on the effect of intensity and duration of this intervention. Twenty-three patients with a clinical condition requiring ICP monitoring were enrolled over a 12-month period. Oral care provided by neuroscience intensive care nurses was observed and videotaped. Characteristics of the intervention were documented including products used, patient positioning, and duration of the intervention. A subjective scale of 1–5 was used to score intensity of oral care. Wrist actigraphy data were collected from the nurses to provide an objective measure of intensity. Patient physiologic data were collected at 12-second epochs 5 minutes before, during, and 5 minutes after oral care. The mixed-effect repeated measures analysis of variance model indicated that there was a statistically significant increase in ICP in response to oral care ($P = 0.0031$). There was, however, no clinically significant effect on ICP. This study provides evidence that oral care is safe to perform in patients in the absence of preexisting elevated ICP. (Szabo, Grap, Munro, Starkweather, & Merchant, 2014)

Fourth Edition

INTRODUCTION TO NURSING RESEARCH

Incorporating Evidence-Based Practice

EDITED BY

Carol Boswell, EdD, RN, CNE, ANEF, FAAN
Professor
Texas Tech University
Odessa, Texas

Sharon Cannon, EdD, RN, ANEF
Regional Dean and Professor
Texas Tech University
Odessa, Texas

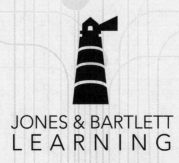

JONES & BARTLETT
LEARNING

World Headquarters
Jones & Bartlett Learning
5 Wall Street
Burlington, MA 01803
978-443-5000
info@jblearning.com
www.jblearning.com

Jones & Bartlett Learning books and products are available through most bookstores and online booksellers. To contact Jones & Bartlett Learning directly, call 800-832-0034, fax 978-443-8000, or visit our website, www.jblearning.com.

Substantial discounts on bulk quantities of Jones & Bartlett Learning publications are available to corporations, professional associations, and other qualified organizations. For details and specific discount information, contact the special sales department at Jones & Bartlett Learning via the above contact information or send an email to specialsales@jblearning.com.

10895-8

Production Credits

VP, Executive Publisher: David D. Cella
Executive Editor: Amanda Martin
Associate Acquisitions Editor: Rebecca Myrick
Editorial Assistant: Danielle Bessette
Production Editor: Vanessa Richards
Senior Marketing Manager: Jennifer Scherzay
VP, Manufacturing and Inventory Control: Therese Connell

Cover Design: Michael O'Donnell
Rights & Media Specialist: Merideth Tumasz
Media Development Editor: Shannon Sheehan
Composition: Integra Software Services Pvt. Ltd.
Cover Image: © VLADGRIN/iStock/Thinkstock
Printing and Binding: Edwards Brothers Malloy
Cover Printing: Edwards Brothers Malloy

Library of Congress Cataloging-in-Publication Data
Introduction to nursing research : incorporating evidence-based practice / edited by Carol Boswell, Sharon Cannon. — Fourth edition.
    p. ; cm.
Includes bibliographical references and index.
ISBN 978-1-284-07965-4 (pbk.)
I. Boswell, Carol, editor. II. Cannon, Sharon, 1940– editor.
[DNLM: 1. Nursing Research—methods. 2. Evidence-Based Nursing. WY 20.5]
RT81.5
610.72—dc23
                                        2015025807
6048
Printed in the United States of America
19 18 17 16 15   10 9 8 7 6 5 4 3 2 1

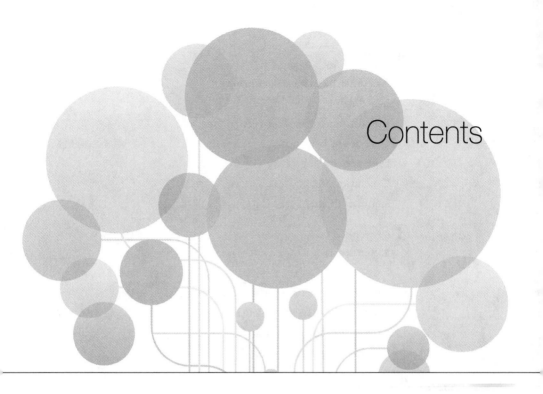

Contents

JoAnn Long, Carol Boswell, and Donna Scott Tilley

Sharon Cannon, Theresa Delahoyde, and Jane Sumner

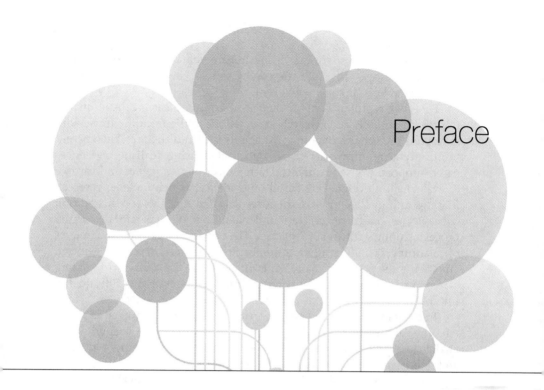

Preface

Research, quality improvement, and evidence-based practice must go hand in hand as nursing knowledge grows and develops. Healthcare changes resulting from the Patient Protection and Affordable Care Act, the Institute of Medicine's 2010 report *The Future of Nursing: Leading Change, Advancing Health*, and other challenges require nurses to embrace and advance nursing knowledge through these different evidence-development formats. Evidence-based practice (EBP) has progressed into a decisive component for authenticating quality health care. The concept of evidence-based practice requires the integration of clinical expertise with investigational corroboration from evidence, which includes research. Nurses must integrate consistent and judicious evidence into policies and procedures. These EBP-based policies and procedures are utilized for the provision of holistic health care. The public expects that each skill or task completed using a particular technique is justified by evidence.

In this text, fundamental research information is presented using evidence-based research examples. Each of the concepts associated with the research process are covered. In addition, the information concerning the interconnectedness of research, EBP, and quality improvement is discussed. Another aspect included in this text is the growth and development of understanding about what makes up the scope of evidence. This undertaking strives to make the information pertinent and appropriate to nurses working in healthcare venues and who are motivated to engage in EBP. Research should be FUN (functional, understandable, and nonthreatening).

This text represents the challenge to communicate realistic quality improvement, EBP, and research expectations to the frontline nurse who is responsible for the ongoing management of health care. The current health arena requires that care be instituted using realistic, evidence-based support. Consequently, the nurse must be competent and capable to evaluate and initiate care based on evidence, which includes research findings and quality improvement results. The stimulus for this edition concentrates on furnishing an understanding of preparatory research processes along with an EBP mind set. The crucial and cardinal techniques of planning, conducting, and reporting research data are depicted employing the perspective of EBP. Every aspect in the delivery of nursing care requires painstaking deliberation and documentation of EBP, quality improvement, and research outcomes for the care provided.

To contemplate these challenges, this edition was organized to facilitate the nurse in the management of analyzing the strengths and challenges evident in research projects, quality improvement reports, and published reports/manuscripts. By acquiring expertise about which aspects indicate strong evidence, nurses can utilize applicable research findings and quality improvement results with other evidence while disregarding inappropriate findings. It was envisioned that this edition would function as the prevailing text in research and EBP courses presented at universities and as a practical and constructive resource for practicing nurses who are engaged in EBP.

For use within this text, two articles are primarily used as examples to illustrate chapter concepts. Each chapter pulls from these articles to showcase the components being discussed within the materials. The qualitative article is:

Iverson, K. M., Huang, K., Wells, S. Y., Wright, J. D., Gerber, M. R., & Wiltsey-Stirman, S. (2014). Women veterans' preferences for intimate partner violence screening and response procedures within the Veterans Health Administration. *Research in Nursing & Health, 37,* 302–311. doi:10.1002/nur.21602.

The quantitative article is:

Hanna, K. M., Weaver, M. T., Slaven, J. F., Fortenberry, J. D., & DiMeglio, L. A. (2014). Diabetes-related quality of life and the demands and burdens of diabetes care among emerging adults with type 1 diabetes in the year after high school graduation. *Research in Nursing & Health, 37,* 399–408. doi:10.1002/nur.21620.

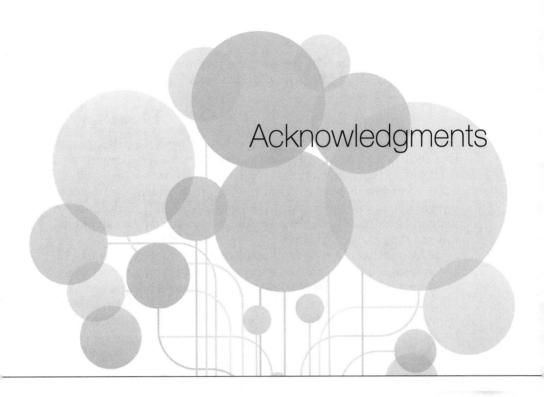

Acknowledgments

We would like to communicate our appreciation and respect for our outstanding colleagues who enthusiastically and cooperatively consented to the management of updating the designated chapters. The significance and usefulness of this text result from the expertise and proficiency of the contributing authors, to whom we are immensely grateful. Several new colleagues have joined us in this edition to provide interesting and applicable information related to the different subjects.

We continue to value the first and previous edition reviewers for their conscientious analysis of the chapters, which provided real-life examples in clinical settings and facilitated the focus of the chapter content. From their observations, we were able to preserve the scholarly level of the text. Comments and suggestions provided by the numerous users of the text provided insights for inclusion into each new edition. The suggestions and recommendations provided by the end-users have been constructive in helping to keep the original intent of this text intact. Within the current edition, we emphasize the idea of evidence being imperative to advancing the field of EBP, quality improvement, and nursing research. We continue our grateful recognition of Mary E. Nunnally, who provided her strong editorial perspective to earlier editions.

Dr. Carol Boswell and Dr. Sharon Cannon

Every once in a while, our lives are enhanced by very special people. One such person is my friend and colleague, Dr. Carol Boswell, who continues to diligently seek new opportunities. Many wonderful colleagues and friends have enriched my life through their loyal support, especially our colleagues who have joined us on this evidence-based journey. I have truly been blessed to know them and try each day to pay forward their many kindnesses.

My family has played a significant part in the shaping of my life. So, I wish to say a special thank you to my parents G. E. and Laurine Cannon (who are always with me in spirit); my family, especially Joe and Lynn Tischner, and Ryan Ganey; my grandchildren, Kelly Tischner, Andrew Ganey, Shelby Ganey, and Shannon Ganey; and my brother and sister-in-law, Gene and Cathi Cannon.

Dr. Sharon Cannon

As this text moves into the fourth edition, the individuals who persist in allowing me to mature, flourish, and stretch for the stars are Dr. Sharon Cannon; Marc E. Boswell; Dwight and Wanda Miller; Michael and Casey Boswell, Jeremy Boswell, and Stephanie Boswell; Matthew Boswell, Kobe Boswell, Kayia Howard, and Caleb Boswell. Each of these individuals keeps me grounded while providing me numerous opportunities to laugh both with them and at myself. They are truly my cheering section; thus, providing me encouragement and support. In addition to these magnificent and astonishing individuals, I want to recognize the awesome colleagues who enter my professional and personal life. These individuals bestow inspiration and passion to continue on a journey to magnify and advance the knowledge related to evidence-based practice, quality improvement, and nursing research. To be challenged to strive for the mountaintops and stars is a treasured and astonishing conviction to embrace. With the inspiration and confidence of my family and friends, I have been able to confront and overcome the insanity and idiocy of the world while welcoming the veracity of a person's humanity.

Dr. Carol Boswell

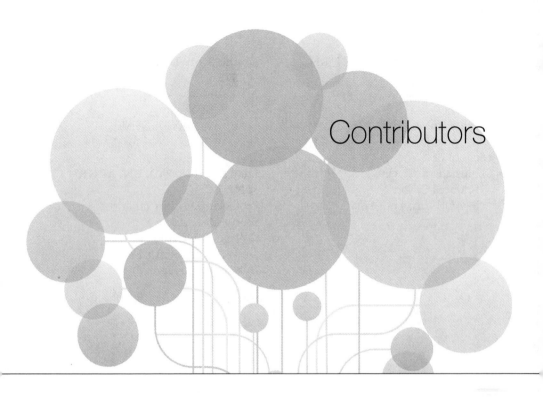

Contributors

Kathaleen C. Bloom, PhD, ARNP, CNM
Associate Professor
School of Nursing
College of Health
University of North Florida
Jacksonville, Florida

Theresa Delahoyde, EdD, RN
Dean of Undergraduate Nursing
Bryan College of Health Sciences
Lincoln, Nebraska

Pam DiVito-Thomas, PhD, RN, CNE
Professor of Nursing
Methodist College UnityPoint Health
Peoria, Illinois

James Eldridge, PhD
Associate Professor
University of Texas of the Permian Basin
Odessa, Texas

Dorothy Greene Jackson, PhD, RN, FNP
Assistant Professor/Director
School of Nursing
University of Texas of the Permian Basin
Odessa, Texas

JoAnn Long, PhD, RN, NEA-BC
Associate Professor
Department of Nursing
Lubbock Christian University
Lubbock, Texas

Margaret Robinson, MSN, RN
Retired
Midland, Texas

Jane Sumner, PhD, RN
Associate Professor of Nursing
School of Nursing
Louisiana State University Health
  Sciences Center
New Orleans, Louisiana

**Donna Scott Tilley, PhD, RN,
  CNE**
Associate Professor
College of Nursing
Texas Woman's University
Denton, Texas

**Lucy B. Trice, PhD, RN, ARNP,
  FNP-BC**
Professor, Director Emeritus
School of Nursing
College of Health
University of North Florida
Jacksonville, Florida

Connection Between Research and Evidence-Based Practice

Carol Boswell and Sharon Cannon

Chapter Objectives

At the conclusion of this chapter, the learner will be able to:

1. Identify the need for research to validate evidence-based practice.
2. Define evidence-based practice.
3. Discuss obstacles to evidence-based research.
4. Examine the nurse's role in evidence-based practice.
5. State how evidence-based practice impacts nursing practice.

Key Terms

Evidence-based practice (EBP)	Research
Obstacle	Research process
PICOT	Research utilization

Introduction

Regardless of the specific healthcare setting a nurse may select for practicing the art and science of nursing care, the overarching principle for the practice is the provision of quality nursing care to all clients without consideration of social, financial, cultural, ethnic, or other individual characteristics. As the nurse initiates contact with the client, the client should be confident that the care provided by that nurse is based on the most current, up-to-date health information available. Having established the currency of the health information to be utilized, the nurse and client must also agree that individualized application of this information is necessary. (Although the healthcare field defines "client" and "patient" differently, for the purposes of this text, these terms are used interchangeably.) Thus, the need for **evidence-based practice (EBP)** is confirmed by our expectations related to nursing care.

The nurse who receives the assignment to care for an elderly woman, a young child, or a critically ill man must come to the nursing practice arena with more than the latest information. The information must be tested and confirmed. To see how this works, let's consider the idea of cardiac information, although any disease process could be utilized for this purpose. Within nursing practice, certain health information concerning the management of cardiac complications such as a myocardial infarction is accepted. The initial question that should be asked by a nurse would be: Is this disease management information corroborated by research results? The answer to this question is frequently an unsure response by the nurse. Too often, the healthcare provider delivers the care because it is the known process or because it has been ordered instead of providing care based upon the evidence found within the profession. Yoder and colleagues (2014) found that "staff nurses perceive finding and using research evidence as an esoteric activity that lies beyond their immediate responsibilities" (p. 35). However, the informational basis for each aspect of the nursing care to be provided should be analyzed to determine its source and the strength of the information. Does the information come from general usage, or is it information that has been established through research or other critical analyses to be accurate?

Having determined the basis for the care to be provided, the nurse must then determine the application of the information based on the individuality of the client situation. The application of the information for each client situation depends on the specifics of the client's needs, the client's expectations concerning health, and many other aspects requiring modification of the confirmed knowledge application. The foundation of nursing care delivery must be research-tested, research-confirmed, and/or critically analyzed knowledge, tempered by an awareness of the unique characteristics of the client and the situation.

Pravikoff, Tanner, and Pierce (2005) describe the process of EBP as including assessing and delineating a problem through verbalization of an identifiable question, pursuing and evaluating the available facts, implementing a practice intervention as a result of the evidence, and evaluating the entire process for effectiveness. Initially, EBP requires the identification of the practice problem, followed by the utilization of tested research and other evidential results to improve the care provided to the clients. According to Conner (2014), the essential assessment questions are interchangeable—whether the clinical question involves treatment, diagnosis, outcomes, or causation:

- Are the conclusions of the study convincing?
- Which outcomes were recognized?
- Will the results facilitate the management of the patient's care?

It was this need to incorporate proven practices into the provision of health care that fostered the expectations and development of EBP in the current healthcare arena. Bucknall (2012) notes that cognitive approaches, intuition, and analysis of information play key roles in how evidence is acknowledged, evaluated, and incorporated into the clinical decision-making process that impacts patient outcomes. Clinical decisions are frequently not corroborated by unambiguous, persuasive evidence. Nurses are asked to make real-world decisions with limited information in a fast-paced environment. Time is valuable to the nurse at the bedside, so any course of action has to be both practical and rational (Cannon & Boswell, 2010). This responsibility to make knowledgeable, well-supported decisions based on sound facts emphasizes the need to become effective and efficient at EBP, quality improvement (QI), and research utilization.

Conner (2014) states that the purpose of QI is to provide "a systematic, data-guided approach to improve processes or outcomes" (p. 3). The idea of QI is directed toward the improvement of patient outcomes. QI does tend to be site specific, which is one of the key aspects where it differs from research. The goal of the results obtained from a QI project is not to have information that is generalizable to another site, nor is it to set up the results as best practices. However, when multiple sites discover the same outcomes from consistent QI projects, the data then move toward best practices.

◼ Providing a Line of Reasoning for EBP and Evidence-Based Research

Health care is a complex system addressing multiple health-related aspects in an attempt to accomplish the anticipated outcome for the client. Throughout the healthcare arena, nursing care is provided to individuals in need of assistance related to their health status. This attention requires nurses to identify a core foundation of information that reflects quality care. Thus, the need for EBP to be developed around a research-centered foundation was envisioned.

Malloch and Porter-O'Grady (2015) suggested that the management of EBP requires the use of unique clinical applications based on accessible, up-to-date research. In the quest for quality nursing care, the nurse must use both reliable clinical knowledge and high-quality clinical information. This process of establishing a core foundation of knowledge has been called many things over the years, such as best practices, evidence-based practice, and quality of care. No matter what the practice is called, the basis for the care to be provided must be grounded in evidence. According to Melnyk and Fineout-Overholt (2015), healthcare providers must be able to locate, analyze, evaluate, and use the significant evidence to ensure that patients are certain and convinced that their providers are basing care on evidence for optimal outcomes. It is this assurance that the care being provided is confirmed from a tested research/evidence foundation that inspires patient confidence in the nurses' commitment to quality health care. Nurses should not rely on unsubstantiated treatment plans, but rather must endeavor to critically analyze aspects of the care to be provided to be sure that quality, tested practices are utilized in the provision of nursing care for each individual.

Three new developments in health care and nursing have had an impact on the understanding of the importance of EBP and research in nursing in the United States. First, in 2010, the Patient Protection and Affordable Care Act (PPACA), also known as the Affordable Care Act (ACA), was passed by Congress and signed by President Barack Obama (Mason, Leavitt, & Chaffee, 2012). Catalano (2015) suggests the ACA will result in nursing responding to societal needs with increased attention while still maintaining the previous nursing focus. While the ACA has a primary focus on affordable, accessible care, an emphasis on supporting research effecting safe, quality patient care is vital at this time. Nurses are being asked to step into the lead roles for community health, along with preventive health management. The Health Resources and Services Administration (HRSA; 2014) confirms this perception by stating that within the new models of health care, innovative roles for nurses with new opportunities for advancement will be realized. As nurses provide patient-centered care, nurses will increasingly find themselves actively engaged in EBP and research projects.

The second development in 2010 came from the Carnegie Foundation recommendation in a report by Benner, Sutphen, Leonard, and Day (2010) calling for radical transformations of nursing education. Two of their recommendations support the need for nurses to have an education grounded in inquiry and research to provide evidence-based care. For the educational community, attention must be given to ensuring that nurses coming out of the programs understand and incorporate EBP into the essence of the practice of providing holistic nursing care.

The third development came from the Institute of Medicine (IOM; 2011) and the Robert Wood Johnson Foundation (RWJF) report regarding the future of nursing. This report urged funding for collaborative nursing projects with other healthcare professionals, so that research can involve nurses in developing models of care and solutions to improve health and health care. They identified eight research priorities for nursing practice and nursing education. The priorities for research included areas such as delivery models, reimbursement, care trends, nurse residencies, and funding for nurses' training. Herlehy (2011) authenticates the ideas set forth by the report to "underscore nurses' unique contributions and capacity to enhance the quality of care through practice, education, and leadership" (p. 519). Nursing brings to the table aptitudes and competences that reinforce and advocate for safe and quality health care for all generations and cultures. The incorporation of EBP, research, and QI provides the fortification and reinforcement of the evidence needed to provide effective and efficient health care in multiple settings.

These three new recommendations require nurses to examine their knowledge, skills and, most important, their values about EBP and research. Each of these three developments has provided further clarification of the expectations for safe, effective care to every individual encountering healthcare issues. By looking at how to best address the burdensome aspects of health care through effective utilization of key providers allows for the successful management of health challenges.

The practicing nurse has to value the ideas of the EBP process, research, and QI to facilitate its complete incorporation and implementation. Nurses must understand the value of integrating carefully analyzed results from research, QI, and other sources with personal experiences and client values when determining the treatment plan

---

❓ THINK OUTSIDE THE BOX

Make a list of tasks that are routinely done by nurses during a typical clinical day. Carefully consider what evidence could be used as the foundation for these tasks. Are the skills for the tasks in your practice setting based on research, personal preferences, clinical guidelines, or traditions?

that best addresses a situation's identified challenges. Even when healthcare providers utilize the most advantageous evidence accessible, each engagement with an individual continues to be distinctive. The treatments and outcomes will change based on the uniqueness of the client's values, preferences, interests, and/or diagnoses. According to Fonteyn (2005), "A bonus of nurses' involvement in EBP activities is their improved ability to think critically and their increased understanding of and comfort with research, all of which seems to perpetuate their interest and success in subsequent EBP pursuits" (p. 439). Nurses are taught, encouraged, and expected to think critically. This process of critical thinking corresponds to the use of EBP on clinical units and in primary care settings. Critical thinking embraces the need for health care to be based on a foundation of proven research and other tested data while including the client's perspective. The use of unconfirmed reports, hearsay, and unfounded information, combined with a lack of client input, does not fit with the provision of sound, quality nursing care at this point in time. The evolution of EBP has moved the focus of client-centered care to the forefront of nursing care.

Fineout-Overholt and Melnyk (2005) state that continuous opportunities for learning EBP must be given to providers to enhance and sharpen EBP skills for posing searchable, answerable questions, locating the optimal evidence that can be accessed, while competently and proficiently evaluating research and evidence reports for establishing significant evidence vital for encouraging an evidence-based environment in which to practice. A key element within the effective provision of EBP is the nurse's expertise. Each nurse brings serviceable knowledge to the practice arena. During the process of providing nursing care to a group of individuals, nurses build an underpinning of knowledge on which they draw when delivering future care. This underpinning knowledge base intensifies and expands with each client encounter that the nurse has. Thus, the knowledge base is not stagnant, but rather increases throughout an individual's nursing career. A competent nurse uses each healthcare encounter to augment and strengthen their knowledge base.

Jolley (2002) articulated the expectation that practicing nurses should retrieve, generate, and use various and diverse categories of evidence, including research, to ascertain appropriate clinical practices. Even if nurses are not actively involved in an actual research project, they must understand the method for accessing published information and assessing it for applicability. Bator, Taylor, and Catalano (2015) propose that nursing research is essential, and nurses educated at all levels must use research and EBP to improve the care of patients. Rolston-Blenman (2009) supports this idea by stating that management must identify the solid foundational truths that every system is intended to accomplish as it attains any identified outcome. We all know that individuals rise to the level to which we expect them to rise: If we set low expectations, they will rise to meet the expected level of performance. If we establish challenging expectations, they will strive to attain them. At times, a knowledge base is unconsciously incorporated, because the nurse seems to manage the nursing care without directly acknowledging the underlying foundation. This process or intuition grows as the nurse gains experience and expertise.

Research is a methodical examination that uses regimented techniques to resolve questions or decipher dilemmas. The conclusions resulting from this focused chain of examination provide a base upon which to build a practice of care that is centered on tested solutions. According to Omery and Williams (1999), research is a scientific process using intrinsic expertise to clarify and envisage as it augments a discipline's capacity to foresee and target relations. This anticipation and guidance are related to a discipline's ability to incorporate into practice the sound evidence derived from valid research endeavors. Although EBP goes beyond research results, the foundation for the practice is the grounded knowledge that comes from the research process and QI. This underpinning allows for the safe and effective provision of quality health care. According to Melnyk and Fineout-Overholt (2015), the publishing of research and other evidence along with the translation into practice to advance patient care takes too long and is a source of anxiety in healthcare organizations and federal agencies. Moving the use of researched evidence into the actual patient care setting requires that nurses become increasingly familiar and comfortable with the process of critiquing and applying the evidence to the practice arena.

Each of these aspects—thought process, client preferences, research, and nursing expertise—is included in the EBP definition used in this text (**Figure 1-1**). Although all of these aspects are required, the actual situation directs the weighting of the aspects, because each situation is unique. Melnyk (2004) acknowledges that a consistent, hard-and-fast weighting of the different pieces—research, patient values, and clinician's expertise—included in EBP is not possible, because the decision-making process is contingent on the situation. In this text, EBP is defined as a process of using confirmed evidence (research and quality improvement), decision making, and nursing expertise to guide the delivery of holistic patient care by nurses. Holistic nursing care encompasses the clinical expertise of the nurse, patient preferences, cultural aspects, psychosocial facets, ethical considerations, and biological components. The research process and scientific data generated serve as the foundation on which the decision-making process for nursing care is based.

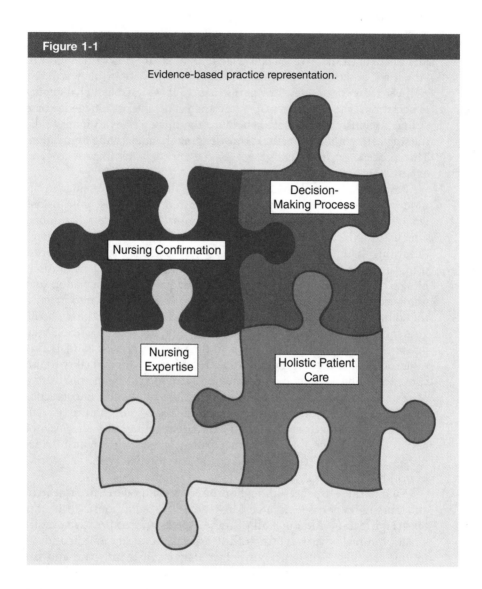

Figure 1-1

Evidence-based practice representation.

Assessing the Need for Research in the Practice Arena

According to Davies (2002), moving research evidence along with other types of evidence into the practice arena is a multifaceted process that requires shifting provider behavior. This process is challenging even when the comparative rewards are compelling and robust. The nurse is essential to the success of the EBP process. Each nurse, whether in the acute care, home health, community health, or other healthcare setting, regularly identifies nursing aspects of care. Those aspects of care may seem to (1) appropriately address the care needs of the client, (2) not fit the current accepted provision of care, or (3) be better addressed via some other method of care. According to Laskowski-Jones (2015), "if nurses don't read and evaluate whether or not research findings have relevance to this work, they run the risk of practicing in a way that's either ineffective or possibly even deleterious to patient care" (p. 6). Most nurses have at some point in their practice identified a situation that needs to be reevaluated. Within the day-to-day provision of nursing care, the question arises about why we perform a procedure a certain way when something else seems to work better. It could also be a question of how the care can be better provided to meet the client's needs and expectations. The healthcare community is also encouraging this line of questioning in an effort to identify the best methods for the provision of care. The expectation behind EBP is that everyone will become involved in the identification, examination, and implementation of research-founded, evidence-tested health care that can result in the provision of effective, validated client care. Nurses must accept the responsibility of being active in providing quality care to their clients. To do so effectively, they must base the provision of care on results that support the care being administered in a wide variety of healthcare settings.

Cronenwett (2002) discussed the slow process for moving evidence of any type into the practice arena results from scientists endeavoring to ascertain initially what works in controlled environments followed by what works in daily clinical practice. Bator, Taylor, and Catalano (2015) suggest it takes more than 20 years for research findings to be accepted into practice. The application of research results in the everyday provision of nursing care takes both time and energy by each and every nurse to ensure that the quality of care is appropriate. All nurses have the responsibility of ensuring that the care they provide to their clients is based on sound nursing knowledge, not just "the way we have always done it." Cronenwett (2002) has further identified the need to challenge clinical community partners to become increasingly involved up front in the recognition of the problem and the development of the intervention, which includes new research opportunities. Practicing nurses must become actively engaged at multiple levels of the different phases of the research endeavor. At each phase, the nurse's clinical expertise should be readily valued as the process moves forward to establish the evidence for use in the clinical setting.

Outcomes research is a growing expectation within health care. The provision of quality health practices requires that individuals strive to comprehend and recognize the outcomes from specific and individual healthcare routines and interventions (Agency for Healthcare Research and Quality, 2000). Outcomes research is viewed as a mechanism for determining which quality care is possible and how to get to that point of significance and usefulness for the patient. The linkage of outcomes experienced with the care expected empowers research to cultivate improved channels for monitoring and improving the quality of care provided within the healthcare arena. Translational research is an endeavor that seeks to move the evidence that has been collected by effective research projects into the actual provision of health care. Nurses at the bedside must become champions for the inclusion of timely, documented, substantiated results into the active provision of health care to benefit clients confronted with the relevant health issues.

Titler, Everett, and Adams (2007) discuss the notion of implementation science as "the investigation of methods, interventions, and variables that influence adoption of evidence-based healthcare practices by individuals and organizations to improve clinical and operational decision making and including testing the effectiveness of interventions to promote and sustain use of evidence-based healthcare practices" (p. S53). It is through the use of concepts such as implementation science that **research** (conducting of research), **research utilization** (application of research), QI, and EBP are coming together for the improvement of healthcare delivery. As nurses learn to appreciate the importance of investigating the different routines, interventions, and obstacles within the provision of quality care, innovative and tested systems of healthcare delivery and skills will become increasingly available and accepted. The idea behind clarifying the process of research is to enable practicing nurses to utilize the scientific thought process to validate and augment the nursing care provided to clients. The entire process of critiquing research articles and conducting research projects is designed to strengthen the nursing professional's critical thinking abilities, thereby allowing for the delivery of the most holistic care possible in the work environment. An indispensable skill required for effective EBP is the capability of professionals to analytically scrutinize all types of results and evidence to clarify the optimal data to employ in the provision of holistic health care on a day-to-day basis. Without this foundation, which enables them to methodically examine the evidence, nurses are left to vacillate among varying interpretations of healthcare information. As mentioned earlier, the ACA, IOM/RWJF, and Carnegie Foundation reports of 2010 leave no room for nurses to ignore the need for research in the practice arena. Having defined research and established the need for research, an examination of EBP is in order.

❓ THINK OUTSIDE THE BOX

Look at the different definitions for evidence-based practice. How do you see patient preferences meshing with research utilization? How can nurses' expertise be effectively incorporated into sound nursing care management?

Exploring EBP in Light of Research

Definitions of EBP

Many different definitions of EBP exist, and each definition tends to add another dimension to the concept of EBP. Each different dimension should be carefully and thoroughly considered as EBP is implemented, to ensure that actual nursing practice is comprehensive. Within each definition, however, certain aspects are consistently identified. The consistent and unique aspects can be visualized as shown in **Table 1-1**.

Melnyk and Fineout-Overholt (2015) conceptualize EBP as a method that allows healthcare providers to deliver the maximum quality of care when addressing the multifaceted requests of their patients and families. In another article by Melnyk (2003), EBP is defined as "a problem solving approach to clinical decision making that incorporates a search for the best and latest evidence, clinical expertise and assessment, and patient preference and values within a context of caring" (p. 149). Both of these definitions reflect the use of problem solving with clinical involvement and patient contribution.

Rutledge and Grant (2002) define EBP as "care that integrates best scientific evidence with clinical expertise, knowledge of pathophysiology, knowledge of psychosocial issues, and decision making preferences of patients" (p. 1). This definition incorporates the ideas of pathophysiology and psychosocial components into the mix.

According to Porter-O'Grady (2006), "Evidence-based practice is simply the integration of the best possible research evidence with clinical expertise and with patient needs. Patient needs in this case refer specifically to the expectations, concerns, and requirements that patients bring to their clinical experience" (p. 1). This definition tends to further emphasize the importance of the patient within the entire process.

Burns and Grove (2009) define EBP as "conscientious integration of best research evidence with clinical expertise and patient values and needs in the delivery of quality, cost-effective health care" (p. 699). Consequently, these authors integrate the idea of cost-effectiveness as an additional consideration when determining the appropriate EBP components.

Magee (2005) defines evidence-based medicine as "the conscientious, explicit, and judicious use of current best evidence in making decisions about the care of individual patients" (p. 73). The entire focus of this definition is evidence-based medicine. It is directed toward physician care, not nursing care.

While definitions from other disciplines can be helpful, nursing needs to take the components presented and apply the concepts to the practice of nursing care. As can be seen, each of these definitions includes a decision-making process with the use of evidence balanced by patient and provider interactions. Another definition that includes this balance submitted by Pravikoff and colleagues (2005) for EBP is "a systematic approach to problem solving for healthcare providers, including RNs,

Table 1-1 Comparison of Qualities Included in Evidence-Based Practice Definitions

Author (Year)	Quality of Care	Multifaceted	Decision-Making Process	Clinical Focus	Foundation of Practice	Client Involvement	Other Aspects
Newhouse, Dearholt, Poe, Pugh, & White (2007)			X	X		X	
Melnyk & Fineout-Overholt (2015)	X	X					
Melnyk (2003)			X	X	Evidence, expertise, assessment	X	
Rutledge & Grant (2002)			X	X	Evidence, expertise, pathophysiology, psychosocial		
Porter-O'Grady (2006)				X	Evidence, expertise	X	
Burns & Grove (2009)	X				Research	X	Cost
Magee (2005)			X		Evidence	X	
Pravikoff, Tanner, & Pierce (2005)			X	X	Evidence	X	
Omery & Williams (1999)			X		Expertise		
DiCenso, Cullum, & Ciliska (1998)			X	X	Evidence, proficiency	X	Assets

characterized by the use of the best evidence currently available for clinical decision making in order to provide the most consistent and best possible care to patients" (p. 40). For their part, Omery and Williams (1999) define EBP as "a scientific process [that], with its inherent ability to explain and predict, enhances a practice discipline's ability to anticipate and guide interventions" (p. 50). Both of these definitions consolidate the idea of systematic processing with that of anticipatory consideration when providing nursing care.

DiCenso, Cullum, and Ciliska (1998) offer a model for evidence-based decision making that integrates research evidence, clinical proficiency, patient choices, and accessible assets. Within this model, each element is weighted differently based on the particular client circumstances. The evidence desired for an EBP process can be accessed via sources as diverse as bibliographical databases or a QI department located within a healthcare agency. The evidence used within this process can include research, integrative reviews, practice guidelines, quality improvement data, clinical experience, expert opinion, collegial relationships, pathophysiology, common sense, community standards, published materials, and case studies. According to Ferguson and Day (2005), the forms of evidence, in descending order of credibility, include the following:

1. Randomized, controlled trials
2. Single randomized, controlled trials
3. Controlled trials without randomization
4. Quasi-experimental studies
5. Nonexperimental studies
6. Descriptive studies
7. Expert consensus
8. Quality improvement data
9. Program evaluation data

While each of these forms of evidence is necessary and functional, the credibility of the evidence must be considered carefully when determining a plan of action. Each evidence format provides information to use in a decision-making process, and the support for the information (evidence) is better in those based on research than in those based on opinion.

Each of the proposed definitions supports the definition identified for this text, in which EBP is viewed as a process of using confirmed evidence (research and quality improvement), decision making, and nursing expertise to guide the delivery of holistic patient care. The four consistent aspects found within all of these definitions are (1) a decision-making process, (2) a clinical focus, (3) nursing expertise, and (4) client involvement (see Figure 1-1).

As evidence-based practice has evolved within the field of health care, the idea of what constitutes appropriate evidence has also matured (**Figure 1-2**).

While research results constitute the strongest category of evidence, other evidence—such as quality improvement results, policy/procedure confirmation, and protocol guideline confirmation—is nevertheless beneficial to the provision of safe and effective health care. Within the realm of EBP, each component of the evidence must be carefully assessed in terms of the strength and applicability of the information to the unique client setting. Each agency and nurse must critically consider the results and evidence available concerning an identified healthcare problem. As the results and evidence are thoroughly examined for practicality and efficiency, nursing care practices can be modified to manage the various aspects of care.

Posing Forceful Clinical Questions

Melnyk and Fineout-Overholt (2015) declared that a key aspect within the process is asking the "right" question. The clarification of the question focuses the search for valid evidence so that it speaks to the issue under examination. According to DiCenso, Guyatt, and Ciliska (2005), "The searchable question requires focus to avoid complicating and time-consuming searches that retrieve irrelevant materials" (p. 23). As the

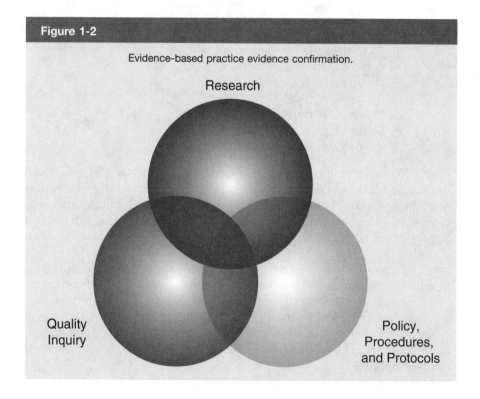

Figure 1-2

Evidence-based practice evidence confirmation.

Research

Quality Inquiry

Policy, Procedures, and Protocols

issue under examination is carefully considered to determine the principal focus for the investigation, two components need to be considered. First, the initial attention should be directed to answering the "what, where, when, why, and how" aspects of the issue. Second, the scrutiny should then turn to the outcome of interest, which reflect the nursing diagnosis and/or research project.

Melnyk and Fineout-Overholt (2015) describe the two types of initial questions as background questions and foreground questions. Background questions address the core knowledge within the healthcare field. Conner (2014) calls this type of question a "knowledge-focused trigger" (p. 3). Knowledge comes from literature, new philosophies, or new regulations. This type of information provides a strong foundation of knowledge related to biological, psychological, and sociological facets of care that can be located in any textbook. Background questions are viewed as broad searches that can frequently be answered by information obtained from textbooks (Echevarria & Walker, 2014). These questions generally begin with the word "what" or "when." These types of questions serve as the underpinnings for other questions. Obtaining answers to these questions does not require access to research databases, because the information is preparatory to the provision of basic holistic care. In contrast, foreground questions address the scientific evidence about diagnosing, treating, or assisting patients as they work to comprehend their healthcare challenges (Melnyk & Fineout-Overholt, 2015). This type of question can be classified as a "problem-focused trigger" (Conner, 2014, p. 3). The problems can come from an identified clinical problem, risk management, finances, or QI. Echevarria and Walker (2014) clarify that foreground questions are used to answer a precise and distinctive clinical issue. At this point in the process of EBP, the search for answers to the identified question focuses on the combination of core knowledge and scientific evidence.

The use of the acronym **PICOT** is helpful in focusing the development of the foreground questions (**Box 1-1**). The PICOT acronym has the following meaning (Melnyk & Fineout-Overholt, 2015):

P Patient population of interest
I Intervention of interest
C Comparison of interest
O Outcome of interest
T Time

❓ THINK OUTSIDE THE BOX

Within every organization, obstacles to incorporating changes such as evidence-based practice are present. Look at an institution. Which obstacles do you see? What can you do to confront and overcome these obstacles?

Examples of Searchable Questions for Research in EBP

Example 1: Labor and Delivery

You are a staff nurse in a rural hospital that performs 120 to 150 vaginal deliveries each year. Within the past 6 months, the institution has hired a certified registered nurse anesthetist (CRNA) to help with anesthesia for the facility. The CRNA and physicians have decided to begin offering epidural anesthesia for routine vaginal deliveries. You offer to seek out studies that address the use of epidural anesthesia in the labor and delivery process.

Preliminary Question: Is epidural anesthesia appropriate for all laboring patients?

Clarification of Question: This question identifies the population and time as all laboring patients and the intervention as the use of epidural anesthesia. It fails to document any comparison with other anesthesia methods or the outcome that the hospital is interested in achieving. Here is the PICOT analysis:

Population: All laboring patients
Intervention: Use of epidural anesthesia
Comparison: Use of narcotic pain management
Outcome: Reduction in labor complications
Time: Individuals in labor

Revised Searchable Question: For all laboring patients, will the administration of epidural anesthesia be more effective in reducing labor complications than other forms of anesthesia administered during the labor process?

Example 2: Routine Checkup

A 50-year-old man comes to the clinic for his yearly physical examination. His blood pressure is recorded as 158/90 mmHg. He complains of frequent headaches during stressful periods. The patient has been fired from his place of employment. When you confer about the findings with him, he asks you about the potential of having a heart attack or stroke. Because these areas are regular potential complications identified within the clinic population, you elect to search for the best evidence to use for discussion with the clinic population.

Preliminary Question: Which type of patient information needs to be included in the teaching related to hypertension and cardiovascular accidents?

Clarification of Question: The limitations of this question include the failure to stipulate the population and to supply adequate particulars about the situation. Here is the PICOT analysis:

Population: Ambulatory clients between the ages of 30 and 60 years
Intervention: Development of cardiovascular symptoms such as hypertension and headaches
Comparison: Ambulatory clients without cardiovascular symptoms
Outcome: Development of cardiovascular complications
Time: Within the initial year following diagnosis

Revised Searchable Question: Within the initial year following diagnosis, are ambulatory clients between the ages of 30 and 60 years who have developed cardiovascular symptoms at an increased risk for developing cardiovascular complications, such as stroke and acute myocardial infarction, compared with ambulatory clients who do not exhibit cardiovascular symptoms?

Example 3: Pediatrics

You work for the pediatric unit at the local hospital. The same children keep getting readmitted for earaches, injuries, and respiratory diseases. You have been assigned to prepare and deliver parenting classes for adolescent parents who have had their children admitted to the hospital. As you are thinking about the classes to be prepared, you question whether the adolescent parents are at greater risk and if they need different information than the general community of parents. You want to provide the most recent and best practices for child rearing.

Preliminary Question: Which type of information must be included in a parenting class for adolescent parents?

Box 1-1

Examples of Searchable Questions for Research in EBP *(continued)*

Clarification of Question: Although the population has been somewhat specified, additional clarification is needed. Other limitations within the preliminary question are the lack of clarification about the interventions, comparisons, outcomes, and time component of the PICOT. Here is the PICOT analysis:

Population: Parents who have had children admitted to the hospital for recurring health problems
Intervention: Parenting classes
Comparison: Age of parents affects the information needed in the classes
Outcome: Reduction in the number of admissions for recurring health problems
Time: Within a 6-month period

Revised Searchable Question: Does the age of the parents (adolescent versus non-adolescent) influence the number of child admissions for recurring health problems within a 6-month period for parents who attend a parenting class program?

Example 4: Cancer-Related Illness

A 75-year-old woman who had been admitted to the hospital for cervical cancer treatment asks to talk with you about general cancer-related issues. She has three children between the ages of 40 and 55 years. She is worried about their potential for developing cancer and wants to know what she should tell them about getting routine checkups. She does tell you that her father died of colon cancer at the age of 71 years.

Preliminary Question: Which type of routine screening examinations should be performed for middle-aged adults who have a family history of cancer?

Clarification of Question: Within this question, the population is briefly delineated. The question does not clearly denote the intervention, the outcome, or the time aspects of a PICOT question. Here is the PICOT analysis:

Population: Individuals with a family history of cancer
Intervention: Scheduling of routine cancer screening examinations
Comparison: No comparison used in this example due to no comparison intervention
Outcome: Early diagnosis of cancer
Time: Routine cancer screening examinations

Revised Searchable Question: For individuals with a family history of cancer, what effect does the timing of routine cancer screening examinations have on the early diagnosis of cancer compared with those individuals who do not have an identified family history of cancer?

Example 5: Staffing

As a new nurse manager on a medical–surgical unit in a large acute care setting, the unit has had a turnover rate of 25% during the last 6 months. The patient satisfaction scores do not reflect good nursing care being provided. The unit is staffed with four BSN-prepared nurses, four AD-prepared nurses, three LVNs, and eight CNAs.

Preliminary Question: What type of nursing model should be used to improve the staff retention on this unit?

Clarification of Question: The question does not adequately define the population nor the intervention for addressing the concerns. It is voiced more as a global type of question. Here is the PICOT analysis:

Population: Full-time nursing staff employees
Intervention: Use of 12-hour shifts with primary care model
Comparison: Use of 8-hour shift with team nursing care model
Outcome: Improved staff retention rate and improved patient satisfaction findings
Time: Not used in this question

Revised Searchable Question: For full-time nursing staff employees, will the use of 12-hour shifts with a primary care nursing model improve the staff retention rate and patient satisfaction findings, when compared to 8-hour shifts using a team nursing approach?

Note: AD = associate degree; BSN = bachelor of science in nursing; CNA = certified nursing assistant; LVN = licensed vocational nurse.

In considering the population aspect within the question, thought is needed to determine specific information about the characteristics of the group under investigation. This description could relate to age, gender, diagnosis, and/or ethnicity. The process needs to be specific enough to provide direction, while not restricting the search too much. According to Dawes and colleagues (2005), "There is a balance to be struck between getting evidence about exactly your group of patients and getting all the evidence about all groups of patients" (p. 13). Care must be given to providing enough specificity to ensure that the search addresses the appropriate population while not excluding relevant information.

The depiction of the intervention for the question is another key aspect that necessitates careful thought and attention. This facet provides the clear determination of the topic under consideration. It does not have to be an action step (and, therefore, an activity), but rather is the key topic for clarification. This aspect of the query should seek to potentially include each and every contact, treatment, patient insight, diagnostic test, and/or predictive aspect (Melnyk & Fineout-Overholt, 2015). Clarification of this aspect within the questioning process reduces the potential for having to backtrack later when the results are not as clearly delineated as anticipated.

The third aspect of the question formation—the comparison of interest—is an optional facet within the questioning process. The comparison is of alternative treatments that can be used for the identified populations. A comparison intervention is a secondary treatment, insight, test, or predictive aspect that can be used as an alternative process of the area of interest. A PICOT question does not need to state that a comparison is the lack of the identified intervention. The only time that a comparison of interest is used in the PICOT format is when a secondary intervention is available that could result in the same outcomes. Within this component, the comparison of different treatment options would be analyzed to reach the desired outcome as identified in the PICOT. In many situations, alternative treatment decisions may not be available. The lack of supplementary preferences does not restrict the development of EBP guidelines.

The fourth aspect for consideration in PICOT questions is the outcome of interest. According to Dawes and colleagues (2005), it is very important to carefully consider this aspect to determine exactly the outcome that is expected. Care must be given to the outcomes that are anticipated by using the identified treatment as compared to the alternate "comparison" treatment. The outcome should be those one or two results that are expected as a consequence of using the intervention treatment. Why is the intervention treatment better for obtaining the results than the other alternative treatments for the population?

The final aspect on which to reflect is time. Timing for the outcome of interest is a principal characteristic to prudently contemplate. While time is not included in all PICOT questions, it is valuable for inclusion on those questions that can be directly affected by the passage of time.

Having presented these considerations for preparing the question(s) for concentrating the evidence-based search, it must be acknowledged that too specific a question can also be a major problem. According to Gennaro, Hodnett, and Kearney (2001), "A one-size-fits-all technical procedural protocol will not help" (p. 236). Because no single way exists to ask a searchable question, care must be given to clarifying the questions prior to moving forward to the investigation of the evidence. The PICOT format fosters clarification of the heart of the area for investigation. The overarching motivation must be the narrowing of the investigation to allow for the effective determination of evidence to strengthen the delivery of holistic nursing care for the client population.

It is interesting that as EBP evolves, PICOT has also evolved. Initially, PICOT was restricted to the four aspects of population, intervention, comparison, and outcome (PICO). As one searches for information about how to develop an EBP question, PICOT can be viewed as PICOTS, which adds setting to the questions, or as PICOT-SD, which incorporates the study design into the statement of the problem (Delfini Group, 2012). These modifications to the question format come from the field of medicine to provide directions for ensuring that the best question can be developed for driving the different types of inquiries.

As our thoughts move to the **research process**, the use of different types of questions for various research types must be clarified. Questions focusing on "how many" or "how much" are frequently answered through the use of quantitative studies. According to DiCenso and colleagues (2005), a quantitative question involves three components— population, intervention/exposure, and outcomes. Questions that are directed toward discovering how people feel or experience a specific state of affairs or environments are answered through the use of qualitative research designs. Qualitative questions are worded to include only two parts—population and situation (DiCenso et al., 2005). These questions focus on characteristics that provide a foundation for composing EBP questions and analyzing research results to confirm EBP practices.

Research Utilization

In the past, lip service has been given to the need for nurses to apply research to practice. More recently, with the emergence and acceptance of EBP, the literature regarding research utilization in the clinical arena has proliferated. The need for improved patient outcomes, decreased healthcare costs, greater patient safety, and higher patient satisfaction are driving forces for the use of scientific data in the decision-making process of nursing care provision (**Box 1-2**).

Box 1-2

Suggested Resources to Support the Retrieval and Appraisal of Evidence

Agency for Healthcare Research and Quality (www.ahrq.gov)

Cochrane Database of Systematic Reviews (www.cochranelibrary.com/cochrane-database-of
-systematic-reviews/index.html)

Institute of Medicine of the National Academies (holds the documents produced by the IOM related to
patient safety; www.iom.edu)

Joanna Briggs Institute (www.joannabriggs.org)

The Joint Commission (http://jointcommission.org)

Medscape (integrated information and educational tools; www.medscape.com/nurseshome)

Morrisey, L. J., & DeBourgh, G. A. (2001). Finding evidence: Refining literature searching skills for the
advance practice nurse. *AACN Clinical Issues, 12*(4), 560–577.

National Comprehensive Cancer Network (www.nccn.org)

National Guidelines Clearinghouse (www.guideline.gov)

National Library of Medicine (allows free searches of MEDLINE through PubMed; www.ncbi.nlm.nih
.gov/pubmed)

Oncology Nursing Society (ONS)—"Putting Evidence into Practice (PEP)" section (www.ons.org
/practice-resources/pep)

Registered Nurses' Association of Ontario (RNAO), Nursing Best Practice Guidelines (http://rnao.ca
/bpg)

Sarah Cole Hirsh Institute for Best Nursing Practices Based on Evidence (http://fpb.case.edu/Centers
/Hirsh)

School of Health and Related Research (ScHARR), University of Sheffield—Information Resources
(www.shef.ac.uk/scharr/sections/ir)

Schulmeister, L., & Vrabel, M. (2000). Searching for information for presentations and publications.
Clinical Nurse Specialists, 16(2), 79–84.

Sigma Theta Tau Virginia Henderson Library (www.nursinglibrary.org/vhl/)

Student BMJ: International Medical Student's Journal (http://student.bmj.com/student/student-bmj
.html)

University of Alberta—Evidence Based Medicine Tool Kit (www.ebm.med.ualberta.ca/ebm.html)

University of North Carolina at Chapel Hill Health Sciences Library, Nursing (http://guides.lib.unc.edu
/nursing)

Note: Access verified July 16, 2015.

As a result of the promotion of the use of research as a basic component in nursing practice, one might ask, "Is nursing research being applied
to nursing practice?" Surprisingly, the answer is both "yes" and "no."
Logic seems to dictate that if EBP can improve patient care, EBP should
be implemented. Most healthcare organizations are attempting to incorporate EBP in their institutions. Unfortunately, obstacles to the use of EBP
often focus primarily on research utilization and understanding EBP.

■ Obstacles to Using Research

Much of the literature discusses barriers to using research for the guidance of practice. Merriam-Webster (2015a) defines a barrier as "a physical
object that blocks the way." A barrier seems to imply a structure that

impedes success. Perhaps another word better defines the challenge of utilization of research in nursing practice—**obstacle**. An obstacle is "something that impedes progress or achievement" (Merriam-Webster Dictionary, 2015b). An obstacle can be overcome. As a result, the term *obstacle* will be used instead of *barrier* when discussing reasons for not employing research utilization in evidence-based nursing care.

The nurse strives to identify ways to overcome each impediment to the path to success; thus, it becomes a challenge to overcome the hindrance and be successful. The use of theories can be viewed as a barrier within the application of research, for example. The complexity of theories and functionality of using theories within the field of research can be perceived as a challenge by the nurse providing care at the bedside. An in-depth discussion of theories is beyond the scope of this text, although it is useful to generate a general dialogue about the use of theories within the research process. Nurses at the bedside do need to understand the connection between theory, research, and practice.

While it may seem simple to apply research to practice, it is actually a complex problem. Three major categories of obstacles deter nurses from readily incorporating research into their practice—education, beliefs/attitudes, and support/resources. Staffileno and McKinney (2011) and Whitmer, Auer, Beerman, and Weishaupt (2011) suggest many nurses don't have enough time, support, mentoring, or sufficient education to use EBP in their practice.

Education

Educational preparation ranks high on the list of obstacles to using research for the guidance of practice. Omery and Williams (1999) suggest that the more education a nurse has, the greater the chance the nurse will use research in providing patient care. The majority of nurses (45.4%) practicing in the United States are prepared at the associate degree (ADN) level, while 20.4% are prepared at the diploma level (HRSA, 2010). Because many of these programs (ADN and diploma) do not focus on research, it is important that care be given to providing further education directed toward EBP and research. If nurses practice as they were taught, then few nurses today have knowledge about research. It is common to hear, "That's the way I was taught." Considering that the average age of nurses is 47, the fallacy of that line of thinking

---

❓ THINK OUTSIDE THE BOX

Discuss the incorporation of clinical expertise in the provision of evidence-based nursing care.

becomes apparent; such a nurse may have been taught 20 to 25 years ago. Research may appear to be too "mystical" and have no relevance to nurses educated during that time period.

Another aspect of educational preparation that influences a nurse's use of research is the way in which research is taught. Even though baccalaureate and graduate programs include research courses in their curricula, many graduates continue to resist engaging in or exploring research. Learning research can be likened to learning a foreign language. Carroll and colleagues (1997) state, "Researchers often present their findings in technical language that is difficult to understand" (p. 209). It is a common misperception that only an academician at a state-of-the-art university can conduct research. The idea that research is practical and beneficial, if linked to clinical practice, appears to be poorly explained to novice nurses. It is therefore no wonder nurses do not understand research, much less want to use it in their practice. Without adequate motivation to use all aspects of an educational program, nurses are unwilling to translate research to practice.

Beliefs/Attitudes

A major portion of the literature attributes the lack of research use by nursing professionals to beliefs and attitudes regarding research. Several authors (Carroll et al., 1997; Cronenwett, 2002; Jolley, 2002; Omery & Williams, 1999; Pravikoff et al., 2005) suggest that negative attitudes concerning the use of research represent obstacles to incorporating EBP into nursing care. This negativity is true of both healthcare organizations and individual nurses. If organizations perceive that research has a lack of value for their operations (Jolley, 2002), little support will exist for EBP within the organization. If nurses feel intimidated (Yoder, 2005) or lack confidence in their ability to use research (Cronenwett, 2002), nurses will not actively incorporate research into their practice.

Support/Resources

The third major category of obstacles to the incorporation of EBP is support and resource availability. Too often, administrators list "cost" as a reason for limiting or hindering the use of EBP. When a nursing shortage exists, staffing becomes a major issue. Allowing staff adequate time to do the requisite reading to update their clinical or EBP knowledge or to attend continuing nursing education offerings is not always possible in such circumstances.

Another problem relates to the lack of access and availability of research materials. Many organizations do not have a library, librarian, or personnel familiar with accessing current research findings. Nurses who lack computer skills may not know how to conduct online searches.

For this reason, without the assistance of a library, librarian, or information technology personnel, nurses may not seek out EBP data. Both new and older generations of nurses have little, if any, expertise in using search engines for obtaining evidence to enhance their practice. Even when a nurse has the requisite knowledge and skills to be able to conduct EBP database searches, state and federal policies may prevent the searches from being conducted within the healthcare organization. For example, privacy issues relating to Health Insurance Portability and Accountability Act (HIPAA) guidelines inhibit access to the World Wide Web from agency computer systems.

One can easily understand why EBP has a steep learning curve, as practitioners struggle to overcome these obstacles. Lack of nursing educational preparation, lack of value assigned to research by organizations and individual nurses, and lack of support/resources must be critically examined. Solutions to these problems must be found if nursing is to promote widespread use of EBP. According to Vratny and Shriver (2007), guidance, eagerness, mentorship, clinical investigation, and insightful practice are what really increase evidence-based practice and help it flourish. An aspect that intensifies thoughts about support relates to mentoring. Kelly, Turner, Speroni, McLaughlin, and Guzzetta (2013) found that empowering staff in the components of inquisitive thinking allows for the development of the skills needed. Terms such as "culture of inquiry," "culture for excellence in nursing research," and "discipline thinking" are now being used and are viewed as a way to clarify and define the idea of mentoring and supporting individuals in a quest for evidence. The formalizing of programs showcases the support and resources available for individuals willing to make the journey. Yoder and colleagues (2014) support the idea of incorporating champions for both research utilization and EBP at all levels within an organization to ensure that EBP is embraced. The use of champions allows for the effective implementation of the concepts of EBP within the daily workings of the unit/agency.

In the future, as agencies support nurses in recognizing the extent of improvement possible in clinical care and patient outcomes through the use of EBP, nurses will seize the opportunity to move nursing care forward and seek empowerment as part of their professional growth. Of course, expecting all organizations and every nurse to conduct research is unrealistic. Nevertheless, use of research in EBP provides the opportunity for research utilization by all.

Responsibility for Using Research

Given the formidable obstacles to research, why do research at all? Few would argue with the premise that having evidence to improve patient outcomes is desirable. As Brockopp and Hastings-Tolsma (2003) say,

"Professional nurses have the responsibility to participate in the promotion of evidence-based practice. Such expectations are both societal and professional" (p. 459). A better-informed consumer will inevitably demand higher-quality care. Thus, given their greater accessibility to healthcare information, today's healthcare consumers expect nurses to use current data to provide quality care. To do so, nurses must continuously explore new evidence and incorporate that evidence into nursing practice. Carroll and colleagues (1997) have suggested, "The possession of a body of knowledge from research is the hallmark of a profession" (p. 208). Fain (2009) recommends that nurses take an active role in developing a body of knowledge. As a relatively new profession, nursing has the responsibility to generate scientific data and to use that data to achieve optimal outcomes. EBP uses the best clinical data available in making decisions about nursing care. Thus, the profession demands that nurses not only be responsible for the use of research, but also participate in research to add to the body of nursing knowledge through EBP.

According to Kitson (2007), "Health administrations across the world are looking to understand how best to improve the quality, effectiveness, and safety of the health care they deliver" (p. S1). Two key movements in health care have led to this quest for excellence: quality/safety initiatives and the evidence-based practice innovation. By striving to acquire a foundation of knowledge while holding fast to honesty, integrity, and respect for the wide variety of perspectives and experiences within the healthcare delivery system, nursing can establish a firm base on which to build the practice of health care for each individual patient encountered.

Overcoming obstacles to the use of research in practice can improve patient outcomes, decrease costs, and increase the body of knowledge for the nursing profession as a whole. Nursing practice leads to research questions, and vice versa. Practice and research as evidence confirmation are inseparable pieces of the puzzle of EBP, as depicted in Figure 1-1. Posing questions about nursing care frequently generates scientific data, which in turn often generate further questions to be explored.

■ The Importance of Generating Evidence

Discovering Significant Evidence

As stated earlier, to practice nursing based on "how we are taught" assumes that no further need to produce evidence is acknowledged. That dangerous assumption was investigated as early as 1975, when Ketefian's study revealed that nurses did not use research for making decisions about nursing care (Polit & Beck, 2008).

Lack of innovation and failure to develop a rationale for nursing care will result in a decrease in respect for nursing as a profession. Currently, consumers of health care list nurses/nursing (82%) as one of the most respected roles in today's society (MacDonald, 2014). Consequently, generating and using scientific evidence can only improve the image of nursing and provide better outcomes from nursing care.

Another force underlying the need for generating evidence, and its incorporation into practice, is the increasing cost of health care. Healthcare costs are spiraling upward at an uncontrollable rate that demands nurses perform their work in the most cost-effective way. As Bucknall (2012) notes, a thorough assessment of the relevancy of the facts along with the anticipated contributions to a particular conclusion are needed for materials to move from simply being facts to serving as evidence. Each and every fact must be carefully gauged to ensure that the cost of delivering the care remains within an acceptable level while still leading to high-quality, high-safety health care. In fact, the nursing profession cannot afford to ignore innovative approaches in nursing care that will reduce costs while simultaneously improving outcomes.

Impact on Practice

The potential impact of using research in evidence-based nursing practice is enormous. No longer can nurses rely on "how I was taught" or a "gut feeling." Research provides tangible scientific data to promote optimal patient outcomes. The nurse at the bedside must be an integral participant in the development of EBP. Nurses are the individuals who observe what works and what does not work in the real world of health care. The expertise that this hands-on practice brings to the research process is of paramount importance to the effective development of a body of nursing knowledge.

Patients interact with nurses and, as Gallup poll (2015) surveys indicate, trust them with their care. As a result, nursing practice that incorporates research also increases patient satisfaction. In turn, assisting a patient to recover health brings satisfaction to the nurse and helps keep the cost of health care at an acceptable level.

Within the current healthcare environment, nurses are expected to embrace continuous performance improvement (CPI) processes such as Six Sigma and the plan–do–check–act (PDCA) cycle. These continuous improvement processes are being driven by the IOM's (2003) "Health Profession Education: A Bridge to Quality," which identified five core areas of concern: providing patient-centered care, working in interdisciplinary teams, employing evidence-based practice, applying quality improvement, and utilizing informatics. According to Finkelman and Kenner (2007), "The [IOM] report recommends (1) adopting transformational leadership and evidence-based management, (2) maximizing the capability of the workforce, and (3) creating and sustaining cultures of safety" (p. 8). As a result, nurses are confronted with the challenges of transforming care at the bedside (TCAB); situation, background, assessment, recommendation (SBAR) communication strategies; electronic medical records (EMR); and other healthcare trends such as the ACA, IOM/RWJF, and Carnegie Foundation reports. Change is imperative for each of us working within the healthcare field. It is our responsibility to become knowledgeable about the evidence that is available as we select mechanisms to address these core areas and national imperatives to change and transform care provided by nurses.

Nurses must ask targeted, concise questions about the nursing care that is being provided. Rolston-Blenman (2009) suggests that success in embracing a culture of change and innovation entails recruiting nurses to advocate for the objectives, resulting in a culture that empowers them to conceive the tools they require for success on the frontline. Settling for the status quo is no longer acceptable. Instead, nurses must take the lead in querying the healthcare delivery venue as to the appropriateness and safety of the care being provided. According to Yoder (2008), "By deploying the broadest range of solutions possible, organizations can significantly improve communication among providers, decrease care delays, and enable clinicians to spend more time with patients, all of which can lead to improved outcomes" (p. 26). Evidence-based nursing practice requires that each nurse develop this "inquiring mind" posture to ensure that the resulting patient outcomes are of high quality, safe, and appropriate in the current healthcare arena.

Nursing is truly both an art and a science. EBP not only provides elements of each aspect, but also contributes to the profession's overall development. As a result, EBP improves everyday practice by providing empirical data to guide nursing interventions. In addition, prompted by national developments mentioned earlier, nurses need to collaborate with physicians and other healthcare providers to improve patient outcomes. Nurses do not work in isolation but rather are essential members of the healthcare team. Generating evidence for use by all professionals requires teamwork and collaboration, as silos of research are no longer the standard approach. As a result, partnerships of individuals and agencies allow for more efficient use of resources and decreased costs.

Summary Points

1. Recent national legislation and reports have had an impact on the importance of EBP and research utilization.
2. A core body of nursing knowledge is derived from the process in which research is incorporated into practice; this process has been called best practice, quality of care, and evidence-based practice.

3. EBP is a process of utilizing confirmed evidence (research and quality improvement), decision making, and nursing expertise to guide the delivery of holistic patient care.
4. The PICOT acronym provides a mechanism for posing forceful, clinical questions to generate scientific questions.
5. Obstacles to research utilization can be categorized into three areas: education, beliefs/attitudes, and support/resources. Lack of time and lack of mentoring are additional obstacles.
6. Generating evidence adds to the core of nursing knowledge, which promotes nursing as a profession.
7. The combination of nursing practice and research is essential to developing EBP.
8. Safe, effective patient care is not a luxury, but rather a necessity.

RED FLAGS

- Within the documentation of a research project, certain decisions concerning the planning and implementation of the process must be supported by rationales. In EBP, randomized controlled trials are viewed as the most powerful evidence. As a result, some research aspects are viewed as stronger designs (quantitative, experimental, and randomized sampling) than other facets of the process. In this text, the designation of a red flag will reflect features of the research project that are less stringent than others. These areas are not strictly forbidden within research, but rather are concerns that need to be taken into account. Within the documentation, these aspects should be supported by rationales reflecting the thought process for utilization of those pieces.

- When a nurse is appraising an article for inclusion in an EBP situation and/ or policy and procedure rationale, the presence of red flags should be seen as an opportunity to assess the justification for the decisions made by the research team. If the research team has provided an adequate justification for its research decisions, a study characterized by multiple red flags can still be a strong study. The documentation of the research report by a researcher is a process of validation and justification of the various judgments made during the planning process. The researcher has the responsibility to document the reasoning for the decisions incorporated into the study such as ethics, sampling, design, and data collection.

- Red flags are areas within the documentation of the study that may raise concerns. These areas are not items that should never be done, but rather are items that should be supported by sound, clear rationales as to why the researcher used the research components.

Multiple-Choice Questions

1. Which of these examples represent an effective application of safe and competent nursing care delivery? The nurse:
   A. Investigates the latest online information in deciding how the care is to be provided.
   B. Reads peer-reviewed nursing research articles to determine the best care to be provided.
   C. Asks a clinical instructor from the university how the care for a client should be given.
   D. Provides care following the instructions provided when attending school.

2. The ACA, IOM/RWJF, and Carnegie Foundation reports are national movements to:
   A. Reaffirm current nursing practice.
   B. Ignore current nursing practice.
   C. Transform current nursing practice.
   D. Eliminate current nursing practice.

3. A nurse is seeking a research article to use as the foundation for a change in the manner in which care is provided. An example of a research article is a manuscript that provides:
   A. An overview of how to provide care.
   B. A discussion of the method used for the research along with recommendations.
   C. A discussion of a case study without any recommendations.
   D. An overview of guidelines for a particular type of case.

4. Which of these forms of evidence carries the highest degree of credibility?
   A. Research study using a nonexperimental study
   B. Intuition
   C. Research study using a random control sample
   D. Research study providing a case study approach

5. A problem-focused trigger would generate which of the following PICOT questions?
   A. Registered nurses have less work stress than other healthcare providers.
   B. Adult cardiac patients involved in bedside rounding compared to multidisciplinary rounding have an increased understanding of their treatment plan.
   C. Palliative care patients enjoy music therapy more than pet therapy when provided by their family members.
   D. Registered nurses can use any nursing theorist to provide sound care.

6. Which of these PICOT questions or statements demonstrates effective development?

    A. What type of care is best used for pediatric patients?

    B. Nurses prefer 12-hour shifts to 8-hour shifts to allow for more time with family.

    C. Individuals using saline for hep-lock flushes have fewer complications.

    D. Hospitalized children have less stress and heal quicker when allowed to use play therapy in comparison to pet therapy while recovering from surgery.

7. You are a BSN-prepared nurse who wants to initiate a research project on your unit. To get the other nurses to participate, you would:

    A. Ask the doctors what they think.

    B. Check the educational level of other nurses on the unit.

    C. Ignore your desire to learn more at this time.

    D. Give a presentation to your peers on the benefits of research.

8. Research is often not valued because:

    A. It costs too much.

    B. Administration wants it.

    C. Search engines are easy to access.

    D. Staffing is not an obstacle.

Discussion Questions

1. You are a public health nurse working in an outpatient hospice facility. You are responsible for clients and their families in a six-county area. During the course of a week, you have from 6 to 10 clients or their families who experience stressful situations related to the disease process. These families and their loved ones experience anguish and guilt as they confront and deal with the terminal nature of the healthcare situation. You have been asked to explore the following question: How do others in this type of situation deal with the numerous stressful challenges? Which type of searchable question could you develop to drive the data search related to this request?

2. As a BSN staff nurse, you are excited that your hospital wants you to participate in an evidence-based project. You have been chosen to chair a taskforce. How would you approach this task?

3. You are an ADN-prepared staff nurse at an acute care facility who has enrolled in an RN-BSN program. One of the key messages presented by the RN-BSN program is the importance of evidence-based nursing practice. In your first course in the program, you are asked to identify an evidence-based topic for development. The faculty members instruct you to select a topic that will be functional in your workplace. Which types of activities would you carry out to aid in the selection of this topic?

Suggested Readings

Harvey, G., Loftus-Hills, A., Rycroft-Malone, J., Titchen, A., Kitson, A., McCormack, B., & Seer, K. (2002, March). Getting evidence into practice: The role and function of facilitators. *Journal of Advanced Nursing, 37*(6), 577–588.

Hewitt-Taylor, J. (2002, December). *Evidence-based practice.* Nursing Standard, *17*(14–15), 47–52, 54–55.

McCormack, B., Allison, K., Gill, H., Rycroft-Malone, J., Titchen, A., & Seers, K. (2002, April). Getting evidence into practice: The meaning of "context." *Journal of Advanced Nursing, 38*(1), 94–104.

Newhouse, R. P. (2006, July/August). Examining the support for evidence-based nursing practice. *Journal of Nursing Administration, 36*(7–8), 337–340.

Rycroft-Malone, J. (2003, July). Consider the evidence. *Nursing Standard, 17*(45), 21.

Rycroft-Malone, J. (2004). The PARIHS framework: A framework for guiding the implementation of evidence-based practice. *Journal of Nursing Care Quality, 19*(4), 297–304.

Rycroft-Malone, J., Kitson, A., Harvey, G., McCormack, B., Seers, K., Titchen, A., & Estabrooks, C. (2002). Ingredients for change: Revisiting a conceptual framework. *Quality and Safety in Health Care, 11*(2), 174–180.

References

Agency for Healthcare Research and Quality (AHRQ). (2000). *Outcomes research fact sheet*, AHRQ Publication No. 00-P011. Retrieved from http://archive.ahrq.gov /research/findings/factsheets/outcomes/outfact/outcomes-and-research.html

Bator, S., Taylor S., & Catalano, J. T. (2015). Nursing research and evidence-based practice. In J. T. Catalano (Ed.), *Nursing now!: Today's issues, tomorrow's trends* (7th ed., pp. 581–610). Philadelphia, PA: F.A. Davis.

Benner, P., Sutphen, M., Leonard, V., & Day, L. (2010). *Educating nurses: A call for radical transformation*. San Francisco, CA: Jossey-Bass.

Brockopp, D. Y., & Hastings-Tolsma, M. T. (2003). *Fundamentals of nursing research* (3rd ed.). Sudbury, MA: Jones and Bartlett Publishers.

Bucknall, T. (2012). Bridging the know-do gap in health care through integrated knowledge translation. *Worldviews on Evidence-Based Nursing, 9*(4), 193–194.

Burns, N., & Grove, S. K. (2009). *The practice of nursing research: Appraisal, synthesis, and generation of evidence* (6th ed.). St. Louis, MO: Saunders Elsevier.

Cannon, S., & Boswell, C. (2010). Challenges and opportunities for teaching research. In L. Caputi (Ed.), *Teaching nursing: The art and science* (2nd ed.). Glen Ellyn, IL: College of DuPage Press.

Carroll, D. L., Greenwood, R., Lynch, K. E., Sullivan, J. K., Ready, C. H., & Fitzmaurice, J. B. (1997). Barriers and facilitators to the utilization of nursing research. *Clinical Nurse Specialist, 11*(5), 207–212.

Catalano, J. T. (2015). *Nursing now!: Today's issues, tomorrow's trends* (7th ed.). Philadelphia: F.A. Davis.

Conner, B.T. (2014). Differentiating research, evidence-based practice, and quality improvement, *American Nurse Today, 9*(6). Retrieved from http://www.americannursetoday .com/differentiating-research-evidence-based-practice-and-quality-improvement/

Cronenwett, L. R. (2002, February 19). *Research, practice and policy: Issues in evidence-based care*. Online Journal of Issues in Nursing [Online serial], *7*(2). Retrieved from http:// www.nursingworld.org/MainMenuCategories/ANAMarketplace/ANAPeriodicals /OJIN/Columns/KeynotesofNote/EvidenceBasedCare.aspx

Davies, B. L. (2002). Sources and models for moving research evidence into clinical practice. *Journal of Obstetric, Gynecologic, & Neonatal Nursing, 31*(5), 558–562.

Dawes, M., Davies, P., Gray, A., Mant, J., Seers, K., & Snowball, R. (2005). *Evidence-based practice: A primer for health care professionals* (2nd ed.). Edinburgh, Scotland: Elsevier Churchill Livingstone.

Delfini Group. (2012). 5 "A"s of evidence-based medicine & PICOTS: Using "population, intervention, comparison, outcomes, timing, setting" (PICOTS) in evidence-based quality improvement work. Retrieved from http://delfini.org/blog/?p=416

DiCenso, A., Cullum, N., & Ciliska, D. (1998). Implementing evidence-based nursing: Some misconceptions. *Evidence-Based Nursing, 1*(1), 38–40.

DiCenso, A., Guyatt, G., & Ciliska, D. (2005). *Evidence-based nursing: A guide to clinical practice*. St. Louis, MO: Elsevier Mosby.

Echevarria, I. M., & Walker, S. (2014, February). To make your case, start with a PICOT question. *Nursing, 44*(2), 18–19.

Fain, J. A. (2009). *Reading, understanding, and applying nursing research: A text and workbook* (3rd ed.). Philadelphia, PA: F. A. Davis.

Ferguson, L., & Day, R. A. (2005). Evidence-based nursing education: Myth or reality? *Journal of Nursing Education, 44*(3), 107–115.

Fineout-Overholt, E., & Melnyk, B. (2005). Building a culture of best practice. *Nurse Leader, 3*(6), 26–30.

Finkelman, A., & Kenner, C. (2007). *Teaching IOM: Implications of the Institute of Medicine reports for nursing education.* Silver Springs, MD: American Nurses Association.

Fonteyn, M. (2005). The interrelationship among thinking skills, research knowledge, and evidence-based practice. *Journal of Nursing Education, 44*(10), 439.

Gallup. (2015). *Honesty/ethics in professions.* Retrieved from http://www.gallup.com/poll/1654/Honesty-Ethics-Professions.aspx

Gennaro, S., Hodnett, E., & Kearney, M. (2001). Making evidence-based practice a reality in your institution: Evaluating the evidence and using the evidence to change clinical practice. *American Journal of Maternal/Child Nursing, 26*(5), 236–244.

Health Resources and Services Administration. (2010). *The registered nurse population: Initial findings from the 2008 National sample survey of registered nurses.* Retrieved from http://bhpr.hrsa.gov/healthworkforce/rnsurveys/rnsurveyfinal.pdf

Health Resources and Services Administration. (2014), *The future of the nursing workforce: National- and state-level projections, 2012–2025.* Retrieved from http://bhpr.hrsa.gov/healthworkforce/supplydemand/nursing/workforceprojections/nursingprojections.pdf

Herlehy, A. M (2011). Nursing's role in the transformation of health care. *AORN, 93*(5), 519–523.

Institute of Medicine (IOM). (2003). *Health professions education: A bridge to quality.* Washington, DC: National Academies Press.

Institute of Medicine (IOM). (2011). *The future of nursing: Leading change, advancing health.* Washington, DC: National Academies Press.

Jolley, S. (2002). Raising research awareness: A strategy for nurses. *Nursing Standard, 16*(33), 33–39.

Kelly, K. P., Turner, A., Speroni, K. G., McLaughlin, M. K., & Guzzetta, C. E. (2013). National survey of hospital nursing research, part 2: Facilitators and hindrances. *JONA, 43*(1), 18–23. doi:10.1097/NNA.0b013e3182786029

Ketefian, S. (1975). Application of selected nursing research finding into nursing practice. *Nursing Research, 24,* 89–92.

Kitson, A. L. (2007). What influences the use of research in clinical practice? *Nursing Research, 56*(4S), S1–S3.

Laskowski-Jones, L. (2015). Research: The path to enlightenment. *Nursing2015,* p. 6.

MacDonald, C. (2014). Nurses top honesty poll. Retrieved from http://nursingethicsblog.com/2014/01/06/nurses-top-honesty-poll/

Magee, M. (2005). *Health politics: Power, population, and health.* Bronxville, NY: Spencer Books.

Malloch, K., & Porter-O'Grady, T. (2015). Innovation and evidence: A partnership in advancing best practice and high quality care. In B. M. Melnyk & E. Fineout-Overholt (Eds.), *Evidence-based practice in nursing & healthcare: A guide to best practice* (3rd ed., pp. 255–273). Philadelphia, PA: Wolters Kluwer.

Mason, D. J., Leavitt, J. K., & Chaffee, M. W. (2012). *Policy & politics in nursing and health care* (6th ed.). St. Louis, MO: Elsevier Saunders.

Melnyk, B. M. (2003). Finding and appraising systematic reviews of clinical interventions: Critical skills for evidence-based practice. *Journal of Pediatric Nursing*, *29*(2), 125, 147–149.

Melnyk, B. M. (2004). Integrating levels of evidence into clinical decision making. *Journal of Pediatric Nursing*, *30*(4), 323–325.

Melnyk, B. M., & Fineout-Overholt, E. (2015). *Evidence-based practice in nursing and healthcare: A guide to best practice* (3rd ed.). Philadelphia, PA: Lippincott Williams & Wilkins.

Merriam-Webster Dictionary. (2015a). Barrier. Retrieved from http://www.merriam-webster.com/thesaurus/barrier

Merriam-Webster Dictionary. (2015b). Obstacle. Retrieved from http://www.merriam-webster.com/dictionary/obstacle

Newhouse, R. P., Dearholt, S. L., Poe, S. S., Pugh, L. C., & White, K. M. (2007). *Johns Hopkins Nursing evidence-based practice: Model and guidelines*. Indianapolis, IN: Sigma Theta Tau International.

Omery, A., & Williams, R. P. (1999). An appraisal of research utilization across the United States. *Journal of Nursing Administration*, *29*(12), 50–56.

Polit, D. F., & Beck, C. T. (2008). *Nursing research: Generating and assessing evidence for nursing practice* (8th ed.). Philadelphia, PA: Lippincott Williams & Wilkins.

Porter-O'Grady, T. (2006). A new age for practice: Creating the framework for evidence. In K. Malloch & T. Porter-O'Grady (Eds.), *Introduction to evidence-based practice in nursing and health care* (pp. 1–29). Sudbury, MA: Jones and Bartlett Publishers.

Pravikoff, D. S., Tanner, A. B., & Pierce, S. T. (2005). Readiness of U.S. nurses for evidence-based practice. *American Journal of Nursing*, *105*(9), 40–51.

Rolston-Blenman, B. (2009). Nurses roll up their sleeves at the bedside to improve patient care. *Nurse Leader*, *7*(1), 20–25.

Rutledge, D. N., & Grant, M. (2002). Introduction. *Seminars in Oncology Nursing*, *18*(1), 1–2.

Staffileno, B. A., & McKinney, C. (2011). Getting "research rich" at a community hospital. *Nursing Management*, *42*(6), 10–14.

Titler, M. G., Everett, L. Q., & Adams, S. (2007). Implications for implementation science. *Nursing Research*, *56*(4S), S53–S59.

Vratny, A., & Shriver, D. (2007). A conceptual model for growing evidence-based practice. *Nursing Administration Quarterly*, *31*(2), 162–170.

Whitmer, K., Auer, C., Beerman, L., & Weishaupt, L. (2011). Launching evidence-based nursing practice. *Journal for Nurses in Staff Development*, *27*(2), E5–E7.

Yoder, L. (2005). Evidence-based practice: The time is now! *Medsurg Nursing*, *14*(2), 91–92.

Yoder, L. (2008). Evidence-based design. *Nursing Management*, *39*(12), 26–29.

Yoder, L. H., Kirkley, D., McFall, D. C., Kirksey, K. M., StalBaum, A. L., & Sellers, D. (2014). Staff nurses' use of research to facilitate evidence-based practice. *American Journal of Nursing*, *114*(9), 26–37.

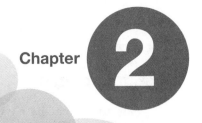

Chapter 2

Overview of Evidence

Pam DiVito-Thomas and Carol Boswell

Chapter Objectives

At the conclusion of this chapter, the learner will be able to:

1. Explain the importance of EBP as key to the provision of quality nursing care.
2. Identify different qualities for classification of information as evidence.
3. Discuss various methods for grading evidence.

Key Terms

Case-controlled

Case report

Case series

Clinical decision making

Consensus

Editorials

Evidence

Evidence-based practice (EBP)

Expert opinion

Forensic science

Ideas

Observations

Opinions

Qualitative research

Quality improvement

Quantitative research

Research

Introduction

In today's media environment, the idea of "evidence" is the primary focus of television series such as Law and Order, NCIS, Elementary, and 60 Minutes. The dramatic storylines' problem-solving and process proceedings are invested to obtain the best available evidence and get as much of the total unbiased information as possible. Resoundingly, the question, "what does the evidence say?" is posed and the answers are systematically sought in order to render the "truth" in findings. Dictionary.com (n.d.) defines **evidence** as "that which tends to prove or disprove something; ground for belief; proof; something that makes plain or clear; an indication or sign." The concept of evidence-based practice has been adopted in the healthcare community and adding clarity and providing the groundwork for understanding is key to the provision of quality nursing care (Schreiber, 2013). Evidence is that foundation on which quality nursing and health care can be based to allow for authentic management of the care provided. As patients and family members realize that the care provided by the healthcare professional is established on trustworthy, responsible, and reliable information, compliance with the plan of care can be supported and embraced. Nursing, as a highly respected discipline, is championing healthcare reform by positioning its professional nursing practice to lead the nation with an evolving **evidence-based practice (EBP)** focused on patient-centered care (Stevens, 2013). Attention given to the development of sound professional care allows for the evolution of effective health care.

The Institute of Medicine (IOM) Health Professions Education Summit (2002) prescribed the future for health professions' education, regulation, policy, advocacy, quality, and industry and developed strategies for restructuring clinical education to be consistent with the principles of the 21st-century health system. The goals set the national agenda that educators, accreditation and licensing agencies, and certification organizations should ensure that students and working professionals develop and maintain proficiency in five core areas: delivering patient-centered care, working as part of interdisciplinary teams, practicing evidence-based medicine, focusing on quality improvement, and using information technology. These core competencies have influenced healthcare policies and governmental funding initiatives that are directed toward clinical and community settings to translate and integrate evidence-based answers to clinical patient care issues (Schreiber, 2013). These interrelated competencies "should be applied in most clinical interactions and lead to improved quality to gather data about outcomes that could be associated with better patient care, the desired goal" (Finkelman & Kenner, 2016, p. 269). Energy and effort must be invested to secure an understanding of these interrelated competencies to move towards evidence-based patient care outcomes.

Currently, evidence-based quality improvement and healthcare transformation are driven by the Affordable Care Act of 2010 (ACA; on June 28, 2012 the Supreme Court rendered a final decision to uphold the healthcare law) that is changing today's healthcare environment based on the supposition that every citizen deserves the right to a healthy and productive life (Nickitas, Middaugh, & Aries, 2016). The ACA sets the stage for the changes anticipated in health care over the next several years. An important provision within EBP emphasizes patient preferences in order to provide the best health outcome for the unique patient-centered situation. Four critical elements have been identified for integrating patient preferences into EBP: (1) healthcare redesign, (2) decision support, (3) empowered organizational culture, and (4) informed and empowered nurses (Burman, Robinson, & Hart, 2013). Hauck, Winsett, and Kuric (2012) support these elements and found that in the acute care setting incorporating EBP outcomes into the strategic plan is essential to creating accountability at the nursing unit level and improving the quality of patient-centered care. Strategies that include the practical implementation goals include the following:

- Establish EBP and nursing research support
- Describe and discuss EBP
- Develop EBP mentors
- Champion EBP in daily patient care using a critical mass of nurses at the unit level
- Promote an EBP culture through nursing leadership
- Disseminate EBP and nursing research outcomes with nurse recognition
- Improve patient outcomes on four nursing-sensitive indicators (these can be found on the National Database of Nursing Quality Indicators website: http://nursingworld.org/Research -Toolkit/NDNQI)

EBP is an integral part of all local, regional, national, and global healthcare environments. Nurses are the largest segment of the nation's workforce; therefore, it is vital that nurses embrace the quest for attaining the best information available for translating EBP into a practice norm for providing quality health care to all patients (Makic, Rauen, Watson, & Poteet, 2014). Nurses should make every effort to develop a spirit of inquiry through problem-solving and decision-making activities that incorporate findings of the best evidence to turn "evidence into action" at the point of providing care. Dogherty, Harrison, Graham, Vandyk, and Keeping-Burke (2013) found positive and negative themes related to factors at the individual, environmental, organizational, and cultural levels. Positive themes that emerged included importance of the issue, development of partnerships and a project team, engagement of key stakeholders, and characteristics of a facilitator—clinical and process expert, broker of knowledge, good communicator, and possession of political savvy. Negative themes included lack of engagement and ownership, dissonance and conflict, and lack of evaluation and sustainability. Organizations and practitioners planning for change in facilitating the implementation of an evidence-based practice can emphasize these positive themes and address the negative barriers that may be encountered. In addition, transformational nursing leadership was found to facilitate incorporating EBP outcomes into the strategic plan, supporting mentors, advocating for resources for education, and outcome dissemination that will empower nurses to include evidence in their practice as they drive organizational change (Hauck, Winsett, & Kuric 2012). Although the process of translating evidence into clinical practice can be challenging, Irwin, Berkman, and Richards (2013) affirm, "evidence-based practice implementation can be a rewarding and inspirational experience for nurses that fosters teamwork and collaboration to improve patient care" (p. 549). Nurses from all areas of practice must embrace the different aspects encompassed for turning evidence into action throughout the healthcare environment.

Foundations for Evidence-Based Practice

As nurses begin the work of understanding EBP, a firm appreciation for the interconnectedness of the different aspects within EBP, research, and quality improvement becomes essential. Each of these aspects has unique characteristics, but all serve to advance the quality of care provided within the healthcare setting. An appreciation for the consistencies and differences among these concepts is important to establish a foundation to use the best evidence to improve healthcare delivery. In answering the question, "What is evidence?", it is important that we differentiate external evidence that is generated through rigorous **research** methodologies and is intended to be used in other settings from internal evidence generated through practice initiatives such as outcomes management of **quality improvement** projects generated from data within organizations to improve clinical care.

The distinction between **quantitative research** that uses the positivist paradigm and **qualitative research** that uses the constructivist paradigm needs to be established. Quantitative researchers use a deductive process, a scientific method that moves in a systematic series of steps according to a prescribed plan beginning with the definition of a problem to the solution of the problem. By gathering empirical evidence that is rooted in objective reality, control of the research situation in minimizing bias, maximizing validity, and generalizing the research findings beyond the study are possible. Using an inductive process, qualitative researchers emphasize the dynamic, holistic, and individual aspects of human life within the context of those who are experiencing them to integrate information to develop a theory or a description of the phenomena under observation (Polit & Beck, 2014). Inquisitive thinking is required for each aspect of both research paradigms to lay the foundations for an EBP. By taking the time and energy to effectively consider research findings, quality improvement outcomes, and EBP activities, nurses can integrate the critical components to allow for the provision of safe and quality health care. According to Melnyk and Fineout-Overholt (2015), evidence-based **clinical decision making** includes critical components of "the external evidence from research, evidence-based theories, opinion leaders, and expert panels; clinical expertise, and internal evidence generated from outcomes management of quality improvement projects, a thorough patient assessment, evaluation and use of available resources; and patient preferences and values" (p. 4). EBP takes on the concept of clinical decision making and processing information rather than conclusions used to guide the process for implementing practice change that leads to improved practice (Schaffer, Sandue, & Diedrick, 2012). By the year 2020, 90% of clinical decisions will be supported by accurate, timely, and up-to-date clinical information and will reflect the best available evidence (Institute of Medicine Roundtable, 2009).

However, Mensik (2011) found that although evidence-based health care results in improved patient outcomes and reduced costs, nurses do not consistently implement evidence-based best practices. Nurses believe in evidence-based care but barriers remain prevalent, including resistance from colleagues, nurse leaders, and managers. Sullivan (2013) concurs with the previous comment, stating, "The movement using evidence-based information has been ongoing but there continue to be dilemmas and challenges" (p. 51). Nurse advocates, leaders, educators, clinicians, and stakeholders must collaborate to create policies and infuse current nursing curricula to provide learning opportunities and facilitate supportive academic and clinical practice environments to achieve the Institute of Medicine's goal that 90% of clinical decisions be evidence-based in 2002.

EBP resonates across nursing practice, education, and research and magnifies the need for redesigning care that includes multiple decision-making efforts for the optimal provision of safe and effective health care in any venue (Stevens, 2013). In line with multiple direction-setting recommendations for safe, effective, and efficient health care, both national experts and nurses have responded to launch initiatives that maximize the valuable contributions that nurses have made, can make, and will make to fully deliver on the promise of EBP (IOM, 2002). Rapidly changing initiatives include practice adoption, education and curricular realignment, model and theory development, scientific engagement in new fields of research, policy change, and development of a national research network to study improvements that will lead in change and advance health.

Nursing, as an evidence-based profession, requires nurses to be able to understand, synthesize, and critique research (Fothergill & Lipp, 2014). Proehl and Hoyt (2012) note that "evidence-based practice involves critical appraisal of the available research, the formulation of recommendations based on the findings of well-designed and executed studies, and an indication of how solid the evidence is to support the practice" (p. 2). In addition, EBP is many sided and involves more than critical appraisals of research, because clinicians need to apply the findings from all evidence pertaining to individual circumstances as part of their clinical decision-making process. Setting EBP throughout healthcare services is a challenging goal. Implementing up-to-date research, research utilization, and quality improvements is a pivotal cornerstone of contemporary nursing practice (Stetler, Ritchie, Rycroft-Malone, & Charns, 2014). To better understand the interconnectedness of EBP and research, reviewing **Figure 2-1** will provide a visualization of the flow for research as it relates to EBP.

Clinical inquiry generated in the work environment leads to pertinent clinical questions, because what works for one patient may not work for other patients even within the same setting (Melnyk & Fineout-Overholt, 2015). Whether research or quality improvement activities are needed, the initial step is always the identification of the clinical question and the problem to be addressed. As a problem is identified, a PICOT (population, intervention, comparison, outcome, time) statement is formed. The PICOT statement is an organized, effective framework for structuring the problem into a manageable format. This PICOT statement drives the review of the literature, with each part of the PICOT statement providing key words and subject headings to narrow the search for relevant articles during the literature review. This attention to the statement allows for a truly in-depth evaluation of the accessible evidence relevant to the problem topic under investigation. While most of the evidence will be available through the literature, other forms of evidence can be accessed and included in this part of the process. All evidence pertinent to the problem topic should be included within the review. Once the literature has been collected and reviewed, gaps and consistencies within the literature can be determined.

Based on these gaps or consistencies, the next step can be taken toward establishing a thorough foundation constructed on the evidence. These gaps and consistencies can either lead to a research study (quantitative or qualitative design) or a quality improvement project. If the evidence indicates that a policy, procedure, or protocol needs to be investigated, a quality improvement process is instituted for that purpose.

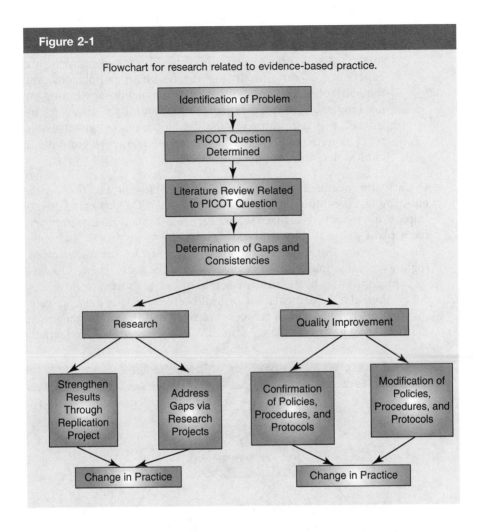

Figure 2-1

Flowchart for research related to evidence-based practice.

Identification of Problem

PICOT Question Determined

Literature Review Related to PICOT Question

Determination of Gaps and Consistencies

Research

Quality Improvement

Strengthen Results Through Replication Project

Address Gaps via Research Projects

Confirmation of Policies, Procedures, and Protocols

Modification of Policies, Procedures, and Protocols

Change in Practice

Change in Practice

Quality improvement is the process of bringing standards of practice to the actual bedside or expanding practice arena. Within this process, the functionality of the standard within a variety of settings is addressed. In bringing forth the quality improvement change resulting from the EBP analysis, new standards are developed for the bedside setting. When the evidence found in a literature review and the evidence analysis reflect that a problem exists, the application of a standard of practice at the bedside setting is the quality improvement action required. In Figure 2-1, the quality improvement can either confirm a policy, procedure, and/or protocol already in place or it can drive their modification. Either way, the change resulting from the EBP analysis is a local change and/or modification rather than a more global alteration.

Hain and Kear (2015) assert:

> In the quest for the Triple Aim of health care—improving the experience of care, improving the health of populations, and reducing per capita costs of health care—nephrology nurses can no longer afford to practice the way we have always done. Instead, it is critical to consider the best available evidence, personal expertise, and patient/family preference when engaging in clinical decision-making. (p. 11)

Quality improvement works to validate the current practices while ensuring that continuity of health care is provided. The process of quality improvement can be visualized within **Figure 2-2**. Many quality improvement plans are available in the literature. The basic process is for the question to be asked, current structures examined, changes made accordingly, and evaluation of those changes within the local venue, followed by communication of the next steps related to the process.

Further, the implementation of healthcare standards must be carefully considered to validate the best practices within the uniqueness of the expanding practice venues. As the ACA has launched the development

Figure 2-2

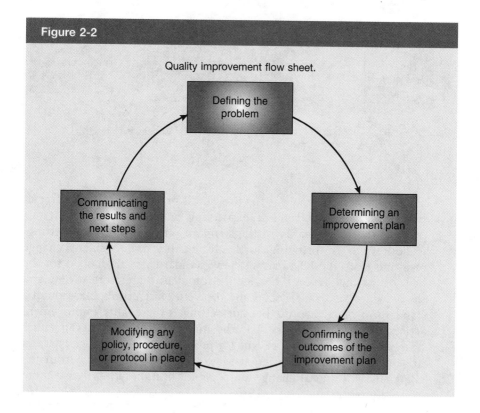

Quality improvement flow sheet.

and dissemination of evidence-based standards throughout the Unites States, the practice roles and responsibilities of nursing are expanding: "Every day, healthcare professionals will need to exercise their clinical judgment, political acumen, and leadership skills to make important and much needed changes that further increase access to and improve the quality and affordability of health care" (Nickitas et al., 2016, p. xv). Importantly, understanding how Medicare and Medicaid reimbursements will affect the outcome of care for a multitude of patient-related expenses including nursing services has generated many questions that are yet to be answered. Some of the questions include: "What is the basis for reimbursement?", "How does Medicare determine payment levels?", "How do patients in different inpatient and outpatient facilities qualify for reimbursement?", "What will be the guidelines for payment levels of healthcare professionals?", and "Will payment be related to productivity and quality outcomes?" (Kander, 2014). Stuart and colleagues (2013) state, "the advent of the Medicare Part D drug benefit presents an opportunity to explore the impact of cost-sharing on patients' use of and adherence with evidence-based medications" (p. 1961). Some settings will have more resources than others to procure quality improvement activities and ensure continuity of health care.

On the other side of the flow sheet (Figure 2-1), the gaps and consistencies may identify the need for further evidence to provide a foundation for the clinical question and the problem to be addressed. If the gaps and consistencies suggest that further research is required to arrive at an answer for the identified problem, a full research project should be planned and implemented. When the evidence is not strong enough to denote the best practice for a problem topic under investigation, additional research projects are required to provide that foundation for the management of the identified challenge. Both aspects of the process are focused on changing and/or improving the practice provided at the bedside or other similar community healthcare settings. If research is the direction in which the nurse should proceed, the best process for arriving at a sound conclusion should be determined (see **Figure 2-3**). As a research endeavor is planned, the methodology for best addressing the problem must be selected. The flowchart in Figure 2-3 identifies the steps commonly followed when conducting quantitative or qualitative research. The steps are similar for both types of research, but they do reflect the uniqueness of the research approaches. At this point, the general flow within the process is strategic for understanding how and why the levels and strengths of evidence are assigned to these types of decision-making processes. Due to the systematic decision-making activities incorporated into the different research methodologies, the assignment of degrees of strength for the resulting evidence/findings has been made through evidence grading methods.

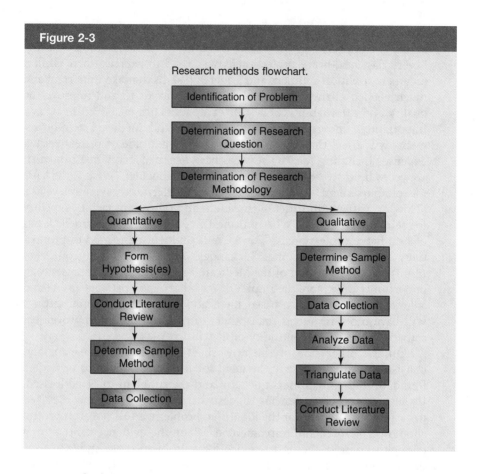

Figure 2-3

Research methods flowchart.

Whether a project is research or quality improvement, the beginning component is assessing the current state of the evidence. Schreiber (2013) poses:

> EBP is an integral part of all healthcare domains: clinical, academic, and research. As with any new thought paradigm, information is produced in significant volume, leading to decision points or crossroads that necessitate a time to reflect and process the current body of knowledge before moving forward. (p. 210)

Individuals directly responsible for the safe and quality care of the patient must embrace the entire process of evidence-based practice for it to become a commonplace tradition within the provision of health care. "What evidence is available?", "How valid and reliable is the evidence?", and "What is the level of the evidence?" are key questions in this context. Understanding what is evidence and determining how to evaluate the evidence is necessary for the process. The querying of evidence to support the different procedures used in the advancement of health care, along with the questioning of the validity and reliability of that evidence, must be foremost and fundamental for each and every provider of care.

Qualities of Evidence

The Agency for Healthcare Research and Quality (AHRQ; 2014) notes that a goal for effective primary care can improve health and cost outcomes and patient, clinician, and staff experience, and evaluations can help determine how best to improve primary care delivery. For example, Nickitas and Mensik (2015) note that integrated staffing models that build the metrics of safety, quality, and patient and nurse engagement will add value to health care, resulting in "better care for individuals, better health for populations, and outcomes at lower per capita costs" (p. 40). Each piece of information being considered for care delivery must be carefully and critically evaluated due to the many varying forms and strengths of the levels of evidence. Nurses are uniquely positioned to evaluate and apply the best evidence within their daily practice to improve patient outcomes (Makic et al., 2014). Nurses must assume the responsibility that is placed on them to provide health care based on the best evidence available.

Within the field of **forensic science**, the idea of evidence is dominant. Evidence is viewed as the data upon which judgments and decisions are made. To be beneficial, evidence has to be established by scrutiny and contemplation of the materials from multiple vantage points. Many accrediting bodies have increased their attention on the use of evidence to make decisions (Lee, Johnson, Newhouse, & Warren, 2013), and regulatory agencies are renowned for using supporting information and benchmarking as evidence of compliance with standards.

Consequently, sound evidence is more than just the simple decisions set forth by one or two individuals. Sound evidence is based on hard and fast particulars, details, and specifics that can be confirmed from different views of the same materials. Within the forensic science discussion of evidence, it is classified as having class and individual characteristics. Class characteristics are established on the physical qualities that are shared by a group of like items. Individual characteristics are those qualities that are unique to the specialized entity. By using the factors and concepts from forensic science concerning evidence, greater latitude in regard to accepting and utilizing other beneficial forms can be exercised.

Within the discussion of evidence, several factors need to be carefully considered. Finkelman and Kenner (2016) support that an EBP review and nursing research are not the same thing and that an EBP review includes evidence from research results, clinical expertise, other sources, and patient's assessment, preferences, and values. In essence, research cannot and will not answer all of the questions concerning health care; however, Wallin, Boström, and Gustavsson (2012) affirm that "EBP is the globally used concept for providing health care grounded in convincing research findings" (p. 140). Evidence must be carefully and thoughtfully considered for each aspect of health care to ensure that the optimal level of health care is being provided.

Nursing care topics must be investigated using the most relevant information for an EBP review. Once the information is collected, the distinctiveness of the results should be focused on that identified topic. The data that are under consideration must represent the wholeness of what is known about a topic. Distinguishing traits of the results along with the topic also need to be evaluated and contemplated. Another important aspect to consider is the frequency that the results are seen. When the same results are observed without regard to person, place, or situation, the results are viewed with increased confidence. When multiple sources in various venues are found to come to the same conclusions about a topic, the reliability of the findings are strengthened. This aspect can also be viewed as the persistence in the result. *Persistence* and *consistency* within the results add support and strength to the quality of the evidence.

A final aspect to carefully consider when contemplating evidence is the likelihood of any alternative explanations for the results obtained. Alternative styles of evidence must be carefully considered so that the justification for the findings yields more power and influence. Improved patient outcomes will follow from the valid results from critical appraisals of the best evidence (Peterson et al., 2014). Within the consideration of all evidence, attention to critically think through the definitive evidence must be given when working in health care.

Other relevant sources of evidential material are case studies, which may provide information that is not reported in the results of clinical trials or survey research (Melnyk & Fineout-Overholt, 2015). The consideration of case studies can have several different dimensions. A case scrutinizes the lives of individuals, dealings, resolutions, episodes, phases, projects, and/or other systems to determine the uniqueness of the situation. Case studies do not follow rigid sets of rules, and the greatest strength of case studies is the depth of the investigation that is possible when using small numbers (Polit & Beck, 2014). The case or situation drives the consideration of specific aspects identified in the case. Case series and case reports can be intermeshed with case studies. Each type of case scenario adds additional depth to the evidence. A **case series** incorporates several case studies that have resulted in similar outcomes. Thus, the findings can be combined to provide additional strength to the results documented. A **case report** is the documentation of the aspects identified within a situation. The strength of this evidence is based on the clarity of the report provided. In addition to the outcomes, the situation and environment where the case occurred lend depth and influence to the resulting materials. A useful resource for case reports on some of the most common medical diagnoses is available through the Cumulative Index of Nursing and Allied Health (CINAHL) library database: "Evidence-Based Care Sheets" that organize "what we know" and "what we can do" with a coding matrix of the references listed in order of strength.

Another form of evidence that can be considered is **expert opinion**. Expert opinion is the furnishing and/or contributing of applicable and significant information by an individual who is viewed as an authority based upon a set of criteria. Different rules can be utilized to identify the expert based upon the materials being sought. While biases are possible due to the nature of the evidence provided by the expert, the expectation is for the expert to qualify any opinion based upon what is known about the topic under investigation.

In conjunction with the topic of expert opinion, the definitions of ideas, editorials, and opinions must be clarified. An idea encompasses thoughts, convictions, and/or principles. An idea can be based upon potentially or actually existing foundations. **Ideas** are considered to be individual work, thus their influence can be minimal.

Editorials are the statements of the opinions of an owner, manager, or similar individual. Again, the weight of this type of evidence is based upon the perceived biases associated with the thoughts and statements. Finally, **opinions** represent a person's beliefs, judgments, and/or values about a designated subject. Opinions can be viewed as evidence, but these have the same caveats as noted with ideas and editorials. Opinions are attitudes and viewpoints that do not rest on adequate foundations to be viewed as completely unbiased because they reflect an individual's world-view.

A third type of evidence that can be considered is **observation**. Observations begin with the individual striving to attentively perceive and/or scrutinize a situation. Following the inspection and surveillance, the observer documents those aspects pertinent to the topic or activity being observed. This process can have biases associated with the observations. To minimize this concern, observations are often placed into the context of when, where, and how the observations were gathered. Documentation of the observation requires the clear determination of what constitutes an observed activity. For example, multiple nonverbal behaviors can be recorded as evidence of noncompliance. By designating which behaviors will be counted and which will not, the quality of the evidence can be increased.

A final example of alternate forms of evidence is a **consensus**. A consensus occurs when individuals involved in the process come to a common understanding. A consensus usually is understood to mean that the majority has reached an agreed resolution. Because the evidence (consensus) is based on a majority and not the complete agreement, the strength of the results can be questionable. With the other forms of evidence, attention to factors and types of evidence must be integrated into the classification of the data. Each and every type and piece of evidence, whether provided by research or via some other avenue, must be thoroughly and unconditionally scrutinized to ensure the validity of the claims being made.

Melnyk and Fineout-Overholt (2015) affirm that the "critical appraisal of evidence is the hallmark of EBP" (p. 80), and the quality of the journey toward that evidence is important. Dogherty and colleagues (2013) support this idea, because "efforts have shifted from focusing on methods for rigorously synthesizing study results into practice recommendations and improving guideline quality toward implementation" (p. 129). The quality of the evidence is becoming increasingly critical, and best practices in health care include diffusing evidence into practice (Makic et al., 2014). The use of evidence, which has a strong foundation to move nursing care forward, is imperative and expected by the public.

In providing care, a nurse may use multiple ways of knowing, classified as four generally accepted patterns of knowledge—empirical, ethical, personal, and aesthetic—and synthesize, or mesh, the four types of knowledge together. These types of knowing the information around us provide various vantage points by which to consider the material put forth as evidence to better understand patients for higher quality care.

Empirical knowledge relates to quantitative explanations, predicting, and explaining (Finkelman & Kenner, 2016). Formal research does hold the position as the strongest form of evidence, and "nursing research is a systematic inquiry designed to develop trustworthy evidence about issues important to nurses and their clients" (Polit & Beck, 2014, p. 2). Using the levels of evidence to help guide the use of the information discovered is vital for effective and competent management of patient-centered care and/or management of patient care and resources. *Aesthetic knowing* embraces those facts and information that reflect emotion and awareness of the beauty and art around us. This term includes the idea that data must be interpreted within the environment in which it was formed or discovered. Removing the information out of that setting can and does modify the application of the findings.

The third form of knowing is *ethical*. The incorporation of ethical knowledge within the venue of evidence brings in the ideas of right and wrong. Finkelman and Kenner (2016) connect ethical knowing with the focus on a person's moral values—what should be done. Nursing can relate this knowing to the professional Code of Ethics for Nurses (American Nurses Association, 2015). Ethical considerations must always be considered when selecting and moving evidence forward toward safe healthcare practices. This ethical aspect incorporates the patient's desires into the utilization of the evidence.

The final type of knowing is *personal* knowledge. Personal knowledge and clinical expertise are critical components within EBP. Personal knowing allows for the participants in the process of healthy living to be actively engaged and involved. These individuals are not passive members but enthusiastic contributors to the consideration of the evidence and the plan of care. The clinical question becomes the key within this process of accessing the evidence. Background questions— asking about general information—are foundational and broader in scope than foreground questions—asking about specific knowledge (Melnyk & Fineout-Overholt, 2015). A well-prepared question with clinical relevance focuses the search for evidence on these types of questions. Notably, the type of question facilitates the types of evidence to be sought. It also promotes the evaluation of that evidence using these different forms of understanding the knowledge bases. For some questions, empiric knowing would be important. For other queries, the ethical and/or aesthetic component could be the driving force toward the level of evidence needed.

As the concept of evidence becomes understandable and transparent, attention must be directed toward classifying the different levels of evidence to allow for consistency within the discussion. Without a uniform means of evaluating the evidence, communication of the nature of the evidence will be confusing and disoriented.

Nurses must become increasingly aware of their current practice— what is and is not known through evidence—and support it with research conclusions appropriate to the distinctive interventions that can be utilized. Lee and colleagues (2013) affirm that EBP in nursing is essential in quality care. Nurses need to embrace a standardized objective approach for use when evaluating evidence of all natures—research, quality improvement, expert opinion, or case studies—to ensure that nursing care is delivered with the best evidence available.

Evidence Grading Methods

One topic drawing an increasing amount of attention as part of the movement toward incorporation of research critiques into EBP is the grading of evidence: "One essential step in examining the evidence is evaluating the strength of the evidence so that the strong evidence is preferentially considered over lower levels of evidence" (Makic et al., 2014, p. 29). A quick Internet search can provide multiple levels for consideration. According to Steelman, Pape, King, Graling, and Gaberson (2011), more than 40 evidence-rating methods were discoverable in 2011. As a result of finding so many rating tools, the Association of periOperative Registered Nurses (AORN) board elected to evaluate the different methods using the AHRQ's three domains of evidence—quality, quantity, and consistency. Within the study conducted by Steelman and colleagues (2011), only eight tools out of the 40 methods were found to address these three domains. Two additional tools were also identified for a total reviewed of 10. Within this scoring of the different methods, the AORN group identified only one method that addressed the five criteria that were evaluated: the Oncology Nursing Society (ONS) Putting Evidence into Practice (PEP) schema.

Peterson and colleagues (2014) affirm that "the purpose of determining the level of evidence and then critiquing the study is to ensure that the evidence is credible and appropriate for inclusion into practice" (p. 59). After the critique of an article is completed, the information assessed is awarded a specific grade based on the strength of the evidence presented in the publication. For the most part, the "levels of evidence" categories developed by the various organizations are compatible, with only minor differences. Each of the formats being used to score and/or grade evidence categorizes the evidence from strongest to least supported evidential materials, but the rating hierarchies are not established to allow for a value judgment about the quality of any study, or to provide clinicians with information about the significance to practice.

Attention must be given to the use of these tools to gain a better understanding of the evidence and be able to defend the rationales used for providing care in different manners based on the individual setting. To score/grade the article by Hanna, Weaver, Slaven, Fortenberry, and DiMeglio (2014), for example, the research methodology would need to be established. The study states that it is part of a larger longitudinal study. No control group was used along with no evidence of randomization within the sample and no intervention resulting in the research methodology being a nonexperimental design. According to **Figure 2-4**, a nonexperimental design would be a level 4 on this hierarchy tool. In contrast, the article written by Iverson and colleagues (2014) states that it is a qualitative research design. Thus, it would classified as a level 5 using the Figure 2-4 tool. In regard to both of these articles in determining the strength of the evidence using **Figure 2-5**, each could be placed at either level A or B depending on the health care provided in the local area.

Each grouping has unique characteristics based upon the agency or organization responsible for the determination of the categories. Numerous organizations, such as the AHRQ, Joanna Briggs Institute, and Cochrane Collaboration, among others, have developed "levels of evidence" hierarchies in an effort to help reviewers categorize the strengths and weaknesses of various studies. One such hierarchy developed by the U.S. Preventive Services Task Force (USPSTF) is shown in Figure 2-4. Within this ladder, quantitative and qualitative types of research design are designated as a specific level within the hierarchy of

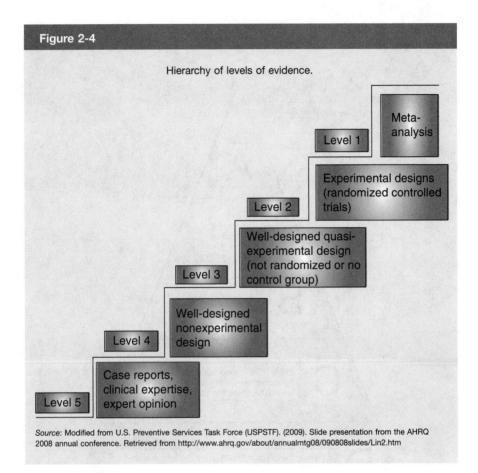

Figure 2-4

Hierarchy of levels of evidence.

Level 1 — Meta-analysis

Level 2 — Experimental designs (randomized controlled trials)

Level 3 — Well-designed quasi-experimental design (not randomized or no control group)

Level 4 — Well-designed nonexperimental design

Level 5 — Case reports, clinical expertise, expert opinion

Source: Modified from U.S. Preventive Services Task Force (USPSTF). (2009). Slide presentation from the AHRQ 2008 annual conference. Retrieved from http://www.ahrq.gov/about/annualmtg08/090808slides/Lin2.htm

research study designs. One drawback with this ranking is the lack of classification of mixed method studies. Reviewers must make their own decisions about classifying such studies as quantitative or qualitative, because no level for mixed method studies has been established. Another concern raised with this hierarchy relates to the four levels given to research results and the classifying of all other types of evidence as level 5. The message from the ordinal ranking of this hierarchy is that research is the only valid evidence mechanism.

The Oncology Nursing Society (ONS) Putting Evidence into Practice (PEP) schema was identified as meeting specific criteria for evaluating the evidence; it can serve as an effective foundation for use within the clinical arena. This tool is used after the selection of articles and evidence is determined. The use of this tool is to aid in the determination of whether the practice should be included in the day-to-day performance of health care (Steelman et al., 2011). Within the schema, specific decision rules for summative evaluation of a body of evidence have been

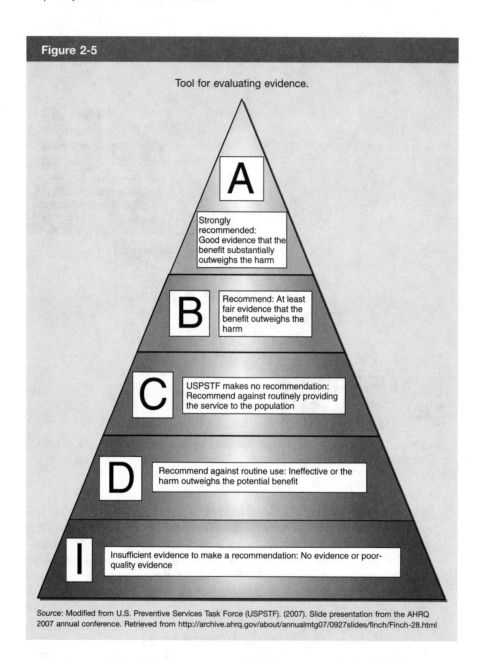

Figure 2-5

Tool for evaluating evidence.

A

Strongly recommended: Good evidence that the benefit substantially outweighs the harm

B

Recommend: At least fair evidence that the benefit outweighs the harm

C

USPSTF makes no recommendation: Recommend against routinely providing the service to the population

D

Recommend against routine use: Ineffective or the harm outweighs the potential benefit

I

Insufficient evidence to make a recommendation: No evidence or poor-quality evidence

Source: Modified from U.S. Preventive Services Task Force (USPSTF). (2007). Slide presentation from the AHRQ 2007 annual conference. Retrieved from http://archive.ahrq.gov/about/annualmtg07/0927slides/finch/Finch-28.html

established to guide the reviewers in making the designations of recommended for practice, likely to be effective, benefits balanced with harms, effectiveness not established, effectiveness unlikely, and not recommended for practice. Each rating tool should be carefully and thoroughly evaluated to determine which one works best in the designated clinical setting.

A more recent revised schema has been developed by the American Association of Critical-Care Nurses (AACN) Evidence Rating System (Armola et al., 2009); it includes experimental evidence at levels A, B, and C, and recommendations at levels D, E, and M (Peterson et al., 2014). A goal of the utility of the AACN Evidence Rating System is that "nurses can determine the strength of research studies, assess the findings, and evaluate the evidence for potential implementation into best practice" (Peterson et al., 2014, p. 58). Each type of scoring tool for evidence has its strengths and challenges. Each agency and/or nurse must carefully consider which format works best in which setting.

Another type of classification for evidence comes from the Trip (formerly Turning Research Into Practice) database. This levelling of evidence provides three basic divisions. Evidence falls into one of three global categories—filtered information, unfiltered information, or background information/expert opinion (Harvey Cushing/John Hay Whitney Medical Library, n.d.). While this process appears to address different levels, the hierarchy shows that six out of the seven levels speak to research endeavors. Again, all other types of evidence are placed into the one lowest level within the structure. This hierarchy does provide an additional designation for the levels of filtered information, which addresses the critical analysis and meta-analysis levels.

The Joanna Briggs Institute (JBI; 2012a, 2012b) has moved toward the use of the FAME (Feasibility, Appropriateness, Meaningfulness, Effectiveness) level of evidence and the AGREE (Appraisal of Guidelines Research and Evaluation) collaboration. Within the JBI approach to levels of evidence, evidence documents are scored based on four criteria: feasibility, appropriateness, meaningfulness, and effectiveness. Effectiveness relates to whether an intervention performs as expected. Appropriateness considers the psychosocial aspects of the intervention. It is concerned with the impact the activity will have on the consumer and whether it will be accepted by the individual. Meaningfulness considers the effect of the intervention on the individual. Within each of these areas, a document would be scored from 1–4. Level 1 is the strongest level of evidence. In addition to these four components, each document is also assessed for economic evidence. The majority of this ranking focuses on meta-synthesis of research. As the AGREE tool and FAME grid are examined, aspects such as **case-controlled**, observations, expert opinion, and consensus can be found only in the lowest levels of the document. In conjunction with the level of evidence ranking, JBI developed a practice focus ranking document that accompanies the AGREE collaboration. This document grades the evidence used within the guideline from level A to level C based on the appropriateness of application to a practice setting. By having this document alongside the levels of evidence (FAME) document, individuals can look toward the application within the practice setting.

AHRQ has also developed a "tool for evaluating the strength of the evidence" (USPSTF, 2009); see Figure 2-5. With this tool, the evidence is assigned a level of strength based on the anticipated benefit and/or harm to the patient. As this rating schedule is used, the process looks at the application of any evidence into the practice arena. None of the five levels speak to the idea of research. Each level clarifies a different amount of benefit or harm for the patient from the use of the service. Differences in classifications using this tool continue to be a problem because individual opinions have to be used to rank or assign the levels.

SUNY Downstate Medical Center (2014) provides an evidence pyramid as a means of classifying and/or ranking evidence. This pyramid has nine levels. Within these levels, the ranking progresses from systematic reviews and meta-analyses at the top to in vitro ("test tube") research at the base. Within the middle range on the pyramid, the levels of case series, case reports, and ideas, editorials, and opinions are listed. While the framework is interesting, the placement of research at both the top and bottom of the pyramid is confusing. Animal research and in vitro research tend to be quantitative research, which is held to be strong evidence by other ranking groups. No rationale was provided as to why the pyramid develops from quantitative research to expert sources, and finally ending back with quantitative research designs.

With the integration of evidence-based practice into the research critique process, the classification of research projects in terms of the "level of evidence" and the strength of the evidence using instruments such as the AHRQ tool seeks to improve the clarity of the information available for making clinical decisions about the modification of policies, procedures, and clinical guidelines.

❓ THINK OUTSIDE THE BOX

1. Look at the different types of evidence. List the strengths and weaknesses for each type of evidence. Can you identify any other types of evidence that should be considered when establishing healthcare practice?
2. Select one or two research articles. Use at least two of the different rating tools to evaluate the evidence and classify it based on each tool. Which tool was easiest to use? Which provided the best review of the evidence? Which tool was difficult to use and why?
3. Debate the use of a rating tool. Do healthcare professionals need to rate all of the evidence they use? Is the rating of evidence just added work that does not meet the needs of the clinical workplace?

◼ Conclusion

The concept of evidence-based practice has been adopted in the healthcare community and adding clarity and providing the groundwork for understanding is key to the provision of quality nursing care (Schreiber, 2013). EBP resonates across nursing practice, education, and research and magnifies the need for redesigning care that includes multiple decision-making efforts for the optimal provision of safe and effective health care in any venue (Stevens, 2013). In providing care, a nurse may use some of these methods of knowing from four generally accepted patterns of knowledge—empirical, ethical, personal, and aesthetic, plus synthesizing (pulling the four types of knowledge together)—to provide an evidence-based practice. Nurses use evidence of levels schema to determine the strength of research studies, assess the findings, and evaluate the evidence for potential implementation into the best practices. Each nurse must accept the challenge of investigating the evidence that is available to support and advance the practice of nursing care and health care in the local setting. Health care can no longer be provided based on the "way we have always done it." Each nurse must recognize and acknowledge the responsibility for advancing the evidence of how and why the interventions are done. Only when this process is done will health care be able to provide quality health management. The careful consideration of evidence quality is based upon logical steps and criteria. Agencies must consider the different formats available to determine which one works best in each setting. The primary responsibility is to question the evidence and not just accept it because it is there. Nurses must be willing to evaluate and confront the data to ensure that the care provided does rise to the appropriate level to advance the quality of the health care provided.

Summary Points

1. Evidence includes that which can be proven and/or disproven. It is an indication or sign related to a topic.
2. Taking the time and energy to effectively consider the evidence is imperative.
3. The proof and/or indications that can be pulled together to determine the best line of action become the driving force, instead of the amount of research that may have been done.
4. A grading process allows one to carefully and cautiously consider the evidence presented in light of a unique clinical environment.
5. A firm appreciation for the interconnectedness of the different aspects within EBP, research, and quality improvement is paramount.
6. A critical appraisal of EBP must consider more than just the available research.

7. Whether an individual is considering research activities or quality improvement efforts, the initial step is always the identification of the problem to be addressed.

8. Each piece of information must be carefully and thoroughly considered concerning what is the foundation on which the outcome is established.

9. Persistence and consistency of results add support and strength to the quality of the evidence.

RED FLAGS

- All evidence must be carefully and thoroughly questioned prior to the acceptance of the validity of the information.
- Sources of evidence should provide enough information concerning the development of the materials along with the outcomes for others to be able to evaluate the quality of the evidence.

Multiple-Choice Questions

1. What does an evidence-based practice provide to an expanding healthcare environment?

   A. Defragmented healthcare provision in acute care settings
   B. Sound foundation for patient-centered care management
   C. Compliance with the medical plan of care
   D. Support and direction for the medical staff

2. What goal of the IOM national proficiency list is fundamental to the provision of safe and effective patient care?

   A. Delivering patient-centered care
   B. Being at the board table
   C. Working in interdisciplinary teams
   D. Practicing evidence-based medicine

3. What critical element most likely impacts the day-to-day positive health outcomes for integrating patient preferences?

   A. Informed and empowered nurses
   B. Healthcare redesign and funding
   C. Empowered organizational culture
   D. Strong administration

4. What type of nursing leadership best serves the expanding healthcare environment and patient-centered care?

   A. Authentic and service leadership
   B. Transformational leadership
   C. Transactional leadership
   D. Relationship-based leadership

5. When a nurse desires to conduct an investigation about decreasing the level of noise in his critical care units due to family complaints, what type of study best serves the purpose of this institutional problem?

   A. Quantitative study
   B. Quality improvement project
   C. Qualitative study
   D. Informative studies

6. Which action best supports the healthcare team rounding together to provide patient-centered care?

   A. New electronic records
   B. Quality improvement projects
   C. Dedicated nursing unit
   D. Working in interdisciplinary teams

7. When the nurse strives to facilitate the implementation of evidence-based practice to change the culture of the institution, what positive theme may emerge during the process?

  A. Lack of engagement and ownership
  B. Development of partnerships
  C. Marginal sustainability and evaluation
  D. Imbedded administration

8. How has the Affordable Care Act most directly impacted the nursing profession?

  A. Expanding nursing roles and responsibilities
  B. Increasing access and affordability of health care
  C. Increased the political prowess of healthcare practitioners
  D. Lower health cost across the healthcare arena

9. What is a notable concern related to scoring or grading the level of evidence with the current tools?

  A. The tools have a marginal measure of value or judgment.
  B. The tools lack classification for mixed method studies.
  C. Clinicians use their discipline-developed tools.
  D. There are too many tools to find one that works.

10. Why is effectiveness an important consideration when determining the level of evidence?

  A. It shows whether an intervention performs as expected.
  B. Psychological aspects of the intervention are included.
  C. The impact on the consumer is measured.
  D. It is easy to determine the level.

Discussion Questions

1. The Institute of Medicine's *Future of Nursing* report identified four central recommendations to advance the nursing profession and health care. The four recommendations are (1) Nurses function at their full extent of knowledge and education, (2) nurses become active at the decision-making table, (3) there must be seamless academic progression for nurses to advance within the educational system, and (4) adequate and reliable data are required to advance health care. Carefully and thoughtfully consider these four recommendations in light of the use of evidence-based practice. How can the nursing profession best address these four central recommendations related to evidence-based practice? How does implementing tools to grade/score evidence provide strength and rationales for using the evidence in daily healthcare practice?

2. Steelman and colleagues (2011) listed the task force recommendations for implementing the use of a rating scale within a site. The recommendations included determining the steps for completing an evidence review, establishing a consensus minimum for those involved in the review, developing educational materials to be used to update staff and committee members on the process, and allocating resources for the process. Based on these recommendations, what guidelines would you develop to be used in your setting to select and incorporate a rating system for evidence review?

Suggested Readings

Goodman, S. N. (2013). Bayesian methods for evidence evaluation: Are we there yet? *Circulation, 127*, 2367–2369.

Gray, M., Bliss, D., & Klem, M. L. (2015). Methods, levels of evidence, strength of recommendations for treatment statements for evidence-based report cards: A new beginning. *Journal of Wounds, Ostomy, and Continence Nursing, 42*(1), 16–18. doi:10.1097/WON.0000000000000104

Oermann, M. H. (2012). Building evidence for practice: Not without dissemination. *MCN: The American Journal of Maternal Child Nursing, 37*(2), 77.

Porritt, K., Gomersall, J., & Lockwood, C. (2014). Study selection and critical appraisal: The steps following the literature search in a systematic review. *AJN, 144*(6), 47–52.

Riley, J. K., Hill, A. N., Krause, L. B., Leach, L. B., & Lowe, T. J. (2011). Examining nurses' attitudes regarding the value, role, interest, and experience in research in an acute care hospital. *Journal for Nurses in Staff Development, 27*(6), 272–279.

Robertson-Malt, S. (2014). Presenting and interpreting findings: The steps following data synthesis in a systematic review. *AJN, 114*(8), 49–54.

Websites

Information on the Future of Nursing
www.iom.edu/~/media/Files/Report%20Files/2010/The-Future-of
-Nursing/Future%20of%20Nursing%202010%20Report%20
Brief.pdf
www.iom.edu/Reports/2003/health-professions-education-a-bridge
-to-quality.aspx

Original Information on the Future of Nursing
www.thefutureofnursing.org/IOM-Report

Information on the Affordable Care Act:
www.hhs.gov/healthcare/rights/law/index.html

Information on the Institute of Medicine Roundtable on Evidence-Based Medicine
www.ncbi.nlm.nih.gov/books/NBK52847/

Cochrane Library Tutorial—PICO: Formulate an Answerable Question
http://learntech.physiol.ox.ac.uk/cochrane_tutorial/cochlibd0e84.php

Information on the Health Resources and Services Administration's Quality Improvement Parts 1–6
www.hrsa.gov/quality/toolbox/methodology/qualityimprovement/

Information on Medicare and the Affordable Care Act
www.medicare.gov/about-us/affordable-care-act/affordable-care
-act.html
www.cms.gov/Medicare/Health-Plans/Medicare-Advantage-Quality
-Improvement-Program/6QIP.html

Information on the American Nurses Association Code of Ethics
www.nursingworld.org/MainMenuCategories/EthicsStandards
/CodeofEthicsforNurses

Information on the Trip Database
www.tripdatabase.com

References

Agency for Healthcare Research and Quality. (2014). Improving primary care practice. Retrieved from http://www.ahrq.gov/professionals/prevention-chronic-care/improve/index.html

American Nurses Association. (2015). Code of ethics for nurses. Retrieved from http://www.nursingworld.org/codeofethics

Armola, R. R., Bourgault, A. M., Halm, M. A., Board, R. M., Bucher, L., Harrington, L., … Medina, J. (2009). AACN levels of evidence: What's new? *Critical Care Nurse, 29*(4), 70–73.

Burman, M. E., Robinson, B., & Hart, A. M. (2013). Linking evidence-based nursing practice and patient-centered care through patient preferences. *Nursing Administration Quarterly, 37*(3), 231–241. doi:10.1097/NAQ.0b013e318295ed6b

Dictionary.com. (n.d.). Evidence. Retrieved from http://dictionary.reference.com/browse/evidence

Dogherty, E. J., Harrison, M. B., Graham, I. D., Vandyk, A. D., & Keeping-Burke, L. (2013). Turning knowledge into action at the point-of-care: The collective experience of nurses facilitating the implementation of evidence-based practice. *Worldviews on Evidence-Based Nursing, 10*(3), 129–135.

Finkelman, A., & Kenner, C. (2016). *Professional nursing concepts: Competencies for quality leadership* (3rd ed.). Burlington, MA: Jones & Bartlett Learning.

Fothergill, A., & Lipp, A. (2014). A guide to critiquing a research paper on clinical supervision: Enhancing skills for practice. *Journal of Psychiatric and Mental Health Nursing, 21*(9), 834–840.

Hain, D. J., & Kear, T. M. (2015). Using evidence-based practice to move beyond doing things the way we have always done them. *Nephrology Nursing Journal, 42*(1), 11–21.

Hanna, K. M., Weaver, M. T., Slaven, J. E., Fortenberry, J. D., & DiMeglio, L. A. (2014). Diabetes-related quality of life and the demands and burdens of diabetes care among emerging adults with type 1 diabetes in the year after high school graduation. *Research Nursing & Health, 37*, 399–408. doi:10.1002/nur.21620

Harvey Cushing/John Hay Whitney Medical Library. (n.d.). Evidence-based practice (EBP) resources. Retrieved from http://guides.library.yale.edu/EBP

Hauk, S., Winsett, R. P., & Kuric, J. (2012). Leadership facilitation strategies to establish evidence-based practice in an acute care hospital. *Journal of Advanced Nursing, 69*(3), 664–674. doi:10.1111/j.1365-2648.2012.06053.x

Institute of Medicine Health Professions Education Summit. (2002). Report of activity. Retrieved from http://www.iom.edu/Activities/Workforce/HealthProfessionsED/2002-Jun-17.aspx

Institute of Medicine Roundtable on Evidence-Based Medicine. (2009). Charter and mission statement. Retrieved from http://www.ncbi.nlm.nih.gov/books/NBK52847/

Irwin, M., Berkman, R., & Richards, R. (2013). The experience of implementing evidence-based practice change: A qualitative analysis. *Clinical Journal of Oncology Nursing, 17*(5), 544–549.

Iverson, K. N., Huang, K., Wells, S. Y., Wright, J. D., Gerber, M. R., & Wiltsey-Stirman, S. (2014). Women veterans' preferences for intimate partner violence screening and response procedures within the Veterans Health Administration. *Research Nursing & Health, 37*, 302–311. doi:10.1002/nur.21602

Joanna Briggs Institute. (2012a). Grades of recommendation. Retrieved from http://joannabriggs.org/jbi-approach.html#tabbed-nav=Grades-of-Recommendation

Joanna Briggs Institute. (2012b). Levels of evidence FAME. Retrieved from http://joannabriggs.org/jbi-approach.html#tabbed-nav=Levels-of-Evidence

Kander, M. (2014). How medical reimbursement works in skilled nursing facilities. *The ASHA LEADER, 19*, 26–27.

Lee, M. C., Johnson, K. L., Newhouse, R. P., & Warren, J. I. (2013). Evidence-based practice process quality assessment: EPQA guidelines. *Worldviews on Evidence-Based Nursing 10*(3), 140–149.

Makic, M. B. F., Rauen, C., Watson, R., & Poteet, A. W. (2014). Examining the evidence to guide practice: Challenging practice habits. *Critical Care Nurse, 34*(2), 28–44.

Melnyk, B. M., & Fineout-Overholt, E. (2015). *Evidence-based practice in nursing & healthcare: A guide to best practice* (3rd ed.). Philadelphia, PA: Wolters Kluwer.

Mensik, J. S. (2011). Understanding research and evidence-based practice: From knowledge generation to translation. *Journal of Infusion Nursing, 34*(3), 174–178.

Nickitas, D. M., & Mensik, J. (2015). Exploring nurse staffing through excellence: A data-driven model. Nurse Leader, *13*(1), pp 40–47. doi:10.1016/j.mni.2014.1.1.006

Nickitas, D. M., Middaugh, D. J., & Aries, N. (2016). *Policy and politics for nurses and other health professionals* (2nd ed.). Burlington, MA: Jones & Bartlett Learning.

Peterson, M. H., Barnason, S., Donnelly, B., Hill, K., Miley, H., & Whiteman, K. (2014). Choosing the best evidence to guide clinical practice: Application of AACN levels of evidence. *Critical Care Nurse, 34*(2), 58–68.

Polit, D. F., & Beck, C. T (2014). *Essentials of nursing research: Appraising evidence for nursing practice* (8th ed.). Philadelphia, PA: Wolters Kluwer/Lippincott Williams & Wilkins.

Proehl, J. A., & Hoyt, K. S. (2012). Evidence versus standard versus best practice: Show me the data! *Advanced Emergency Nursing Journal, 34*(1), 1–2.

Schaffer, M. A., Sandue, K. E., & Diedrick, L. (2012). Evidence-based practice models for organizational change: Overview and practical applications. *Journal of Advanced Nursing, 69*(5), 1197–1209. doi:10.1111/j.1365-2648.2012.06122.x

Schreiber, J. A. (2013). Beyond evidence-based practice-achieving fundamental changes in research and practice. *Oncology Nursing Forum, 40*(3), 208–210.

Steelman, V. M., Pape, T., King, C. A., Graling, P., & Gaberson, K. B. (2011). Selection of a method to rate the strength of scientific evidence for AORN recommendations. *AORN Journal, 93*(4), 433–444.

Stetler, C. B., Ritchie, A., Rycroft-Malone, J., & Charns, M. (2014). Leadership for evidence-based practice: Strategic and functional behaviors for institutionalizing EBP. *Worldviews on Evidence-Based Nursing, 11*(4), 219–226. doi:10.1111/wvn.12044

Stevens, K. (2013). The impact of evidence-based practice in nursing and the next big ideas. *OJIN: The Online Journal of Issues in Nursing, 18*(2), 4.

Stuart, B., Davidoff, A., Erten, M., Gottlieb, S. S., Dai, M., Shaffer, T., Zukerman, I. H., Simoni-Wastila, L., Bryant-Comstock, L., & Shenolikar, R. (2013). How Medicare part D benefit phases affect adherence with evidence-based medications following acute myocardial infarction. *Health Services and Educational Trust, 48*(6, Pt 1), 1960–1977. doi:10.1111/1475-6773.12073

Sullivan, D. H. (2013). A science perspective to guide evidence-based practice. *International Journal of Childbirth Education, 28*(1), 51–56.

SUNY Downstate Medical Center. (2014). *Guide to research methods.* Retrieved from http://library.downstate.edu/EBM2/2100.htm

U.S. Preventive Service Task Force (USPSTF). (2007). Slide presentation from the AHRQ 2007 annual conference. Retrieved from http://archive.ahrq.gov/about/annualmtg07/0927slides/finch/Finch-28.html

U.S. Preventive Services Task Force (USPSTF). (2009). Slide presentation from the AHRQ 2008 annual conference. Retrieved from http://www.ahrq.gov/about/annualmtg08/090808slides/Lin2.htm

Wallin, L., Boström, A. M., & Gustavsson, P. (2012). Capability beliefs regarding evidence-based practice are associated with application of EBP and research use: Validation of a new measure. *Worldviews on Evidence-Based Nursing 3rd Quarter, 9*(3), 139–148.

Chapter 3

Overview of Research

Sharon Cannon and Margaret Robinson

© VLADGRIN/iStock/Thinkstock

Chapter Objectives

At the conclusion of this chapter, the learner will be able to:

1. Discuss the evolution of evidence-based practice, nursing research, and current healthcare trends.
2. Identify the value of using models and frameworks in nursing research.
3. Differentiate between basic and applied research.
4. Delineate sources for nursing research.

Key Terms

Applied research

Basic research

Best practice

Bundling

National Center for Nursing
  Research (NCNR)

National Institute of Nursing
  Research (NINR)

National Institutes of
  Health (NIH)

■ Introduction

The roots of research utilization can be traced back to the time of Florence Nightingale in the mid-1800s. Over the past 150 years, nursing research has encompassed a variety of models, settings, and foci. The following historical perspective illustrates the trajectory of nursing research.

■ Historical Perspective

Evolution from Nightingale to Present Time

Florence Nightingale's work on sanitation in the 1800s was one of the early efforts at linking environmental variables to clinical outcomes. In the early 1900s, the focal point of nursing research was on nursing education. In the 1940s, the concentration shifted to the availability of and demand for nurses in time of war. A major milestone occurred in 1952 when the first edition of the journal *Nursing Research* was published. In the 1970s, clinical outcomes again reemerged as a focus for nursing research, and the *Nursing Studies Index* by Virginia Henderson was produced. Today, through evidence-based practice (EBP), the focus is on the application of research findings to clinical decision making in an effort to improve individual patient outcomes.

Florence Nightingale's (1858) *Notes on Matters Affecting the Health, Efficiency and Hospital Administration of the British Army* was one of the first published works that outlined the clinical application of nursing research (Florence Nightingale Museum Trust, 2003; Riddle, 2005). Florence Nightingale created a polar-area diagram (or coxcomb) to display data related to the causes of mortality in the British Army during the Crimean War (**Figure 3-1**). This early pie chart used color graphics to depict deaths secondary to preventable disease, war injuries, and all other causes. Using these data, Nightingale calculated the mortality rate for contagious diseases such as cholera and typhus. Her statistical analysis demonstrated the need for sanitary reform in military hospitals.

❓ THINK OUTSIDE THE BOX

Explore the various approaches used to generate knowledge in your practice area. For example, which information has been used to determine the method of catheterizing a laboring mother? Which information serves as the basis for the range of blood sugars used in elderly patients who are newly diagnosed with diabetes?

Figure 3-1

Polar-area diagram.

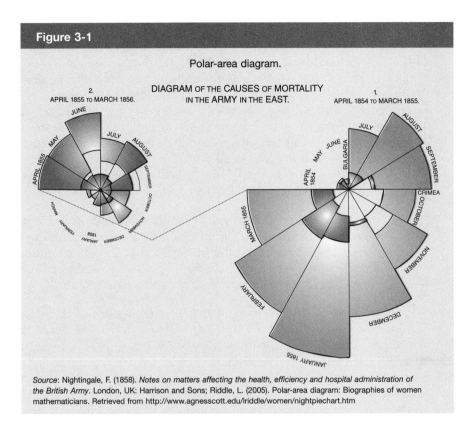

2.
APRIL 1855 TO MARCH 1856.

DIAGRAM OF THE CAUSES OF MORTALITY
IN THE ARMY IN THE EAST.

1.
APRIL 1854 TO MARCH 1855.

Source: Nightingale, F. (1858). *Notes on matters affecting the health, efficiency and hospital administration of the British Army*. London, UK: Harrison and Sons; Riddle, L. (2005). Polar-area diagram: Biographies of women mathematicians. Retrieved from http://www.agnesscott.edu/lriddle/women/nightpiechart.htm

The American Nursing Foundation, established in 1955, was devoted exclusively to the promotion of nursing research:

> The primary objectives of the foundation were to increase public knowledge and understanding of professional nursing, practical nursing and the arts and sciences on which the health of the American people depended. The foundation was to conduct studies, surveys and research; provide research grants to graduate nurses; make grants to public and private nonprofit educational institutions; and publish scientific, educational and literary works. (Kalisch & Kalisch, 1986, p. 651)*

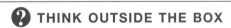

❓ THINK OUTSIDE THE BOX

What would Florence Nightingale say about nursing research and evidence-based practice today?

---

*Reprinted by permission of Wolters Kluwer.

Federal support for nursing research began in 1946, with the creation of the Division of Nursing within the Office of the Surgeon General. In 1955, the **National Institutes of Health (NIH)** established the Nursing Research Study Section. A 1983 study entitled *Nursing and Nursing Education: Public Policy and Private Actions*, published by the Institute of Medicine (IOM), recommended that nursing research be included in the mainstream of health-related research. With growing public support, the Health Research Extension Act of 1985 authorized the development of the **National Center for Nursing Research (NCNR)** at the NIH. The NIH Revitalization Act of 1993 elevated NCNR to an NIH Institute and established the **National Institute of Nursing Research (NINR)** (n.d.).

> The National Institute of Nursing Research supports basic and clinical research to establish a scientific basis for the care of individuals across the lifespan—from the management of the patient during illness and recovery to the reduction of risks for disease and disability, and the promotion of healthy lifestyles. (NINR, 2013)

The strategic planning process at NINR identified areas of focus for prospective nursing research (**Box 3-1**). In April 1993, the Board of Directors of the American Nurses Association (ANA; 1993) adopted a position statement that acknowledged, "research based practice is essential if the nursing profession is to meet its mandate to society for effective and efficient patient care" (p. 1). It went on to identify the role of nursing research for the associate degree in nursing (ADN), bachelor of science in nursing (BSN), master of science in nursing (MSN), and doctoral-

---

Box 3-1

Areas of Focus for Nursing Research

Leading Reform in Nursing Education

Education-Practice Linkage
Domain Specific Knowledge
Technology in Nursing Education

Advancing the Science of Nursing Education

Robust Research Designs
Educational Measurement and Evaluation
Research Scholar Development

Developing National and International Leaders in Nursing Education

Nursing Education Workforce Diversity
Building Capacity

Source: National Institute of Nursing Research (NINR). (2015). NLN research priorities in nursing education 2012-2015. Retrieved from http://www.nln.org/docs/default-source/default-document-library/researchpriorities.pdf?sfvrsn=2. Permission to reproduce granted by the NLN.

Box 3-2

Research Roles at Various Levels of Nursing Education

Associate Degree

Helping to identify clinical problems in nursing practice
Assisting with the collection of data within a structured format
Using nursing research findings appropriately in clinical practice in conjunction with nurses holding
more advanced credentials

Baccalaureate Degree

Identifying clinical problems requiring investigation
Assisting experienced investigators to gain access to clinical sites
Influencing the selection of appropriate methods of data collection
Collecting data and implementing nursing research findings

Master's Degree

Collaborating with experienced investigators in proposal development, data collection, data analysis,
and interpretation
Appraising the clinical relevance of research findings
Creating a climate in the practice setting that promotes scholarly inquiry, scientific integrity, and
scientific investigation of clinical nursing problems
Providing leadership for integrating findings into clinical practice

Source: American Nurses Association (ANA). (1993). Position statement: Education for participation in nursing
research. Retrieved from http://nursingworld.org/MainMenuCategories/Policy-Advocacy/Positions-and-Resolutions
/ANAPositionStatements/Archives/rseducat14484.html. Courtesy of American Nurses Association. This is a retired
position statement and is no longer ANA's official position on the issue.

---

prepared practitioner. The position statement outlined a process whereby clinicians identify relevant clinical problems for investigation and researchers design studies to address these problems (**Box 3-2**).

Early nursing research focused on the development of the profession of nursing, not the clinical practice of nursing. In 1970, a study conducted by Lysaught

> revealed that little nursing research has been conducted on the actual effect of nursing interventions and that nursing had few definitive guidelines for its practice. The study recommended that investigation of the impact of nursing care on the quality, effectiveness and economy of health care be conducted. (Polit & Hungler, 1978, p. 11)

Thus began a new era in which clinical practice emerged as a priority for nursing research.

 THINK OUTSIDE THE BOX

Discuss the barriers you might encounter when trying to implement evidence-based practice and research utilization in your area.

In the 1980s, clinical pathways were introduced into nursing practice. Clinical pathways are a plan of care developed by a multidisciplinary team that outlines the sequential care that should be provided to a predictable group of patients. Early clinical pathways focused on high-volume admissions in the acute care setting, such as elective surgeries and routine obstetrical care. Clinical pathways should incorporate the applicable research. However, the intent of a clinical pathway is to manage the progression of an individual patient through a clinical event. These pathways emerged in response to shifting payment methods for health care and focused on the critical path whose steps must be accomplished for the patient to have a cost-effective and timely discharge. Measures of success were, generally, a reduction in the total cost to provide care and a reduction in the average length of stay for each patient. In the late 1990s, a growing concern arose that many hospitals had adopted clinical pathways without strong evidence that they were clinically or economically effective.

The emergence of EBP takes the application of research one step further to focus on outcomes-based practices. The emphasis is now on the assessment and evaluation of clinical practices that have demonstrated their ability to improve morbidity and mortality for patients. Frequently, multiple interventions have been identified that together enhance the clinical outcome; this practice has come to be known as **bundling**. A bundle is a group of interventions related to a disease or care process that, when executed together, result in better outcomes than when the interventions are implemented individually. Evidence suggests that consistently implementing these practices with all patients who have a specific disease or procedure can improve patient outcomes (Institute for Healthcare Improvement, 2006). In 2005, the Institute for Healthcare Improvement introduced care bundles for the prevention of central-line infection and ventilator-acquired pneumonia as part of the 100,000 Lives Campaign. In this case, the outcomes-based practices focus on a single aspect of care that is known to have serious complications.

Blending evidence-based research and applying it to clinical practice and patient outcomes were goals of the work of the IOM (1999) in its landmark publication *To Err Is Human: Building a Safer Health System*. In the preparation of this report, research in human factors was applied to health care in an attempt to understand where and why systems or processes break down. Specifically, the report's authors looked at how practices in healthcare settings could be made safer so as to prevent adverse outcomes for patients.

In 2004, the IOM expanded on its original work to look at the work environment of nurses in its publication *Keeping Patients Safe: Transforming the Work Environment of Nurses*. This report further described the need for bundles of mutually reinforcing patient safety defenses as part of the effort to reduce errors and increase patient safety. It described "bundles of changes" that are needed within four aspects of care—(1) leadership and management, (2) the work force, (3) the work process, and (4) organizational culture—to strengthen patient safety.

As EBP emerged, a major shift occurred beginning in 2010. National trends began to emphasize patient outcomes, cost containment, and reimbursement related to hospital readmissions. In addition, demand for patient involvement in healthcare decision making has been emphasized ever more; no longer would health care be "doing for" the patient, but rather it would be "doing with" the patient. The importance of EBP and research is currently focused on patient-centered care. As a result of the Affordable Care Act (ACA), the recent establishment of the Patient-Centered Outcomes Research Institute (PCORI) is a prime example of efforts to make the patient the center of care and the provision of outcomes specific to the patient (National Pharmaceutical Council, 2012). In addition, the IOM established 10 priorities for research that include specific diagnostic criteria and treatments for current and future health issues.

Along with recommendations of the IOM, the Agency for Healthcare Research and Quality (AHRQ) continues to provide extensive review of evidence for patient care (Bator, Taylor & Catalano, 2015; Ciliska, DiCenso, Milnyk, & Stetler, 2005). AHRQ focuses on the quality and safety of patient care and designs processes to speed up the usage of EBP in practice (Bator et al., 2015).

Recent changes in Medicare/Medicaid reimbursement have also forced healthcare organizations to reexamine how services are provided. Gold (2014) indicates the ACA is also the impetus for the provision of accountable care organizations (ACOs) that are regulated by the Centers for Medicare and Medicaid Services (CMS). A major area of concern for CMS is quality reporting and performance of ACOs, which include: "(1) patient experience of care; (2) care coordination; (3) patient safety; (4) preventive health; and (5) at-risk population/frail elderly health" (Gordon, 2011, p. 2).

Obviously, research and EBP will play a significant role in patient-centered care and ACOs in the future. Quality assurance/quality improvement (QA/QI) initiatives will provide the necessary evidence for generating knowledge about what does and does not work. Nursing EBP and research will be heavily involved in the years to come.

The major rationale for conducting research is to build a body of nursing knowledge, thereby promoting improvement in patient outcomes. This building of knowledge is accomplished by using results of research in the provision of nursing care that is based on scientific data rather than on a hunch, gut feeling, or "the way I was taught." As a profession, nursing must hold its members accountable for providing safe, cost-effective, and efficient care. EBP that incorporates research findings is a model for nurses to use in their practice.

Theory, Research, and Practice

Parker and Smith (2010) define theories as "organizing structures of our reflections, observations, projections and inferences" (p. 7). Fain (2009) defines research as "a systematic inquiry into a subject that uses various approaches (quantitative and qualitative methods) to answer questions and solves problems" (p. 5). Polit and Beck (2008) define research as "a systematic inquiry that uses disciplined methods to answer question or solve problems" (p. 3). Research can be more readily considered a specific explanation. Fawcett and Garity (2009) have an interesting approach to theories and EBP. They suggest, "theories can be thought of as evidence" (p. 6). The theory becomes evidence to guide practice. Research is therefore equal to theory development.

When considering the relationship between theory and research, one could conclude that theory gives direction to research, which in turn guides practice. As a result, many nursing research projects include a nursing theory/theoretical framework and concepts to guide the research and provide implications for nursing practice.

The evolution of the relationship of theory to research to practice has been ongoing since the days of Florence Nightingale. The current emphasis in research is on translational research and implementation science. These changes move theory into a new dimension for application to practice. If translational research is seen as a method to move a theory into another dimension, and if implementation science is perceived as supporting EBP and research utilization, then the relationship to practice is further enhanced and becomes stronger. Thus, implementing research (evidence) and theory into practice (translation) optimizes EBP.

It is beyond the scope of this text to examine theory in depth. Sometimes a theory is not identified for a research or evidence-based project; however, a theory is still important. The researcher or nurse using evidence to guide nursing care must, at the very least, incorporate a model, framework, plan, or system that gives direction to the project.

❓ THINK OUTSIDE THE BOX

Which model and/or theoretical frameworks do you think can be most appropriate for a medical/surgical unit?

Van Achterberg, Schoonhoven, and Grol (2008) connect models to research and theories for implementation of EBP.

Models and Frameworks

Nursing research provides a way to explain and predict the care that nurses provide, including the underlying rationale. As a result, models of nursing care and their frameworks provide ample opportunities for the generation of new nursing knowledge. As Malloch and Porter-O'Grady (2006) indicate, "Professional Care Models give nurses responsibility and authority to provide patient care. In addition, nurses are accountable for coordinating care and ensuring that continuity of care is provided across the continuum. Patients' unique needs are addressed to achieve outcomes" (p. 236).

Webster's II New College Dictionary (1999) defines a model as "a preliminary pattern serving as the plan from which an item not yet constructed will be produced; a tentative description of a theory or system that accounts for all its known properties" (p. 704). Many nursing care models and research models are problem-solving processes that begin with a question. Nurses ask clinical questions on a daily basis and often conduct research on an informal basis. When a nurse observes the same phenomena occur with multiple patients having the same diagnosis over time, a pattern emerges. The nurse has, through experience, validated his or her observations, just not in a formal, structured research model. As Burns and Grove (2009) state, "A framework is an abstract, logical structure of meaning. It guides the development of the study and enables you to link the findings to the body of knowledge used in nursing" (p. 126). When a theory is not used, a care model, plan, or system is needed in evidence-based practice and research. A model, plan, or system then functions as a framework.

Validation of Best Practices

Best practice is a term used by many different types of professionals in many different settings. The definition of best practices varies depending on the meanings assigned to the words best and practices. Bator and colleagues (2015) suggest "best practice is defined as clinical nursing actions

---

❓ THINK OUTSIDE THE BOX

Most of the research projects associated with evidence-based practice tend to be examples of applied research. Brainstorm about some possible projects that would be classified as basic research.

that are based on 'best evidence' available from nursing research" (p. 593). In this text, best practices is defined as those nursing actions that produce the most desirable patient outcomes through scientific data.

For best practices, research utilization supports decision making for nursing practice through a problem-solving process. Reaffirmation through scientific data validates the desired outcomes and reinforces best practices. This reaffirmation is an excellent example for reality testing. While a wealth of information is available, nurses have little time to look for it, and therefore often practice as they were taught. At times, a nurse thinks or feels that the result of an action is accurate, when it actually is not. Burns and Grove (2001) cite an example related to patient consumption of oxygen. The nurse's sense might be that getting a patient up to the bedside commode results in more oxygen consumption than when the patient uses a bedpan. However, research has shown this is not accurate. Thus, reality can be tested through scientific inquiry, which leads to validated best practice.

Fineout-Overholt and Melnyk (2005) suggest that *best practice* is a term used by more than healthcare providers. According to these authors, "without well-designed research, best practices cannot claim universal application" (p. 27); consensus builds best practices that are achieved through evidence.

Simpson (2005) suggests that through EBP, nurses could overlook the truth about nursing practice. Nurses need to look at what practice is and what is really done. Perhaps, research and practice need to merge to have a major impact on practice. Through this merger, practice and research would combine to actually become a validated best practice. Hopp and Rittenmeyer (2012) promote the term "best available research evidence" for making decisions based on the best evidence (p. 13).

Basic Versus Applied Research

Basic research can be defined as research to gain knowledge for knowledge's sake (Brockopp & Hastings-Tolsma, 2003; Burns & Grove, 2009; Fain, 2009). Another way to look at basic research is that it tests theories (Fawcett & Garity, 2009). Sometimes basic research is also called bench research, such as laboratory experiments intended to elucidate cell structure. Simply stated, basic research is often useful later when, for example, a researcher addresses how a new drug being tested

---

❓ THINK OUTSIDE THE BOX

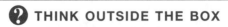

Using Florence Nightingale's ideas about preventable diseases, apply these ideas to research and evidence-based practice.

affects a cell's structure. Fain (2009) indicates that basic research is conducted with little concern for how it might ultimately be applied to practice.

In contrast, **applied research** directly impacts practice and modifies current practice. Most nursing research is applied research that assists in decision making related to nursing care. Applied research occurs in multiple settings and with diverse populations. This type of research can also include the development of new approaches for care. Modification, development, and evaluation of nursing care through best practice form the heart of EBP. Applied research builds a body of knowledge for nursing practice and guides the nurse in providing patient care. An example of applied research in nursing would be a study that generates new information about the use of soap and water versus hand cleansing gels in preparation for a sterile dressing change. An applied research project might indicate that soap and water are more effective in preventing potential wound infections. The nurse would then use the applied research results in preparation for doing a sterile dressing change.

As can be seen, basic research differs from applied research primarily in terms of its focus and intent. Basic science (also known as bench science) is conducted in a laboratory and seeks to add to the knowledge base. Applied research is grounded in the practice area and its application to practice. Fain (2009) suggests that while basic research and applied research are quite different, they can be considered to form a continuum where basic research is required for interpretation of findings of applied studies. One might say that basic research in nursing is building a body of knowledge (theory) and that applied research is the application of the theory to the clinical arena (practice).

■ Sources for Nursing Research

Most nursing research comes from two primary sources: academia and healthcare settings. One might expect that nurses doing research in academic settings would focus only on educational research and that those conducting research in health care would focus only on practice settings. Although that distinction may hold true in some cases, most often both arenas produce research for both education and practice, because they are closely aligned with each other. This intertwining is most evident in the nursing position papers published by two major nursing organizations.

Academia

A major thrust of research in education is the evaluation of programs, technologies, and instructional design. Research in education flourished from the mid-1980s until about 2001, when funding for nursing educa-tion withered. An act of Congress specified that no funding from the NCNR could be distributed for research in nursing education (Diekel-mann, 2001). As a result, nurse educators had to seek funding outside the discipline, where the competition was intense. Consequently, little nursing education research was conducted. Nurse-educator researchers turned to research in clinical practice. Although that effort translated into some positive gains for clinical practice, it drastically affected the research needed to support innovative programs, teaching/learning activities, and other aspects of nursing education.

Since 2000, when the National League for Nursing (NLN) was reor-ganized, increased emphasis and financial support have been directed toward research in nursing education. In its reorganization, the NLN (n.d.) recognized the need for a "quality nursing education that prepares the nursing workforce to meet the needs of diverse populations in an ever changing healthcare environment ... and change the landscape related to funding for nursing education research ... to lead in promoting evidence-based teaching in nursing" (p. 1). This commitment to nursing education research is also expressed in the NLN's mission and goal state-ments. Nurse educators have recognized the need to continue seeking external funds from outside the discipline. Grant funding has also come from several government agencies and foundations. The current impetus for obtaining funding from outside sources is a direct result of the nursing shortage and reports on health care generated by agencies such as the IOM. Due to the nursing shortage that appears destined to last for years to come, research in nursing education has a promising future. The relationship with EBP will likely remain in the forefront when such research in nursing education is carried out.

Healthcare Settings

For healthcare settings to serve as a source for nursing practice, a process for research is necessary. In the *Overview of Evidence* chapter, Figure 2-3 details the steps to commonly follow when conducting quantitative or qualitative research in healthcare settings. The flowchart assists the nurse in identifying the best process for obtaining a sound conclusion for the best method to address the problem. Using the flowchart, the nurse would identify the problem and determine the research question and the

 THINK OUTSIDE THE BOX

There are many nursing theories available within the literature. Search the literature to find evidence of nursing research utilization of a selected theory.

research methodology (either quantitative or qualitative). It is important to note that outcomes of research and EBP determine what works and what doesn't work. In many ways, the research process is similar to the nursing process of assess, plan, implement, and evaluate. According to Cronenwett (2002), in 1999 Marita Titler observed that outcomes achieved in a research study might not be replicated with multiple caregivers in the natural clinical setting. The variable demands on the bedside nurse and multiple comorbidities that exist in the hospitalized patient can make it difficult to replicate findings. Cronenwett (2002) has noted, "evidence for practice mounts slowly over time, as scientists discover first what works in controlled environments and second what works in daily clinical practice" (p. 3). Today, it is our challenge to move from a focus solely on research development to the use of valid and reliable evidence in clinical practice. Nurses have been identified as champions in the adoption of EBP. It is equally important that healthcare institutions implement mechanisms that diffuse available evidence into the practice environment.

Summary Points

1. Florence Nightingale's work emphasized clinical applications of nursing research through the creation of a polar-area diagram.
2. From 1900 to 1940, nursing research focused on nursing education.
3. In the 1950s, the first issue of Nursing Research was published with the notion to share research information with colleagues. Also, the American Nursing Foundation was established to promote nursing research.
4. The 1960s focused on models and frameworks of nursing practice.
5. In the 1970s, Virginia Henderson introduced the Nursing Studies Index.
6. In the 1980s, the Institute of Medicine recommended that nursing research be included in health-related research. In addition, the National Center for Nursing Research was established.
7. In the 1990s and 2000, both the National League for Nursing and American Nurses Association developed position papers on research-based practice.
8. In 2004, the Institute of Medicine published Keeping Patients Safe: Transforming the Work Environment for Nurses, which focused on the need for bundles of mutually reinforcing patient safety defenses as part of the effort to reduce errors and increase patient safety.
9. Recent national trends such as the ACA have had a major impact on the way care is delivered and emphasizes the importance of QA/QI.
10. Models and frameworks of professional practice are validated through research.

11. EBP incorporates research as a professional care model.
12. Basic research is gaining knowledge for knowledge's sake.
13. Applied research directly impacts practice.
14. Sources for research in nursing can be found in academic and healthcare settings.
15. The research process can be defined by a series of detailed steps.

RED FLAGS

- Research projects should be grounded by a model or theoretical framework to anchor the concepts identified within the project.
- Assumptions about best practices must be based on scientific evidence, rather than just on everyday consensus of opinion or intuition.

Case Scenario

Incorporation of EBP into bedside nursing generally requires a change in nursing practice. Change theory models point out that each change process inevitably has potential barriers to effective implementation of the desired change. To more effectively implement EBP, one must identify these barriers to implementation of change. Fink, Thompson, and Bonnes (2005) conducted a nursing research project in an attempt to better understand barriers to implementation of nursing research among inpatient nursing units at a large, university-affiliated Magnet hospital:

> The purpose of this study was to examine the effect of multifaceted organizational strategies on registered nurses' (RNs) use of research findings to change practice in an academic hospital. The specific aims were to (1) identify nurses' attitudes and perceptions about organizational culture and research utilization, (2) identify perceived barriers and facilitators to nurses' use of research in practice, and (3) determine which factors are correlated with research utilization. (Fink et al., 2005, p. 121)

Survey tools, including the BARRIERS to Research Utilization Scale and the Research Factor Questionnaire, were used to gather data. The majority of respondents (83%) were registered nurses who held a baccalaureate or advanced degree in nursing. The results demonstrated an improvement in nurses' perception after implementation of multifaceted interventions. The authors also identified journal club participation as a major strategy to facilitate the use of research in clinical nursing practice.

Case Scenario Questions

1. How might the findings vary in an academic teaching facility that was not a Magnet hospital?

2. How might the findings vary in a community-based hospital setting?

3. How might the findings vary in an outpatient or procedural-based nursing practice?

4. How might the findings vary in a hospital setting that has primarily ADN graduates?

5. What would you anticipate would be the findings in your own clinical practice environment?

6. If you implemented a journal club, do you believe that it would increase the use of research findings in your clinical practice area? Why or why not?

Multiple-Choice Questions

1. The research role of the BSN nurse includes:

   A. Identifying clinical problems that require investigation, assisting experienced investigators to gain access to clinical sites, and collecting data.

   B. Creating a climate in the practice setting that promotes scholarly inquiry, scientific integrity, and scientific investigation of clinical nursing problems.

   C. Collaborating with experienced investigators in proposal development, data collection, data analysis, and interpretation of results.

   D. Providing leadership in integrating research into practice.

2. Potential areas of nursing research identified by the National Institute of Nursing Research include:

   A. Stem cell research.

   B. Application of pharmaceuticals in clinical practice.

   C. Chronic illness, health promotion, disease prevention, and end-of-life care.

   D. Healthcare literacy.

3. What year was the first issue of *Nursing Research* published?

   A. 1858

   B. 1952

   C. 1985

   D. 1992

4. The *Nursing Studies Index*, the first annotated index of nursing research, was the work of:

   A. Florence Nightingale.

   B. Virginia Henderson.

   C. Marita Titler.

   D. Dorothea Orem.

5. The American Nurses Association position statement acknowledges that:

   A. Researchers identify clinical problems and study them.

   B. Faculty members identify clinical problems and study them.

   C. Clinicians identify clinical problems and researchers design them.

   D. Faculty members and researchers identify clinical problems and study them.

6. Clinical pathways are developed by:

   A. Nursing teams.

   B. Physician teams.

   C. Educator teams.

   D. Multidisciplinary teams.

7. A bundle is a group of interventions related to a disease or care process that:

   A. Results in better outcomes than when the interventions are implemented together.
   B. Results in diverse outcomes when the interventions are implemented individually.
   C. Results in confusing information about a single disease or care process.
   D. Provides insufficient evidence to alter clinical practice related to individualized interventions.

8. Professional care models give nurses:

   A. Accountability.
   B. Authority.
   C. Responsibility.
   D. All of the above.

9. Best practice is an excellent example of which kind of testing?

   A. Cognitive
   B. Reality
   C. Didactic
   D. Evaluation

10. Basic research is also known as bench research and is defined as research to gain knowledge for:

   A. Use in academia.
   B. Use in clinical practice.
   C. Knowledge's sake.
   D. Use in biochemistry.

11. Applied research builds a body of knowledge for nursing practice because it is the basis of:

   A. Evidence-based practice.
   B. Clinical pathways.
   C. Nursing processes.
   D. Nursing diagnoses.

12. Sources for nursing research come primarily from two sources:

   A. Business and occupational settings.
   B. Academic and healthcare settings.
   C. Urban and rural settings.
   D. Pharmaceutical and business settings.

13. Best practices in nursing can be defined as:

   A. A well-written plan of nursing care.
   B. A systems approach to nursing care.
   C. Nursing actions that produce desirable patient outcomes.
   D. A way for nurses to justify their care.

14. The Institute of Medicine's publication *Keeping Patients Safe* focuses on:

   A. Building a safer health system.
   B. Processes to report medication errors.
   C. Transforming the work environment for nurses.
   D. Healthcare reform.

15. Theories are:

   A. A guide for research and practice.
   B. Considered to be a specific explanation of an idea.
   C. Not essential to research or EBP.
   D. Static and do not change over time.

16. QA/QI data are now considered:

   A. Valid research to guide practice.
   B. Valid evidence to guide practice.
   C. Generalizable to all practice.
   D. Unlimited to any practice.

17. The research process allows for:

   A. The best method to address the problems.
   B. Little comparison of outcomes.
   C. Limited measures of evaluation.
   D. Extra time for the nurse at the bedside.

Discussion Questions

1. Identify potential opportunities for you to use EBP in your current clinical setting.

2. Identify barriers to implementing EBP in your clinical setting.

3. Identify three clinical problems requiring investigation in your nursing practice. What steps might you take to begin to explore these identified problem areas?

4. Compare your QA/QI data to national standards.

Suggested Readings

Booth, W. C., Colomb, G. G., & Williams, J. M. (2003). *The craft of research* (2nd ed.). Chicago, IL: University of Chicago.

Dimsdale, K., & Kutner, M. (2004). Becoming an educated consumer of research: A quick look at the basic methodologies of research design. Retrieved from http://www.air.org/files/Becoming_an_Educated_Consumer _of_Research.pdf

Gerrish, K., & Lacey, A. (2006). *The research process in nursing* (5th ed.). Oxford, UK: Blackwell.

Gold, J. (2014). FAQs on ACOs: Accountable care organizations explained. Retrieved from http://khn.org/news/aco-accountable-care -organization-faq/

Johnson, B., & Webber, P. (2005). *An introduction to theory and reasoning in nursing* (2nd ed.). Philadelphia, PA: Lippincott Williams & Wilkins.

Kilbom, J., & Cogdill, S. (2004). Writing abstracts. St. Cloud State University and LEO: Literacy Education Online. Retrieved from http://leo .stcloudstate.edu/bizwrite/abstracts.html

Shirey, M. R. (2006, July/September). Evidence-based practice: How nurse leaders can facilitate innovation. *Nursing Administration Quarterly, 30*(3), 252–265.

van Meijel, B., Gamel, C., van Swieten-Duijfjes, B., & Grypdonck, M. H. F. (2004). The development of evidence-based nursing interventions: Methodological considerations. *Journal of Advanced Nursing, 48*(1), 84–92.

References

American Nurses Association (ANA). (1993). Position statement: Education for participation in nursing research. Retrieved from http://nursingworld.org/MainMenuCategories/Policy-Advocacy/Positions-and-Resolutions/ANAPositionStatements/Archives/rseducat14484.html

Bator, S., Taylor, S., & Catalano, J. T. (2015). Nursing research and evidence based practice. In J. Catalano (Ed.), *Nursing Now!: Today's issues, tomorrow's trends* (7th ed., pp. 581–674). Philadelphia, PA: F.A. Davis.

Brockopp, D. Y., & Hastings-Tolsma, M. T. (2003). *Fundamentals of nursing research* (3rd ed.). Sudbury, MA: Jones and Bartlett Publishers.

Burns, N., & Grove, S. K. (2001). *The practice of nursing research: Conduct, critique, and utilization* (4th ed.). Philadelphia, PA: W. B. Saunders.

Burns, N., & Grove, S. K. (2009). *The practice of nursing research: Appraisal, synthesis, and generation of evidence* (6th ed.). St. Louis, MO: Saunders Elsevier.

Ciliska, D., DiCenso, A., Melnyk, B. M., & Stetler, C. B. (2005). Using models or strategies for evidence-based practice. In B.M. Melnyk & E. Fineout-Overholt (Eds.), *Evidence-based practice in nursing and health care.* (pp. 39–70). Philadelphia, PA: Lippincott Williams & Wilkins.

Cronenwett, L. R. (2002, February 19). Research, practice, and policy: Issues in evidence-based care. *Online Journal of Issues in Nursing, 7*(2). Retrieved from http://www.nursingworld.org/MainMenuCategories/ANAMarketplace/ANAPeriodicals/OJIN/Columns/KeynotesofNote/EvidenceBasedCare.aspx

Diekelmann, N. (2001). Funding for research in nursing education. *Journal of Nursing Education, 40*(8), 339–341.

Fain, J. A. (2009). *Reading, understanding, and applying nursing research* (3rd ed.). Philadelphia, PA: F.A. Davis.

Fawcett, J., & Garity, J. (2009). *Evaluating research for evidence-based nursing practice.* Philadelphia, PA: F.A. Davis.

Fineout-Overholt, E., & Melnyk, B. (2005). Building a culture of best practice. *Nurse Leader, 3*(6), 26–30.

Fink, R., Thompson, C., & Bonnes, D. (2005). Overcoming barriers and promoting the use of nursing research in practice. *Journal of Nursing Administration, 35*(3), 121–129.

Florence Nightingale Museum Trust. (2003). The passionate statistician. Retrieved from http://www.florence-nightingale.co.uk/cms/index.php/florence-royal-commission

Gold, J. (2014). FAQs on ACOs: Accountable care organizations explained. Retrieved from http://khn.org/news/aco-accountable-care-organization-faq/

Gordon, J. H. (2011, April). Overview, issues raised, and probable controversies. *Accountable Care News*, pp. 2, 4. Retrieved from http://www.communityoncology.org/UserFiles/pdfs/accountable-care-news-review.pdf

Hopp, L., & Rittenmeyer, L. (2012). *Introduction to evidence-based practice: A practical guide for nursing.* Philadelphia, PA: F.A. Davis.

Institute for Healthcare Improvement (IHI). (2006). 100K lives campaign. Retrieved from http://www.ihi.org/engage/initiatives/completed/5millionlivescampaign/documents/overview%20of%20the%20100k%20campaign.pdf

Institute of Medicine (IOM). (1983). *Nursing and nursing education: Public policies and private actions.* Washington, DC: National Academies Press. Retrieved from http://www.nap.edu/openbook.php?isbn=0309033462

Institute of Medicine (IOM). (1999). *To err is human: Building a safer health system.* Washington, DC: National Academies Press.

Institute of Medicine (IOM). (2004). *Keeping patients safe: Transforming the work environment of nurses.* Washington, DC: National Academies Press.

Kalisch, P. A., & Kalisch, B. J. (1986). *The advance of American nursing* (2nd ed.). Boston, MA: Little, Brown.

Malloch, K., & Porter-O'Grady T. (2006). *Introduction to evidence-based practice in nursing and health care.* Sudbury, MA: Jones and Bartlett Publishers.

National Institute of Nursing Research (NINR). (n.d.). Important events in the National Institute of Nursing Research history. Retrieved from http://www .ninr.nih.gov/aboutninr/history#.VgMEVo9VhBd

National Institute of Nursing Research (NINR). (2013). Mission statement. Retrieved from http://www.ninr.nih.gov/AboutNINR/NINRMissionandStrategicPlan

National Institute of Nursing Research (NINR). (2015). NLN research priorities in nursing education 2012-2015. Retrieved from http://www.nln.org/docs /default-source/default-document-library/researchpriorities.pdf?sfvrsn=2

National League for Nursing (NLN). (n.d.). NLN mission statement. Retrieved from http://www.nln.org/about/mission-goals

National Pharmaceutical Council. (2012). *The patient-centered outcomes research institute resource guide.* Retrieved from http://www.npcnow.org/Public/Research___Publications /Publications/pub_cer/The_Patient_Centered_Outcomes_Research_Institute _Resource_Guide.aspx

Nightingale, F. (1858). *Notes on matters affecting the health, efficiency and hospital administration of the British Army.* London, UK: Harrison and Sons.

Parker, M. E., & Smith, M. C. (2010). *Nursing theories and nursing practice* (3rd ed.). Philadelphia, PA: F.A. Davis.

Polit, D. F., & Beck, C. T. (2008). *Nursing research: generating and assessing evidence for nursing practice.* Philadelphia: Lippincott Williams & Wilkins.

Polit, D. F., & Hungler, B. P. (1978). *Nursing research: Principles and methods.* Philadelphia, PA: J. B. Lippincott.

Riddle, L. (2005). Polar-area diagram: Biographies of women mathematicians. Retrieved from http://www.agnesscott.edu/lriddle/women/nightpiechart.htm

Simpson, R. L. (2005). Leader to watch. *Nurse Leader, 3*(6), 10–14.

van Achterberg, T., Schoonhoven, L., & Grol, R. (2008). Nursing implementation science: How evidence-based nursing requires evidence-based implementation. *Journal of Nursing Scholarship, 40*(4), 302–310.

Webster's II new college dictionary. (1999). Boston, MA: Houghton Mifflin.

Chapter **4**

Overview of Quality

Sharon Cannon and Carol Boswell

Chapter Objectives

At the conclusion of this chapter, the learner will be able to:

1. Define quality improvement and quality assurance.
2. Review the history of quality improvement.
3. Describe the purpose of quality improvement.
4. List sources of quality improvement.
5. Identify settings for quality improvement.
6. Apply principles for guiding improvement to nursing practice in relation to research and evidence-based practice.

Key Terms

Hospital Care Quality Information from the Consumer Perspective (HCAHPS)	Quality assurance (QA)
	Quality improvement (QI)
	Research

■ Introduction

Quality assurance (QA) and **quality improvement (QI)** are terms used every day in all types of healthcare facilities. In fact, the terms are often used interchangeably, although the terms are defined differently. According to Boswell and Cannon (2014), QA is "an orderly practice of examining a product or service to determine if it meets precise requirements" (p. 450). Merriam-Webster (n.d.) defines QA as a program to monitor and evaluate projects, services, or a facility to ensure standards are met. Boswell and Cannon (2014) state that QI is "a process utilized to investigate a policy, procedure, or protocol to determine if it addresses an aspect identified through an evidence-based practice process and works to validate current practice" (p. 450). Obviously, the definitions have some overlap, but keep in mind that both emphasize the necessity of meeting standards through a process that assures benchmark standards are met, while continuously trying to make the standards even better by analyzing the evidence (data). An example of a QI initiative is the **Hospital Care Quality Information from the Consumer Perspective (HCAHPS)**, which measures high-quality service via patient satisfaction.

■ History of Quality Improvement

The history of quality improvement goes back to medieval European times when guilds were used by craftsmen (American Society for Quality, n.d.). Over the years, many notable names have been connected with the ideas and concepts of quality assurance, quality improvement, and continuous improvement. These include Ignaz Semmelweis, Florence Nightingale, Ernest Codman, and W. Edwards Deming, who are well-known individuals who sought to lay the foundation for quality care at all levels of engagement. Much of the work currently housed within QI in the healthcare arena has been taken from the work done within other fields such as the automobile industry, aeronautics, and computer technology. The efforts and/or principles related to improvement from one unrelated area can segue into other areas such as health care to advance the work within that discipline. This transition from one thing to another smoothly and without interruption has benefited the public as a whole.

Within health care, Parry (2014) noted that evidence was found that only 54.9% of patients within healthcare settings in the United States received the recommended care for the health problems identified. QI was noted to be a major concern within the United States due to this finding. The Institute of Medicine (IOM; 2001) defines quality as "the degree to which health services for individuals and populations increase the likelihood of desired health outcomes and are consistent with current professional knowledge" (para. 3). In 1965, the push for quality improvement efforts was emphasized more within health care. In this year, Congress embarked on the formation of the Medicare and the Medicaid programs using Title XVIII and Title XIX of the Social Security Act (Marjoua & Bozic, 2012). While neither of these programs directly discussed QI, they did set out conditions of participation within the different programs that set the benchmark for the quality expected. Although the initial efforts resulting from legislative efforts did move the focus forward, the process was slow.

In 1966, Dr. Avedis Donabedian established a framework for quality that was based on "the elements of structure, process, and outcomes to examine the quality of care delivered" (Marjoua & Bozic, 2012, p. 267). The Donabedian Model provided the foundation for care processes that undertake to move patient outcomes to the forefront of health care. As a result of this advancement in the field, the IOM was established in 1970, followed by the establishment in 1989 of the Agency for Health Care Policy and Research (currently called the Agency for Healthcare Research and Quality [AHRQ]; Marjoua & Bozic, 2012). Both of these agencies have been strong advocates for healthcare quality. Between 1995 and 2000, multiple initiatives and taskforces embraced the sentinel reports being published.

As a result of these efforts, the Leapfrog Group was formed by the Joint Commission. Coming from this group and the efforts during this time, the National Quality Forum (NQF) was created in 1999; its mission is to advance and upgrade health care within the United States. The NQF has been successful in launching national goals and priorities for health-care quality. An endorsement by the NQF has "become the 'gold standard' for healthcare performance measures" (Marjoua & Bozic, 2012, p. 268). The forum has membership from stakeholders, hospitals, healthcare providers, consumer groups, purchasers, accrediting bodies, research organizations, and healthcare QI organizations. All of these groups are focused toward the goal of improving the health care of all individuals.

■ Purpose of Quality Improvement

As evident in the review of the history of QI, efforts to improve health care have lagged behind other industries. However, with the Joint Commission and other accreditation agencies' requirements to implement QI strategies and the push from a 1999 IOM report, the purpose of QI in health care and nursing specifically has been clearly delineated. The major thrusts of QI are to:

- Eliminate errors
- Decrease sentinel events
- Improve patient care and patient safety
- Decrease the financial costs of health care

- Promote health
- Focus on patient-centered care

To understand the purpose of QI as listed here, let's examine an initiative that demonstrated the purpose of QI. Saidleman (2015) discussed the 2000 founding of the Leapfrog Group, which is supported by Robert Wood Johnson Foundation. According to Saidleman (2015), "the Leapfrog Group's mission is to promote giant leaps forward in the safety, quality, and affordability of health care by:

- Supporting informed healthcare decisions by those who use and pay for health care, and
- Promoting high-valued health care through incentives and rewards" (p. 380).

■ Sources of Quality Improvement

Marjoua and Bozic (2012) stated "the ubiquity of health care challenges in the United States is often attributed to the problems of underuse, overuse, and misuse of resources" (p. 3). The lack of accountability related to inadequate management of care along with the challenges of rising healthcare costs has resulted in incomplete and inadequate information on healthcare outcomes. Another critical area related to the management of quality health care lies in the area of "incentivized payment systems that encourage volume without regard to value" (Marjoua & Bozic, 2012, p. 267). The healthcare community has embraced the changes currently being proposed. These productive steps have united the healthcare community, stakeholders, patients, and consumers to demand advancement toward an improved healthcare delivery environment. Each group has accepted the challenge to ascertain their role to distinguish quality care, resulting in the expectation that quality is the foundation for health, not a byproduct.

Two key publications have formed the foundation for the recent advancements in QI: *To Err is Human: Building a Safer Health System* (IOM, 1999) and *Crossing the Quality Chasm: A New Health System for the 21st Century* (IOM, 2001). Both of these publications were instrumental in bringing the challenges and inconsistencies within quality improvement of health care to the forefront of the public. These publications along with subsequent reports have shaped the strategic directions for QI toward redesigning care-delivery opportunities, ensuring that patients are cared for in a safe environment, furthering measurement and informed purchasing aspects, and reforming the health professional education processes.

As resources related to QI are reviewed and considered, a clear understanding of the differences and similarities between **research**, evidence-based practice, and quality improvement becomes essential. **Table 4-1** provides

Table 4-1

Research, Evidence-Based Practice, and Quality Improvement: Comparison Grid

Category	Research	Evidence-Based Practice	Quality Improvement
Definition	Prescribed, methodical, and meticulous technique of investigation	A process of using confirmed evidence (research and quality improvement), decision making, and nursing expertise to guide the delivery of holistic patient care	Appraise the efficiency of clinical interventions and furnish guidance for achieving quality outcomes, productivity, and cost containment
Purpose	Confirms and filters accessible knowledge while generating new knowledge	Supplies an underpinning for optimal patient care by assimilating the strongest evidence accessible; transforms research into practice; advances stability and reliability within practice	Champions pressing workflow enhancement in the practice setting; equates organizational standards with benchmarks and guidelines; contemplates cost efficacy; transforms processes for efficient management of care
Commonalities and differences	Systematic problem-solving method driven by inquiry	Systematic problem-solving method driven by evidence	Systematic problem-solving method driven by data
IRB approval needed	IRB required before implementation of engagement with participants	IRB not usually required unless dissemination of results is anticipated that could expose participants	IRB not usually required unless dissemination of results is anticipated that could expose participants
Supervision	Compliance with local, state, and federal law required usually through IRB approval	Institutional	Institutional
Limitations	Theoretically based; dependent on statistical analysis; time consuming; some topics are not researchable	Begins with clinical/practice question; outcome dependent on "best" evidence" located	Not theoretically based; cause-and-effect outside the scope; numerous internal validity threats possible; rapid cycle; integrated into practice in a timely manner

(continues)

Table 4-1 Research, Evidence-Based Practice, and Quality Improvement: Comparison Grid *(continued)*

Category	Research	Evidence-Based Practice	Quality Improvement
Generalizability	Yes; based on research design used	Probable; dependent on organizational context	No; results are specific to unit and/or agency
Opportunities for knowledge dissemination	Expected following completion of research	Increasingly common	Expected within agency but not usually beyond agency
Influence on practice	Generation of new knowledge for practice	Seeks to improve practice through translation of evidence	Seeks to improve practice on unit and within organization; incorporates knowledge
Methods	Quantitative Qualitative Mixed method Systematic reviews Meta-analysis	PICO, PICOT, PICOTS, PICOT-DM Iowa Model of EBP ACE Star Model of Knowledge	Plan-Do-Check-Act (PDCA) Plan-Do-Study-Act (PDSA) Six Sigma Lean Six Sigma

Sources: Data from North Dakota Center for Nursing. (2014). *Comparison of quality improvement, evidence-based practice, and nursing research.* Retrieved from http://www.ndcenterfornursing.org/wp-content/uploads/2013/02/Comparison-of-QI-EBP-and-Nursing-Research-Final-Document.pdf; Shirey, M. R., Hauck, S. K., Embree, J. L., Kinner, T. J., Schaar, G. L., … McCool, I. A. (2011). Showcasing differences between quality improvement, evidence-based practice, and research. *The Journal of Continuing Education in Nursing, 42(2),* 57–70.

a comparison grid for these three processes. Each of the processes are contrasted in regard to the definition, purpose, commonalities and differences, internal review board (IRB) approval needed, supervision, limitations, generalizability, opportunities for knowledge dissemination, influence on practice, and methods. By viewing them in a grid format, a comparison of the concepts and values assumed under each process can be carefully and systematically contemplated.

Weston and Roberts (2013) provided the goals addressing the quality initiatives established by the National Quality Strategy. These three aims encompass the current expectations for quality and performance improvement and include better care for all members of society, healthy people living in healthy communities, and affordable care for all levels of the population. Each of the aims provides a clear vision of the expectations for health care both in the United States and globally. These aspirations are achievable through "improvements in nursing care efficiency, patient engagement, and access to knowledge" (Weston & Roberts, 2013). Within the contemporary healthcare landscape, excellence and performance strategies will be foundational for advancing the healthcare agenda. Each member within the healthcare profession will be expected to endorse and strengthen the progression toward the appropriate level of quality improvement at all levels of health.

Melynk and Fineout-Overholt (2015) sum up the ideas of QA as involving "planned, systematic processes which should have been established using evidence, that is, the how of practice" (p. 521). By using a systematic process in the investigation of the evidence and the healthcare setting, the resulting outcome will demonstrate quality and appropriate management of the health encounters. QA and QI are the attempt by the healthcare community to pledge to provide competent, effective healthcare management while certifying that the care provided has been based on "best practices." QI efforts are best accomplished by multiple groups evaluating the same phenomena and arriving at the same unambiguous results.

New tools are being used to evaluate the quality of care being provided. Nursing has taken the challenge to evaluate the quality of nursing care: "The American Nurses Association (ANA) has developed nursing-sensitive indicators including nursing staffing information and patient care outcomes such as pressure ulcers, patient falls, and nosocomial infections" (Izumi, 2012, p. 2). These indicators have been labeled as the National Database of Nursing Quality Indicators (NDNQI). Hospital administrators along with accreditation organizations are using these indicator results to provide a thorough picture related to the nursing care provided within the participating agencies. The NDNQI results are used in conjunction with the core indicators developed by other agencies to provide a transparent view of the quality of care being provided within health care throughout the country.

■ Settings

QI in health care takes place in multiple settings. The following list includes but is not limited to:

- Long-term care
- Schools
- Clinics
- Outpatient surgery centers
- Pharmacies
- Medical equipment companies
- Home healthcare agencies
- Industrial sites
- Correctional facilities
- Acute care facilities

As described earlier, QI is a primary concern for all healthcare venues. Nursing is an essential component in all of them. Interaction through interdisciplinary QI activities is an expectation. The nurse plays a central role in all aspects of QI, whether it is on a single unit or for the organization as a whole. In particular, nurses are positioned well to impact and improve services provided to the client regardless of the setting, healthcare system, or the processes used to improve the quality of care.

■ Application of Quality Improvement

Acute Settings

Draper, Felland, Liebhaber, and Melichar (2008) acknowledge, "nurses are pivotal in hospital efforts to improve quality" (p. 2). Nurses are key to the activities and engagement at the bedside. They are readily available to assist and implement measures with patients. As the Affordable Care Act (ACA) has been implemented, a variety of entities, "such as accreditation and regulatory bodies, quality improvement organizations, medical specialty societies, state hospital associations, and health plans" (Draper et al., 2008, p. 2), have all become increasingly interested in the quality of care provided within healthcare settings. As health care has embraced the ideas laid out within the ACA, core quality measures have been determined and established. Hospitals must utilize the core quality measures as they strive to maximize their revenue streams. Medicare, Medicaid, and insurance groups are utilizing the core quality measures to determine the reimbursement rates to be used for different hospitals and healthcare agencies. The public has become progressively more aware of these core measures as they seek to select healthcare providers. Hospitals with sound core quality measure levels are viewed as safer and better healthcare agencies to use, thus improving the reimbursement levels for those institutions. These "report cards" gain in importance as agencies are feeling the impact from the ACA implementations. Nurses are called upon to step up and assist with these quality measures. According to Draper and colleagues (2008), the following five key strategies are needed to foster quality improvement within this healthcare setting:

- Accommodating hospital leadership that takes an active role in the process
- Establishing expectations for all staff members to seek quality as a shared responsibility
- Requiring staff to be accountable within the process
- Employing the idea of champions within the staff
- Furnishing appropriate, valid, and ongoing resources to utilize the staff successfully

To be effective within this process, the majority of the staff must accept individual ownership for the development and management of patient safety and quality efforts. Without each member realizing the role that they play within the process, holes within the quality will develop and expand.

According to the Health Resources and Service Administration (HRSA; 2011), QI must be viewed as a team process. Each member of the team within the acute care setting has a role to play within the process to ensure patient safety and effective management of healthcare interventions. Because the process of QI is understood to be a complex, multidisciplinary activity, a team approach to the process is imperative. Each discipline has a responsibility during the process to advance the management of effective and safe health care for each individual within the acute care setting.

In addition to the work done within the acute care setting, the idea of QI is rapidly moving toward continuous quality improvement that moves from home care to acute care back to home care. All aspects across the continuum must be included within the plan for quality. Health care is no longer only in one segment, but is a comprehensive and extensive management of the healthcare needs of the individual in a holistic manner. Healthcare providers cannot look at only the physical aspects within the current environment. The total picture that impacts the patient must be considered as the treatment options are investigated.

Community Settings

Just as in acute care, nurses in community settings such as clinics, schools, outpatient centers, or home health must be prepared to work as team members of other professionals. Every level and every department must be involved, regardless of the size or type of organization. In many instances, team members may not all be in the healthcare profession. Those who are comprehend the healthcare system. Those who are not healthcare providers will need to be informed about QI and health care to provide appropriate feedback and processes necessary in QI activities. Frequently, this evolution becomes an essential component in the nurses' role in QI in community settings.

In 2011, the HRSA published guidelines for QI that is composed of modules for a QI process/system. The modules discuss the importance of QI, roles in QI, improvements for sustainability of the QI program, references, and additional resources, including tips and a tool kit. The program is designed for and can be used in all healthcare settings.

❓ THINK OUTSIDE THE BOX

1. Visit Medicare's Hospital Comparison website: www.medicare.gov/hospitalcompare/. Once you are at this site, select three hospitals to compare. Look at the comparison. Discuss how a patient and/or patient family might use this information. On a second note, after looking at this information, how might you use it to select the agency that you want to work in or do not want to work in?
2. Go to the HRSA website's QI page: www.hrsa.gov/quality/toolbox/methodology/qualityimprovement/. How could you use the information in your setting?

Summary Points

1. The history of quality improvement goes back to the medieval European times when guilds were used by craftsmen (American Society for Quality, n.d.).
2. Ignaz Semmelweis, Florence Nightingale, Ernest Codman, and W. Edwards Deming are examples of well-known individuals who sought to lay the foundation for quality care at all levels of engagement.

3. Two key publications that have formed the foundation for the recent advancements in QI are *To Err is Human: Building a Safer Health System* (IOM, 1999) and *Crossing the Quality Chasm: A New Health System for the 21st Century* (IOM, 2001).
4. Medicare, Medicaid, and insurance groups are utilizing the core quality measures to determine the reimbursement rates to be used for different hospitals and healthcare agencies.
5. Each member of the team within the acute care setting has a role to play within the process to ensure patient safety and effective management of healthcare interventions.
6. QI is conducted in multiple healthcare settings.
7. The nurse plays a pivotal role in QI, regardless of the setting.
8. All levels and departments of an organization must be involved.
9. The HRSA has published a guide for QI programs in health care.

RED FLAGS

- Quality improvement is a must. All members of the healthcare team must take an active role in the determination and management of quality improvement within health care.

Multiple-Choice Questions

1. The management of quality care is known by several different names. Which of these names is not used when discussing quality improvement?

A. Quality assurance

B. Continuous improvement

C. Managed care

D. Quality improvement

2. What two federal funding sources helped to advance the efforts of quality improvement in 1965?

A. Title XVIII and Title XIX

B. Affordable Care Act and Medicaid

C. Title XIX and Title XX

D. Advancement in insurance and Title XVIII

3. What agency was successful in launching national goals and priorities for healthcare quality resulting in having their endorsement viewed as the "gold standard" for healthcare performance measures?

A. Leapfrog Group

B. National Quality Forum (NQF)

C. Agency for Healthcare Research and Quality (AHRQ)

D. American Nurses Association (ANA)

4. What are the three aims encompassed within the current expectations for quality and performance improvement as established by the National Quality Strategy?

A. Better care for all members of society, healthy people living in healthy communities, and affordable care for all levels of the population

B. Continuing care for selected members, healthy people living in rural communities, and prohibitive care for the upper levels of the population

C. Management of costs for health care, adequate nursing staff to care for the population, and equality for rural and urban communities

D. Appropriate care for selected members, individualized care for rural communities, and inexpensive outpatient care

5. Which of these groups is not directly interested in advancing quality improvement efforts for the nation?

A. Accreditation and regulatory bodies

B. Medical specialty societies

C. State hospital associations

D. National academic regulatory bodies

6. What strategy could be used to foster quality improvement within the acute healthcare setting?

    A. Accommodating hospital leadership that takes an active role in the process

    B. Establishing expectations for nursing staff only to seek quality as a shared responsibility

    C. Requiring physicians and administration only to be accountable

    D. Furnishing inapt and null resources to force the staff to take responsibility

Discussion Questions

1. As health care becomes more involved with core measurements, the report cards for agencies will be available to carefully compare the work done by the different agencies. Visit www.medicare.gov/hospitalcompare/. Identify which of the different aspects could be most valuable to patients and their families. Develop a tool to use with a patient/family population to make them aware of the materials provided from this site and others like it.

2. Carefully consider Draper and colleagues' (2008) five key strategies that are needed to foster quality improvement within the healthcare setting. What type of resources and programs would need to be in place to successfully incorporate some or all of these strategies? Prioritize the five strategies as to which order you think they should be in to facilitate the development of a high level of quality within the health agencies in your area.

3. You are a school nurse in your local school district and have been asked to develop a QI program. How would you begin? What resources would you need? Who should be on the QI team?

Suggested Readings

Centers for Medicare and Medicaid Services. (2015). Hospital Compare. Retrieved from http://www.cms.gov/Medicare/Quality-Initiatives-Patient -Assessment-Instruments/HospitalQualityInits/HospitalCompare.html

Kovner, C. T., Brewer, C. S., Yingrengreung, S., & Fairchild, S., (2010). New nurses' views of quality improvement education. *The Joint Commission Journal on Quality and Patient Safety,* 36(1), 29–35.

Warshaw, G. (2013). Quality improvement. *Annals of Long-Term Care,* 21(7). Retrieved from http://www.annalsoflongtermcare.com/article /quality-improvement

References

American Society for Quality. (n.d.). History of quality. Retrieved from http://asq.org/learn-about-quality/history-of-quality/overview/overview.html

Boswell, C., & Cannon, S. (2014). *Introduction to nursing research: Incorporating evidence-based practice* (3rd ed.). Burlington, MA: Jones & Bartlett Learning.

Draper, D. A., Felland, L. E., Liebhaber, A., & Melichar, L. (2008). The role of nurses in hospital quality improvement. *Center for Studying Health System Change Research Brief, 3*, 1–8.

Health Resources and Services Administration. (2011). Quality improvement. Retrieved from http://www.hrsa.gov/quality/toolbox/methodology/qualityimprovement/index.html

Institute of Medicine (IOM). (1999). *To err is human: Building a safer health system.* Washington, DC: National Academies Press.

Institute of Medicine (IOM). (2001). *Crossing the quality chasm: The IOM health care quality initiative.* Washington, DC: National Academies Press. Retrieved from http://iom.nationalacademies.org/Global/News%20Announcements/Crossing-the-Quality-Chasm-The-IOM-Health-Care-Quality-Initiative.aspx

Izumi, S. (2012). Quality improvement in nursing: Administrative mandate or professional responsibility. *Nurse Forum, 47*(4), 260–267. doi:10.1111/j.1744-6198.2012.00283x

Marjoua, Y., & Bozic, K. J. (2012). Brief history of quality movement in US healthcare. *Current Reviews in Musculoskeletal Medicine, 5*(4), 265–273. doi:10.1007/s12178-012-9137-8

Melnyk, B. M., & Fineout-Overholt, E. (2015). *Evidence-based practice in nursing & healthcare: A guide to best practice* (3th ed.). Philadelphia, PA: Wolters Kluwer.

Merriam-Webster. (n.d.). Quality assurance. Retrieved from http://www.merriam-webster.com/dictionary/quality%20assurance

North Dakota Center for Nursing. (2014). *Comparison of quality improvement, evidence-based practice, and nursing research.* Retrieved from http://www.ndcenterfornursing.org/wp-content/uploads/2013/02/Comparison-of-QI-EBP-and-Nursing-Research-Final-Document.pdf

Parry, G. J. (2014). A brief history of quality improvement. *Journal of Oncology Practice, 10*(3). 196–199. doi:10.1200/JOP.2014.00436

Saidleman, V. (2015). Ensuring quality care. In J. T. Catalano, *Nursing now!: Today's issues, tomorrow's trends* (7th ed., pp. 376–410). Philadelphia, PA: F.A. Davis.

Shirey, M. R., Hauck, S. K., Embree, J. L., Kinner, T. J., Schaar, G. L., Phillips, L. A., … McCool, I. A. (2011). Showcasing differences between quality improvement, evidence-based practice, and research. *The Journal of Continuing Education in Nursing, 42*(2), 57–70.

Weston, M., & Roberts, D. W. (2013). The influence of quality improvement efforts on patient outcomes and nursing work: A perspective from chief nursing officers at three large health systems. *Online Journal of Issues in Nursing, 18*(3), Manuscript 2. doi:10.3912/OJIN.Vol18No03Man02

Chapter **5**

Quantitative Research Design

Sharon Cannon

Chapter Objectives

At the conclusion of this chapter, the learner will be able to:

1. List characteristics of quantitative designs.
2. Discuss descriptive designs.
3. Identify control for quantitative designs.
4. Compare experimental, nonexperimental, time-dimensional, and quasi-experimental designs.
5. Compare and contrast research design, quality improvement programs, and root cause analysis.
6. Select a quantitative design for research utilization in an evidence-based practice clinical situation.

Key Terms

Comparative design	Descriptive design
Control	Experimental design
Correlational design	Independent variable
Dependent variable	Manipulation

Meta-analysis	Randomization
Meta-synthesis	Research design
Nonequivalent control group	Root cause analysis
Nonexperimental design	(RCA)
Quality improvement (QI) project	Secondary analysis
Quantitative design	Sentinel events
Quasi-experimental design	Time-dimensional design

■ Introduction

The most commonly used **research design** is a quantitative design. But precisely what is a quantitative design? This question, as well as the characteristics and types of designs for use in evidence-based practice (EBP) clinical situations, are discussed in this chapter.

Before exploring the characteristics of a study design, it is necessary to define quantitative research. Quantitative research is often identified with the traditional scientific method that gathers data objectively in an organized, systematic, controlled manner so that the findings can be generalized to other situations/populations (Brockopp & Hastings-Tolsma, 2003; Burns & Grove, 2009; Fain, 2009; Polit & Beck, 2008). A design is a plan on how to proceed; thus, a quantitative research design can be defined as an objective, systematic plan or blueprint to gather data that has application to other situations/populations. **Quantitative design** may be (1) experimental, (2) nonexperimental, or (3) quasi-experimental. Studies utilizing an **experimental design** use treatment and control groups, those with a **nonexperimental design** generate questions for experimental design, and studies having a **quasi-experimental design** lack randomization or may not include a control group.

■ Characteristics of Quantitative Research Design

The characteristics of quantitative design center on the why, where, who, what, when, and how questions. The quantitative researcher must state why (purpose) the study is being done, where (setting) the study is being conducted (e.g., laboratory, hospital, or clinic), who (subjects) is being studied (e.g., animals or humans), what type of data is being collected, when the data are to be collected, and how (design) the data are to be collected.

Within the framework of these questions, quantitative research looks for cause and effect in an experiment. When considering potential causes and effects, different groups participating in the study are viewed in terms of being either treatment or control groups. **Control** is one of the most common and important characteristics of quantitative design. To understand the concept of control, it is necessary to understand variables. A variable can be a quality, characteristic, attribute, or property of a person, thing, or situation (Burns & Grove, 2009; Polit & Beck, 2008). The two types of variables found in quantitative research are dependent and independent variables. The **dependent variable** is the outcome caused or influenced by the independent variable; the **independent variable** is a treatment, intervention, or experiment. Consider the situation in which a nurse researcher studies the effect of patient teaching (independent variable) about wound care in an attempt to reduce the likelihood of wound infection (dependent variable) when the surgical patient is discharged from the hospital. In this example, the teaching is what affects the rate of wound infection.

Closely connected to the issue of control is **manipulation** of the independent variable. The researcher wants to make sure that the treatment is the only explanation for the outcome. In the previous example, the nurse researcher wants to ensure that the patient education on wound care delivered prior to discharge is the reason why the rate of wound infections in discharged surgical patients decreases. Control or manipulation in this situation would involve providing patient education to surgical patients who are not taking antibiotics when discharged from the hospital. Patients who are taking antibiotics would be least likely to develop a wound infection and the use of antibiotics would be a variable that might skew the results.

Another important characteristic of quantitative research is randomization. **Randomization** is the assignment of subjects to a group in such a manner that each subject has an equal opportunity of being selected to participate in the study. In the wound care example, the researcher might have two groups: The control group would include those subjects who did not receive any wound care education, whereas the experimental group would include those subjects who did receive patient education. Randomization would occur when the patients were assigned to either

---

? THINK OUTSIDE THE BOX

Considering these examples, which type of research design could be used to provide the strongest methodology possible:

1. What information has been used to determine the method of catheterizing a laboring mother?
2. What information serves as the basis for the range of blood sugars used within elderly persons who are newly diagnosed with diabetes?
3. What nursing model would be useful in a critical access type of agency?

group in a way that each patient had an equal opportunity for inclusion in either group. This sampling could be done by selecting every third patient discharged to be a member of a group. Another way to randomize the sample might be to give each patient a number, draw the numbers out of a hat, and alternate assignment to the groups. Randomization helps to eliminate bias. For example, the nurse who thinks that only her patients should be in the treatment group would be biased; randomization of subjects would eliminate that possibility. Although randomization strengthens a study, be aware that not all studies can be randomized. Randomization can be costly and time-consuming, and there may not be enough participants to randomize them effectively.

In any quantitative research study, it is important to control the influence of extraneous variables, such as gender, age, and ethnicity. Randomization provides for internal validity of a study because the groups are equal at the beginning of the study. External validity is achieved when the outcome can be applied (generalized) to the target population; generalization helps strengthen the study results. Using the wound care example, control of the extraneous variable could involve not providing patient education to pediatric patients, but rather providing it only to adult patients.

Manipulation, control, and randomization are three essential characteristics of quantitative research design. These characteristics enable the researcher to be confident that the outcome is caused by the intervention and not by other variables, and that it can be generalized to a target population.

Descriptive Design

Descriptive design examines the characteristics of just one sample population. According to Burns and Grove (2009), this type of research design may be used for theory development, practice problems, rationale for current practice, generating hypotheses, or clinical decision making based on what others are doing. Examples of descriptive design include comparative (looking at differences in two or more groups), time-dimensional (occurring over an extended period of time), cross-sectional (stages of development simultaneously), trends and events, and correlational (relationships) designs. A descriptive design delineates or explains the variables being studied and provides flexibility in examining a problem from many different angles. However, be aware that data obtained in quantitative, descriptive designs are limited to participant responses to things such as blood pressure equipment or scores on a survey. The two most commonly used types of descriptive designs are comparative and correlational.

The **comparative design** involves no manipulation or control of the independent variable, with the dependent variable being the only variable measured in two or more groups (Brink & Wood, 2001). This type of design can also be retrospective in nature. Using the wound care example, a comparative design would assign patients with wounds to a group of surgical patients or to a group of patients with wounds resulting from trauma to compare the rates of post-discharge infections. The research question might be, "Is the rate of infection higher in trauma patients than in surgical patients?" The patients' past histories would then be examined for prior surgeries or trauma wounds. Cause and effect remain the focus of this design, in that the two groups being compared for infection rates are identified according to the type of wound.

Perhaps the most widely used type of descriptive design is the correlational study. Simply stated, a **correlational design** examines the relationships between two or more variables within a situation without knowing the reason for the relationship. The researcher may use this design when there is uncertainty about whether the variables are related and, if so, how they are related. However, the researcher assumes that the variables are related and seeks to discover and explain that relationship. Correlational designs do not conclude that only one variable causes another, because the independent variable cannot always be controlled (Polit & Beck, 2008).

Another aspect of a correlational design is that it is *ex post facto*, meaning "from after the fact" (Polit & Beck, 2006). For example, a study that compares a variable occurring in the past with a variable occurring currently would be characterized as using a retrospective correlational design. In other words, a study that looks at a variable after the fact is a retrospective study. For instance, the nurse researcher might conduct a chart review on all discharged surgical patients to determine if any patient education on wound care occurred prior to discharge from the hospital and then to check whether any of those patients were readmitted for a wound infection.

Prospective correlational designs are usually considered stronger than retrospective designs, because the researcher may be able to control or rule out explanations for some outcomes (Polit & Beck, 2008). These designs require the researcher to assume cause and effect and to implement the study under those assumptions.

Correlational designs may also be predictive in nature. In this type of study, one variable occurs prior to another variable—that is, the independent variable occurs prior to the dependent variable. Again using the wound care example, a predictive correlational study research statement might be, "The rate of wound infection will decrease 1 week

❷ THINK OUTSIDE THE BOX

Explore the idea of control within a quantitative design methodology. Which aspects of the study design are important to consider and why?

post-discharge after receiving the wound care educational program in the outpatient clinic."

Experimental Design

Experimental design looks for cause and effect (outcome). Obviously, a preceding cause must be present. A relationship between the cause and the outcome without any influencing variables to warrant the conclusion that a cause-and-effect relationship exists is also expected.

Several issues related to experimental design should be addressed before discussing the designs themselves. The first issue is that not all variables can be manipulated. In the prior wound care example, not every patient has a wound. As such, the researcher cannot inflict a wound on all individuals so as to obtain a larger random sample.

Another issue is that of ethics. Consider the famous Tuskegee Syphilis Study (Centers for Disease Control and Prevention, n.d.), an experiment that was conducted over 40 years to examine the progress of syphilis in adult black males. Many of the subjects in this study were not even aware that they were participants. Also, even though an effective treatment for syphilis (penicillin) was available, not all subjects with syphilis in this study were given penicillin. To satisfy ethical concerns, some variables should not be manipulated.

Feasibility is another issue in experimental design. Some experiments may be too expensive, require cooperation from individuals from multiple key areas, require too much time, or not have enough subjects for participation. When considering the feasibility of a proposed study, careful attention should be given to what types of resources might be needed to conduct the research project.

In experimental design, another significant issue is the Hawthorne effect. Simply stated, the Hawthorne effect arises when the subjects know that they are part of the study and change their behavior accordingly; that is, the act of observing changes the observed subject's behavior. While it is not possible to prevent the Hawthorne effect from occurring, thought needs to be given to how to minimize the influence that attention has on the outcome to the study.

Keeping in mind these issues, we now move on to an examination of experimental design. The most classic experimental design is a pre-test/post-test design. With this approach, subjects are assigned to one of two groups: a control (comparative) group that does not receive the treatment (intervention) or an experimental group that does receive the treatment. In the wound care example, patients would be assigned to a group that receives no specific wound care instructions (control group) or to the group that receives patient education regarding wound care (experimental group).

Figure 5-1

Experimental design examples.

Pre-test/Post-test

$\quad$ R $\quad$ O_1 $\quad$ X_1 $\quad$ O_2

$\quad$ R $\quad$ O_1 $\quad$ X_2 $\quad$ O_2

Two-Group Post-test Only

$\quad$ R $\quad$ X_1 $\quad$ O_1

$\quad$ R $\quad$ X_2 $\quad$ O_1

Three Groups

$\quad$ R $\quad$ X_1 $\quad$ O_1

$\quad$ R $\quad$ X_2 $\quad$ O_1

$\quad$ R $\quad$ O_1

Four Groups

$\quad$ R $\quad$ O_1 $\quad$ X_1 $\quad$ O_2

$\quad$ R $\quad$ X_1 $\quad$ O_2

$\quad$ R $\quad$ O_1 $\quad$ X_2 $\quad$ O_2

$\quad$ R $\quad$ X_2 $\quad$ O_2

Note: O = outcome/measurement; R = random assignment; X = treatment/intervention.

Another experimental design of considerable importance in the health-care arena is the randomized controlled trial (RCT). The RCT is considered the true experiment. This design may involve two, three, or four groups. The tests used may involve both a pre-test and post-test, a post-test only, or repeated measures (**Figure 5-1**).

■ Nonexperimental Design

Some studies do not lend themselves to an experimental design; that is, manipulation of variables is not possible, nor is randomization controlled. Studies with this kind of nonexperimental design occur in the here and now and are observational rather than interventional in nature. Two types of nonexperimental designs used in EBP are secondary analysis and meta-analysis.

Secondary analysis follows the course implied by its name: It examines data obtained in another study and allows researchers to examine large and small data sets collected via different approaches. A secondary analysis asks new questions about data previously collected for another purpose. For example, a nurse researcher interested in the effects of patient education on decreased wound infection rates might examine one or several previously conducted studies. By analyzing a variable that had not been studied previously, such as the age of the patient, a secondary analysis might show a relationship to wound healing, especially for geriatric patients.

Meta-analysis also looks at previous studies and, as indicated by Bator, Taylor, and Catalano (2015), it is a way to rank similar study results. Brockopp and Hastings-Tolsma (2003) indicate that meta-analysis, through calculation of statistics, can help researchers establish the existence of bias and confounding variables in the cause-and-effect relationship identified in multiple studies. Polit and Beck (2006) suggest that a data set is "the total collection of data for all sample members for analysis" (p. 642). The data set analysis carried out as part of a meta-analysis is similar to that performed for individual studies through statistical tests. The key facet of meta-analysis is the application of statistics to multiple studies looking at the same phenomenon (Burns & Grove, 2009). Stated another way, meta-analysis for quantitative designs is intended to "to utilize statistical methods to merge the outcomes of independent projects" (Hopp & Rittenmeyer, 2012). Meta-analysis for quantitative designs focuses on statistical methods and is not to be confused with **meta-synthesis** of qualitative designs, which focuses on individual studies that are pooled.

Although secondary and meta-analyses are of particular importance for research utilization in EBP, caution should be taken when considering their findings. Not all studies focus on the same subject, and information may even be missing from some studies. Care should be taken before drawing conclusions or making generalizations in applying findings to specific populations because bias can result, especially in studies with small sample sizes. The researcher should keep in mind the adage that "one size does not fit all."

❓ THINK OUTSIDE THE BOX

If you have elected to use a nonexperimental design, how can you strengthen the confidence in the research project's findings?

Time-Dimensional Design

When establishing a research project, attention must always be given to the dimension of time. The determination of when and how long data are to be collected is an essential component to any research design, and this process is termed **time-dimensional design**. If data have already been collected, then the study is considered to utilize a retrospective design. An example of a retrospective design would be that of a chart review. Perhaps a new procedure has been implemented to decrease length of stay (LOS). The nurse might go to the medical records department and conduct a chart review for the average LOS for patients who did not receive the new procedure versus those who did receive it.

A second type of time-dimensional design comprises a cross-sectional design. The cross-sectional design measures only what is currently in existence; it does not examine anything that happened in the past or future. An example of this design could be a retrospective chart review of lung cancer patients for the past five years to discover how long they had smoked cigarettes. Many cross-sectional studies are retrospective in nature, but they all collect data at a specific point in time.

The third type of time-dimensional design is the longitudinal study. As is implied by the name, a study with a longitudinal design relies on data that are collected at various intervals over time. The times for data collection may be short or long depending on the rate of change. This design is useful to examine changes that occur over time and assist in determining causality (Polit & Beck, 2008). Longitudinal designs are considered stronger than cross-sectional study designs because longitudinal designs allow for the possibility that changes and trends might emerge. An example of a longitudinal study is that by Hanna, Weaver, Slaven, Fortenberry, and DiMeglio (2014), which was conducted over a period of 12 months. They examined emerging adults with type 1 diabetes at high school graduation and at 3, 6, 9, and 12 months later. However, longitudinal studies also face the extra danger of having subjects drop out over time, and they are generally more expensive to manage. For example, in the Hanna and colleagues (2014) study, three subjects withdrew, two died, and two did not complete the study.

Each of the time-dimensional designs has its own set of advantages and disadvantages that must be considered by the researcher. In addition, the strengths and weaknesses of each study design must be considered before the results of the studies are applied to practice.

Quasi-Experimental Design

Given that randomization is often not possible in research studies, quasi-experimental design is the most frequently used quantitative research design. With this approach, the independent variable is still manipulated, but there is no randomization or control group. The purpose of quasi-experimental design is to examine causality, though it is acknowledged that this design is not as strong as the experimental design, which has a control group and randomization. Nevertheless, quasi-experimental design is considered stronger than descriptive design, and it is more practical when true experimental design is not possible.

Types of quasi-experimental design include (1) post-test only with nonequivalent groups, (2) one-group pre-test/post-test, (3) untreated control group with pre-test/post-test, (4) removal treatment and reversal treatment, (5) nonequivalent control group, and (6) time series. The two most commonly used designs—nonequivalent control group and time series—are discussed here.

The **nonequivalent control group** design (sometimes called a comparison group) compares two groups that are not randomized. The initial baseline measurement (O1) is used to determine if the subjects assigned to groups are similar. A treatment/intervention (X) is applied, and then a second measurement (O2) is performed to see if the outcome is a result of the treatment/intervention (**Figure 5-2**).

Using the prior example of wound care, all patients would be assigned to group 1 or group 2. A pre-test assessment would be conducted. The intervention (patient education program) would then be implemented. Each group would then be tested to see if its members experienced a decreased infection rate (outcome). When using this type of study design, the nurse researcher should keep in mind potential confounding factors such as the Hawthorne effect as well as the threat of history. History, in this instance, refers to some other variable that might have occurred. In the wound care experiment, an example of the history variable might be the patients who received additional instruction by the doctor's office staff prior to undergoing surgery or again after the educational program was administered.

The second quasi-experimental design to be discussed is the time-series design. This type of study may be conducted over a long period, in which case it is also called a longitudinal study. With a time-series design, participants are not randomized, nor is a control group used. Data are collected at various intervals prior to the treatment as well as after the treatment (see Figure 5-2). Returning to the wound care example, in a time-series design, the first observation might be on days 2 and 3 post-operatively, with a subsequent observation being recorded on the day of discharge. The educational program would then be conducted. The next three measurements might be on days 5, 7, and 9 postoperatively.

Figure 5-2

Quasi-experimental design examples.

Nonequivalent Control Group

O_1 X O_2

O_1 O_2

Note: O_1 = baseline measurement; X = treatment/intervention; O2= outcome measurement.

Time Series (Simple)

O_1 O_2 O_3 X O_4 O_5 O_6

Note: O_1, O_2, O_3 = baseline measurements at various levels; X = treatment/intervention;

O_4, O_5, O_6 = outcome measures at various intervals.

A variable that should be considered as an alternative explanation for the outcome measurement within time-series studies is maturation. Maturation refers to change that occurs throughout the entire span of time that the experiment is conducted. It might be a result of the repetition of testing, which might influence the scores that follow. For instance, if the patients were tested about wound care knowledge prior to receiving the educational program, they might become aware of what was needed for wound care to prevent infection just because of the questions used to test their baseline knowledge.

Another area of concern with the time-series design is the potential for attrition of subjects. The study occurs over time and subjects may drop out of the study for various reasons. As a result, the sample size may be too small when the study ends, causing the study's findings not to be generalizable to other situations or populations.

❓ THINK OUTSIDE THE BOX

Discuss how you would use the ranking of research designs' strength in evidence-based practice.

The two quasi-experimental designs discussed here offer a practical approach when an experimental design is not possible. Nurse researchers should be alert to the possible threats of the quasi-experimental design that can lead to other reasons for the study's outcomes.

■ Control

As indicated earlier in this text, control of variables is critical when the researcher is seeking to determine the extent of a cause-and-effect relationship for the treatment/intervention applied as part of a study. Randomization helps control extraneous variables, both internal and external, to a research project, especially when the study employs an experimental design.

In studies using nonexperimental and quasi-experimental designs, which do not have randomization or control groups, using subjects who are similar helps control extraneous variables that can influence the outcome. As a result, history, maturation, and attrition threats must be considered when designing the research project so as to maintain control. Variables can be controlled through the establishment of specific inclusion/exclusion criteria for selection of subjects, timing of test intervals, use of scripts for data collectors, and the setting in which the study is conducted.

■ Research Design, Quality Improvement Projects, and Root Cause Analysis

Care must be taken when designing quantitative research. Even though research and **quality improvement (QI) projects** or activities are focused on patient outcomes, they are different processes (Kring, 2008). QI results can provide direction for improving practice but are not necessarily considered true "scientific inquiry." For example, chart reviews may reveal a trend but do not inspire the same level of confidence as results produced from a quantitative retrospective research design. QI projects can and often do contribute additional evidence that may even give significance to previous findings. Nevertheless, research designs take a more rigorous approach toward producing results and have more significant implications for practice. Both research design and QI projects may have implications for evidence-based practice, however, and their relationship should be considered within the totality of quantitative research design.

Root cause analysis (RCA) began in 1949 when the U.S. military wanted to examine system and equipment failures. Other industries, such as the space, manufacturing, and automotive industries, then began to realize the importance of RCA (Dunn & Renner, 2012). Simply stated, RCA identifies whether a failure is due to system-related or human error. For instance, when a plane crashes, the RCA determines whether there was a system/equipment error or pilot error. In health care, RCAs have been used to investigate adverse events or **sentinel events** since the Joint Commission mandated the use of RCAs in 1997 (Agency for Healthcare Research and Quality [AHRQ], 2012). RCAs have a significant impact for designing research and QI projects to eliminate errors and provide safer health care to patients. Examples of errors can range from nurse staffing issues to incorrect dosage calculations, and from amputations of the wrong limb to lack of appropriate policies/procedures. Research design and QI projects can provide evidence for RCA and thus improve patient safety.

▮ Evidence-Based Considerations

Utilization of quantitative research design in EBP requires the nurse to be able to comprehend the various designs and understand both their benefits and their shortcomings. Whether the nurse is participating in research or is applying research findings in practice, the type of design is essential to guide clinical decision making. The concepts of randomization and control in quantitative research provide information about generalization of outcomes in experimental, nonexperimental, and quasi-experimental studies to current practice.

If a nurse wants to look at the relationship between an educational program and the rate of wound infections, a correlational design would be appropriate. In contrast, if a nurse wants to examine the effect of a wound care educational program in producing a decreased rate of wound infections, the appropriate quantitative design would be experimental or quasi-experimental. Use of a secondary analysis or meta-analysis is another way a nurse might use quantitative research to validate existing practice or the need to change practice.

Manipulation, control of variables, and randomization are essential components of quantitative research. Extraneous variables in the practice setting must be examined carefully so that the evidence obtained will be

---

❓ THINK OUTSIDE THE BOX

What could an RCA reveal about a patient who had the wrong leg amputated? What could be considered a system failure? What could be considered a personnel failure? What research design would be most appropriate to investigate this type of error?

applicable to nursing practice. Thus, knowing whether the research design is experimental, quasi-experimental, or nonexperimental influences the strength and generalizability of a study's findings to the current practice being considered. This point is of particular significance when conducting a secondary analysis or meta-analysis of research for the purpose of making clinical decisions.

Quantitative research design and QI projects are important when examining evidence to improve practice. Nurses need to make sure they fully understand the distinctions between QI and quantitative research designs, as well as how both are relevant in EBP.

Summary Points

1. Quantitative research is often identified as corresponding with the traditional scientific method, which gathers data objectively in an organized method to allow findings to be generalized to other situations/populations.
2. A quantitative research design is an objective, systematic plan to gather data.
3. Characteristics of quantitative designs center on why, where, who, what, when, and how questions.
4. Quantitative research examines relationships for cause and effect in an experiment.
5. Manipulation of the independent variable, control of extraneous variables, and randomization are essential to quantitative research.
6. In comparative designs, there is no manipulation or control of the independent variable.
7. The most commonly used descriptive design is the correlational design, which examines relationships between two or more variables within a situation without knowing the reason why the relationship exists.
8. Correlational designs may be *ex post facto*, prospective, or predictive.
9. Experimental designs look for cause and effect (outcome).
10. Issues such as ethics, inability to manipulate all variables, feasibility, and the Hawthorne effect must be addressed when considering studies with experimental designs.
11. The most classic experimental design is the pre-test/post-test design.
12. The RCT is considered to be a true experimental design.
13. Two types of nonexperimental designs are used in EBP: secondary analysis and meta-analysis. Both look at previously completed studies and create data sets from those earlier studies to be analyzed in a different approach.

14. Quasi-experimental designs are used most frequently because the independent variable can still be manipulated even when no randomization or control group is possible.
15. The two most commonly used quasi-experimental designs are the nonequivalent control group and time-series designs.
16. The nonequivalent control group design compares two groups whose members are not randomized.
17. The time-series design is not randomized, and there is no control group. Data are gathered at various intervals.
18. Control of threats such as history, maturation, and attrition is of prime importance in quantitative designs and is of significance when making clinical decisions based on outcomes from quantitative research.
19. Understanding the implications for utilization of quantitative research in EBP requires a working knowledge of quantitative design.
20. Quality improvement projects and quantitative research are important in confirming evidence for EBP.
21. RCA and QI have a relationship with research design and EBP.

RED FLAGS

- For a study to be classified as an experimental (quantitative) design, the design must incorporate control, randomization, and an intervention.
- Experimental (quantitative) design is considered to be the strongest research design. Quasi-experimental (quantitative) design has less strength, and non-experimental (quantitative) design has the least strength.
- When a small sample size is used for a quantitative study, the results of the study need to be examined closely for their generalizability to other populations.
- Prospective designs are stronger than retrospective design formats.
- Control of variables is critical when results are related to cause and effect.
- A comparative design does not involve any manipulation or control of the independent variable.
- Sentinel/adverse events require an RCA to improve.

Multiple-Choice Questions

1. Which of the following characteristics is not part of a quantitative research design?

   A. Randomization
   B. Manipulation
   C. Saturation
   D. Control

2. Which of the following is not an independent variable?

   A. Outcome
   B. Treatment
   C. Intervention
   D. Experiment

3. Quantitative research is often identified with which method of gathering data?

   A. Triangulation
   B. Saturation
   C. Ethnography
   D. Scientific method

4. Nonexperimental designs generate _____ for _____ designs.

   A. Answers; quasi-experimental
   B. Questions; experimental
   C. Solutions; quantitative
   D. Problems; experimental

5. Which of the following is one of the most common and important characteristics of a quantitative design?

   A. The dependent variable
   B. The independent variable
   C. Control
   D. The relationship

6. Manipulation of which variable is connected to control?

   A. Independent
   B. Dependent
   C. Extraneous
   D. Attribute

7. What does randomization helps to eliminate?

A. Confounding data
B. Ethics
C. Subjects
D. Bias

8. Generalization can _____ a study.

A. Weaken
B. Strengthen
C. Shorten
D. Lengthen

9. A comparative design has:

A. No manipulation and control of the dependent variable.
B. Only measurement of the dependent variable.
C. No manipulation and control of the independent variable.
D. Both B and C.

10. A correlational study looks at the:

A. Cause of two or more variables.
B. Relationship of two or more variables.
C. Effect of two or more variables.
D. Both A and C.

11. Issues related to experimental design include:

A. Manipulation of all variables, ethics, and feasibility.
B. The Hawthorne effect, ethics, and sample size.
C. Treatments, interventions, and no manipulation of variables.
D. Feasibility, the Hawthorne effect, and research questions.

12. An example of a randomized controlled trial (RCT) design is as follows (where R = randomization, O = measurement, and X = treatment):

A. R O X O
B. O X O
C. O O X O O
D. O O O X O O O

13. Meta-analysis is the examination of multiple studies through statistical analysis to establish:

A. The nonexistence of bias.
B. New data sets for analysis.
C. The nonexistence of confounding variables.
D. Correlation of the variables.

14. A quasi-experimental design is one in which:

    A.   The dependent variable is manipulated with randomization and a control group.

    B.   The independent variable is manipulated with randomization and a control group.

    C.   The independent variable is manipulated with no randomization and no control group.

    D.   The dependent variable is manipulated with no randomization and no control group.

15. The initial baseline measurement in a nonequivalent control group is used to determine if the subjects assigned to the group are:

    A.   Different.

    B.   Equal.

    C.   Bonded.

    D.   Similar.

16. What is the research design that collects data at various intervals called?

    A.   A long study

    B.   A time-series study

    C.   An experimental study

    D.   A nonexperimental study

17. What is an area of concern in a time-series design?

    A.   Randomization

    B.   Control

    C.   Manipulation

    D.   Maturation

18. Some ways of controlling variables for nonexperimental or quasi-experimental designs are:

    A.   Timing of test intervals and the setting.

    B.   Randomization of subjects and control groups.

    C.   Flexible inclusion and exclusion criteria.

    D.   Control of history and maturation.

19. In evidence-based practice, a nurse using quantitative research for clinical decision making must be most knowledgeable about how:

    A.   To calculate statistics.

    B.   To write research reports.

    C.   The study design applies to practice.

    D.   To design a research study.

20. Using research in practice requires the nurse to be most aware of:

    A. Limited funding.

    B. Generalizability of the results to current practice.

    C. Exclusion of subjects.

    D. The credentials of the researcher.

21. Quality improvement (QI) projects are considered:

    A. The same as scientific inquiry.

    B. Different from scientific inquiry.

    C. To focus on only patient satisfaction.

    D. A rigorous approach for research.

22. Root cause analysis (RCA) had its origin in:

    A. Dental industry.

    B. Mechanical engineering.

    C. Military industry.

    D. Business industry.

23. In what year did the Joint Commission mandate RCAs?

    A. 1967

    B. 1977

    C. 1987

    D. 1997

Discussion Questions

1. You are a nurse in a preoperative holding area in which all patients are classified as nil per os (NPO), meaning "nothing by mouth," after midnight to prevent possible aspiration. You wonder why that policy is necessary, and you and a surgical team want to design a research project to investigate the potential for providing at least some liquid nourishment to preoperative patients. The team decides to do a two-group, post-test only design.

   a. Using the previous example (all surgical patients being NPO after midnight), how would you and the surgical team conduct a meta-analysis?

   b. Using a nonequivalent control group design in the NPO scenario, explain how this design would be constructed.

2. A medication error resulted in a sentinel event on your unit. How would you go about implementing a root cause analysis (RCA)?

Suggested Readings

Bott, M., & Endacott, R. (2005). Clinical research: Quantitative data collection and analysis. *Intensive & Critical Care Nursing, 21*(3), 187–193.

Chulay, M. (2006). Good research ideas for clinicians. *AACN Advanced Critical Care, 17*(3), 253–265.

Freshwater, D. (2005). Integrating qualitative and quantitative research methods: Trend or foe? *Journal of Research in Nursing, 10*(3), 337–338.

Kinn, S., & Curzio, J. (2005). Integrating qualitative and quantitative research methods. *Journal of Research in Nursing, 10*(3), 317–336.

Onwuegbuzie, A., & Leech, N. (2005). Taking the "Q" out of research: Teaching research methodology courses without the divide between quantitative and qualitative paradigms. *Quality & Quantity, 39*(3), 267–295.

Walker, W. (2005). The strengths and weaknesses of research designs involving quantitative measures. *Journal of Research in Nursing, 10*(5), 571–573.

Yoder, L. (2005). Evidence-based practice: The time is now! *MedSurg Nursing, 14*(2), 91–92.

References

Agency for Healthcare Research and Quality (AHRQ). (2012). Patient safety primers: Root cause analysis. Retrieved from http://psnet.ahrq.gov/primer.aspx?primerID=10

Bator, S., Taylor, S., & Catalano, J.T. (2015). Nursing research and evidence based practice. In J. Catalano (Ed.), Nursing now!: Today's issues, tomorrow's trends. (7th ed., pp. 581–674). Philadelphia, PA: F.A. Davis Company.

Brink, P. J., & Wood, M. J. (2001). Basic steps in planning nursing research from question to proposal (5th ed.). Sudbury, MA: Jones and Bartlett Publishers.

Brockopp, D. Y., & Hastings-Tolsma, M. T. (2003). Fundamentals of nursing research (3rd ed.). Sudbury, MA: Jones and Bartlett Publishers.

Burns, N., & Grove, S. K. (2009). The practice of nursing research: Appraisal, synthesis, and generation of evidence (6th ed.). St. Louis, MO: Saunders Elsevier.

Centers for Disease Control and Prevention (CDC). (n.d.). The Tuskegee timeline. Retrieved from http://www.cdc.gov/tuskegee/timeline.htm

Dunn, E. J., & Renner, C. (2012). Root cause analysis: Faculty development [Presentation slides]. Retrieved from http://www.med.cornell.edu/risk-management/best_practices/RootCauseAnalysis.ppt

Fain, J. A. (2009). Reading, understanding, and applying nursing research (3rd ed.). Philadelphia, PA: F.A. Davis.

Hanna, K. M., Weaver, M. T., Slaven, J. E., Fortenberry, J. D., & DiMeglio, L. A. (2014). Diabetes-related quality of life and the demands and burdens of diabetes care among emerging adults with Type 1 diabetes in the year after graduation. Research in Nursing and Health, 37(5), 399–408.

Hopp, L., & Rittenmeyer, L. (2012). Introduction to evidence-based practice: A practical guide for nursing. Philadelphia, PA: F.A. Davis.

Kring, D. L. (2008). Research and quality improvement: Different processes, different evidence. MedSurg Nursing, 17(3), 162–169.

Polit, D. F., & Beck, C. T. (2006). Essentials of nursing research methods, appraisal and utilization (6th ed.). Philadelphia, PA: Lippincott Williams & Wilkins.

Polit, D. F., & Beck, C. T. (2008). Nursing research: Generating and assessing evidence for nursing practice (8th ed.). Philadelphia, PA: Wolters Kluwer/Lippincott Williams & Wilkins.

Chapter 6

Qualitative and Mixed Research Methods

JoAnn Long, Carol Boswell, and Donna Scott Tilley

© VLADGRIN/iStock/Thinkstock

Chapter Objectives

At the conclusion of this chapter, the learner will be able to:

1. Define qualitative and mixed methods research.
2. Describe the various qualitative research methodologies.
3. Describe the various mixed methods research methodologies.
4. Discuss analysis of qualitative and mixed method study data.
5. Contrast the goals and distinctive features of qualitative and mixed methods research.
6. Discuss the advantages of qualitative and mixed methods research.
7. Discuss issues of methodological rigor in qualitative and mixed methods research.

Key Terms

Action research	Content analysis
Bracketing	Convergent validity
Case study	Ethnography

Grounded theory

Mixed methods research

Nesting

Phenomenology

Purposeful sampling

Qualitative research

Rigor

Saturation

■ Introduction

As the United States moves to implement the Affordable Care Act (ACA), nurses must increase their competency in all areas of research (Carnegie Foundation Report, n.d.). Knowledge of qualitative and mixed methods research is an important competency for nurses engaged in evidence-based care and is the focus of this chapter. Human beings are by nature complex. What drives human decision making and behavior is difficult to understand and measure. Understanding in depth the complex nature of how people perceive what they have experienced is a challenging task. Qualitative research methods are based on the assumption that truth is fluid and offers an avenue for exploration of elements of humanity that are not best understood using quantitative research methods. Qualitative methods use narrative to understand meaning. Mixed methods research offers a joint approach to research, which values and draws upon both objective numbers and subjective knowledge. Mixed methods research blends the qualitative and quantitative perspectives and can profoundly enhance insight into the environment in which nurses practice (Siddiqui & Fitzgerald, 2014). This chapter presents an overview of qualitative research methods and mixed methods research. It provides a brief history of qualitative research in nursing; compares quantitative and qualitative research paradigms; presents an overview of the most commonly used qualitative designs in nursing research; discusses sampling, data collection, and data analysis for both qualitative and mixed methods research; and guides the reader in the application to one's nursing practice.

■ Qualitative Research

The word "qualitative" means that one is examining the quality of something rather than the quantity, amount, intensity, or frequency. Examining the quality of something implies a level of subjectivity. Denzin and Lincoln (2011) note that the qualitative researcher considers the socially constructed nature of reality, the relationship between the research and the subject of the research, and the situational factors that shape inquiry. In other words, the social experience shapes the meaning of reality.

Nursing has traditionally focused on the person as a whole. This holistic approach to the person lends itself well to qualitative methods. As a result, qualitative methods have become increasingly common in nursing research. Qualitative methods continue to gain recognition as being valuable to the science of nursing, as these studies contribute to areas in which little research has been done or variables for quantitative research have yet to be defined. With the increased use of these methods, efforts to design qualitative methodologies that offer holistic understanding of persons while still offering reliability and validity are also improving.

A Brief History of Qualitative Methods

Research, as we know it, was founded in the natural sciences with a positivist approach. Simply stated, the positivist approach requires objectivity and neutrality to logically test theories and hypotheses. The underlying assumption is that truth is something that can be known and measured.

Alternatively, **qualitative research** methods are rooted in the disciplines of sociology, anthropology, and philosophy with the underlying assumption that truth can only be approximated. In the 1920s and 1930s, social scientists such as Mead (1935) and Malinowski (1922) put structure to what had previously been an unstructured process of qualitative research. Researchers at the Chicago School, in adopting and formalizing processes of qualitative social study, gave credibility to this new qualitative paradigm of research (Holloway & Wheeler, 2010). Qualitative research carefully investigates those aspects that are not quantifiable.

In the 1960s, qualitative research saw increased use when new qualitative approaches, such as grounded theory (Glaser & Strauss, 1967), were introduced. In the 1970s, it was increasingly common to see journals exclusively publishing qualitative research reports. Nurse researchers began adopting the qualitative paradigm to inform their practice. Today, well over 100 journals are publishing only qualitative research, many of which are specific to nursing. Reputable research journals worldwide routinely publish research drawn from both the quantitative and qualitative paradigms. Further, recent trends illustrate the growing appreciation of publishing synthesized findings from both qualitative and quantitative paradigms (Joanna Briggs Institute, 2015). Qualitative research has come of age and is now accepted as a viable method for discovering new perspectives.

■ Comparing Qualitative and Quantitative Methods

It is not uncommon for both researchers and consumers of research to have strong opinions about the value of quantitative or qualitative methods. Those individuals who favor quantitative methods may be skeptical about qualitative studies, citing limitations in reliability, validity, and structure. Those researchers who favor qualitative methods may claim that quantitative studies are shallow or do not paint a complete and accurate picture of a phenomenon. In truth, both types of research have great scientific merit. The research question informs the type of research method selected.

Three characteristics distinguish the qualitative research approach from the quantitative approach (Morse, 1991). First, qualitative research approaches phenomena from the "emic" perspective. That is, the viewpoint of the participant provides the source of meaning rather than the perspective of the researcher. Second, qualitative research makes use of a holistic approach to the participant. The participant brings values and life experiences that affect his or her perspective on the phenomenon of interest. Although quantitative methods often seek to minimize the impact of these values and experiences, qualitative methods embrace these individual differences. Finally, qualitative methods are inductive and interactive rather than deductive. Quantitative methods require that the researcher not deviate in the data collection process from one subject to another; qualitative methods allow the researcher the flexibility to adapt his or her inquiry as understanding of the phenomenon grows.

The consumer of research may also note that research participants are described differently in these two types of studies. Quantitative researchers typically refer to the individual of interest in a study as a subject. Qualitative researchers may refer to the individual of interest in a study as an informant or a participant; however, the terminology for individuals participating in a study overlaps in quantitative and qualitative methods.

Qualitative and quantitative methods differ significantly in acceptable sample size. Sample sizes in qualitative studies are generally much smaller than in quantitative studies. Because the focus of the qualitative data is on the quality of the data collected, each participant is a source of a large volume of data. Thus, a smaller sample size is reasonable and common.

The differences between qualitative and quantitative methods are significant, but, in many cases, combining both methods is a viable option for researchers. When quantitative and qualitative research methods are combined, a mixed methods design is the result. A researcher might choose to combine methods in order to supplement the data, validate the data, or determine in pilot studies the best approach to data collection with a larger group.

■ Approaches to Qualitative Research

Many rich and varied designs from which to choose when planning a qualitative study are available (Smythe, 2012). The more commonly used designs are discussed here. Many qualitative designs share common features, particularly with regard to sampling strategies, data collection techniques, and data analysis.

Case Study

A **case study** is an in-depth examination of individuals or groups of people. A case study may be used when insight into a unique situation is needed (Rosenberg & Yates, 2007). For example, a researcher interested in end-of-life issues could conduct a case study of a person recently diagnosed with terminal cancer. The investigator might choose to conduct a case study of nurses at a hospice agency. An examiner might also choose to examine a series of similar cases in order to inquire about the phenomenon, population, or general condition. This type of study would be called a collective case study (Stake, 1998). When a study is focused on the phenomenon and telling the participant's story, a case study approach is a realistic method to employ.

The researcher engaging in a case study is typically seeking to understand what is common about a case and what is unique about a case (Stake, 1998). Stake (1998) stated that in order to fully understand commonalities and unique features of a case, the researcher is likely to explore case features such as the following:

- The nature of the case
- The historic background of the case
- The physical setting
- Other contexts, including economic, political, legal, and aesthetic
- Other cases through which this case is recognized
- Those informants through whom the case is known

A case study might include data such as temperatures or pain ratings (quantitative), along with data about the person's experience of pain and discomfort (qualitative). Together, such data paint a more complete picture of the disease experience.

Data analysis in case studies, as with other qualitative methods, involves **content analysis**, in which the researcher looks for patterns and themes. For example, the researcher might identify the themes of "social isolation" and "mistrust and jealousy" in a case study of an adult male who has abused his spouse (Scott Tilley, Rugari, & Walker, 2008). As the research team endeavors to appreciate the theme more completely, the case takes on merit for understanding the unique nature of the experience.

The readers or consumers of a case study should expect to be able to apply the findings from a case to their practice when the researcher has clearly delineated the case by defining the object of the study, identified patterns of data, and developed generalizations or assertions about the case. They should avoid applying findings from a case to their practice when the case is single or is a poor representation of a population, or when a single case as a negative example is applied to general populations. For example, a single case about intractable pain that is poorly managed should not be used to guide policy. Conversely, several cases illustrating effective management of pain through the use of guided imagery might well be used to guide policy about the use of guided imagery in a hospice agency.

Ethnography

Ethnography involves collection and analysis of data about groups. The ethnographer seeks to understand the culture of the group or to gain an understanding of the values, norms, and rules that characterize the group. For ethnography, groups of interest may be organizational, experiential, ethnic, and geographic. Ethnography is an excellent way to understand the norms of groups of interest to nursing. For example, outstanding ethnographies of organizations such as groups of patients or caregivers with specific illnesses (e.g., HIV and AIDS) and specific healthcare delivery settings (e.g., nursing homes, critical care units) are key to understanding the intricacies of the group.

Data collection for ethnography is usually accomplished through reading of documents within the culture, conducting interviews, observation, or a combination of all these methods. Key informants or people who are most knowledgeable about the culture are usually a primary source of interview data.

The reader or consumer of studies based on this method might find practice applications if the ethnography informs one how to:

- Behave when with a certain group
- Approach a person within the group
- Recognize and respond to needs of a person within the group

For example, a nurse might find ethnographic data of the experiential group of parents of children with cystic fibrosis (CF) helpful in the provision of care to a child with the disease. This ethnography might provide the nurse with insight about the needs of the parents, how the parents can access assistance within the community of parents of children with CF, and what experiences and feelings are common among the parents of children with CF.

Grounded Theory

Grounded theory is a general methodology for developing new theory that is inherent in data systematically gathered and analyzed (Denzin & Lincoln, 1998). An explicit expectation of theory development and theory verification in this method exists.

Data analysis in grounded theory is systematic and deliberate. The process begins with open coding, which involves categorizing the information and examining properties and dimensions of the data (Strauss & Corbin, 1998). The next step is axial coding, in which the researcher identifies relationships between categories and subcategories. Selective coding, the final step in data analysis, is the integration of concepts around a core category and the filling in of categories in need of further development and refinement (Strauss & Corbin, 1998). **Saturation** is a concept of relevance in data analysis and data collection, in which the researcher continues data analysis until no new codes or categories emerge.

The final product of the grounded theory method is a theory that is established in data about the phenomenon of interest. The consumer of grounded theory research could expect to apply the model while developing interventions for a population. For example, reading a grounded theory about the attachment patterns of elderly adults might guide the nurse who is assisting a family in relocating their aging parent from a home environment to an assisted-living environment.

Narrative Inquiry

Narrative inquiry, sometimes known as storytelling, is a qualitative research method that seeks to understand the meaning that participants ascribe to their experiences. Telling the story of their experience, say with illness or provision of health care, allows the participant to reflect on the experience from their own point of view to inform others about the experience. Meanings are derived by both the participant and the researcher. Narrations can come from patients, lay or professional care providers, parents, or other parties with stories that can serve to inform practice.

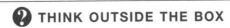 **THINK OUTSIDE THE BOX**

Carefully consider the idea of saturation. Discuss how you can determine that saturation has occurred within a research project.

Phenomenology

As the name implies, **phenomenology** is the study of events and trends from a human perspective. Phenomenology seeks to develop an understanding of lived experience. The firsthand report or description of one's experience of the phenomenon is central to understanding the phenomenon. The meaning one creates in the world is socially constructed and is rooted in the experiences of the person.

Data collection in phenomenology is done through unstructured interviews and inductive analysis. The guiding question in a phenomenological study typically centers on the essence, structure, or lived experience of a phenomenon. Data analysis occurs simultaneously with data collection. The researcher is identifying patterns and themes and developing new questions as data emerge. The reader or consumer of a phenomenological study can use the findings to understand the experiences of clients who are experiencing a similar event.

Comparative Analysis

Qualitative comparative analysis (QCA) is used in the social sciences; however, it is a less well-known approach to collection of narrative data in nursing that allows the researcher to compare elements of interest. Donnelly and Wiechula (2013) used QCA to explore the relationship between nursing education and the clinical placement experience of students. The researchers were interested in understanding how these choices influence the competence of graduate nurses. In QCA, principles of Boolean algebra (a deductive logical technique where variables are limited to two values, true or false; Dictionary.com, n.d.) and the construction of "truth tables" are used to analyze the data from a number of cases. The QCA method is considered an innovative approach to nursing research that combines qualitative and quantitative data that may be particularly useful in small studies (Donnelly & Wiechula, 2013). The QCA method is an innovative research process to explore narrative data in interesting ways.

■ Sampling Strategies in Qualitative Research

In contrast with quantitative research, which requires a careful sample plan that is designed before the study commences and seeks homogeneity of subjects, the sampling strategy in qualitative research is often an intra-project process that seeks to maximize variation of participants, saturation of data, and verification of data (Strauss & Corbin, 1998). Each of these components is discussed in detail in this chapter.

Researchers in qualitative studies often sample for variation. Even when a homogeneous sample is sought—for instance, patients with breast cancer—researchers often seek informants with slightly different experiences who can provide diverse perspectives. Sometimes also called criterion sampling, **purposeful sampling** is designed to select participants who are able to inform the researcher on elements of the phenomenon that remain poorly understood (Strauss & Corbin, 1998). With this sampling method, the researcher strives to identify individuals who reflect both sides of the issue to provide a complete picture of the situation under investigation.

Sample sizes are rarely decided upon before commencing a qualitative study. Rather, a reasonable sample size may be estimated based on similar studies. Sampling is continued until data saturation is reached. The qualitative researcher knows that data saturation has been attained when no new themes or concepts arise or redundancy of data is determined. Consumers of qualitative research may perceive that a small sample size in a qualitative study is a serious limitation of the study. In truth, sample sizes in qualitative studies are often expected to be small. Vast amounts of data are generated in a qualitative study, and analyses of these data from hundreds of participants may not be feasible or necessary. Given the longer time researchers often spend with participants, data saturation may be reached with a small number of subjects. Depending on the study design, goal of the study, phenomenon of interest, and other factors, a reasonable sample size for a qualitative study might be as small as five or six participants.

To verify data, qualitative researchers will often seek out negative cases as they near completion of data collection. This process is similar to the notion of purposeful sampling, but the researcher seeks participants or cases in which the emerging theory or emerging interpretations of data can be challenged. Seeking negative cases is both a sampling strategy and a method of assuring rigor in qualitative research.

■ Approaches to Qualitative Data Collection

The most common approaches to data collection in qualitative studies are interviews and observations. Interviews may occur once or be done in a series. In general, interviews are not neutral in nature. The interviewer naturally introduces a variable into interviews by virtue of his or her race, class, ethnicity, gender, education, and experience. Structured interviews may follow a script of questions established prior to beginning data collection. Structured interviews allow little room for variation in response. The interviewer must remain neutral in the structured interview. The semi-structured interview is commonly used in qualitative research. Using a semi-structured interview, the researcher uses a list of fairly broad questions with prompts. Rather than being an interested listener, the interviewer may engage in the conversation more than in a structured interview.

Interviews of groups, or focus groups, require a researcher who is experienced in the conduct of focus groups. Like individual interviews, group interviews can be structured or semi-structured. Group interviews are not meant to replace individual interviews. They are an alternative way to collect data and should be conducted only when the question is appropriate or as a way to determine a direction for semi-structured interview questions for individuals. For example, in a study investigating women veterans' preferences for intimate partner violence (IPV) screening, data were collected from 24 women during 5 focus groups (Iverson et al., 2014). The researchers performed content analysis of the focus group data by categorizing the narrative responses into themes describing participant attitudes and preferences (Iverson et al., 2014). Focus groups provide different ideas that build on each other to provide a clearer understanding of the situation being investigated.

Observation is an acceptable but less common method of data collection in qualitative research. Elements that may be observed include:

- Appearance
- Clothing
- Interactions
- Roles
- Exits
- Routines
- Rituals
- Temporal elements
- Organization
- Interpretations

Bracketing is a concept common to all qualitative methods, though all researchers may not describe using this process in their study. Bracketing is also known as phenomenological reduction. In bracketing, the researcher identifies his or her own personal biases and beliefs about the phenomenon and sets them aside in order to fully understand the experience of the informants. Bracketing typically commences during data collection and continues through the data analysis process. For example, researchers interested in the phenomenon of preconception health practices of women in abusive relationships would likely bracket by making a conscious decision to temporarily suspend their beliefs and attitudes about how women should plan for pregnancy and what they believe about the experience of being in an abusive relationship. They would make a decision to be open to what the participants had to say about this phenomenon without making prejudgments or assumptions about the phenomenon.

Approaches to Qualitative Data Analysis

Qualitative data analysis is often a tedious and time-consuming process. With most qualitative methods, the data collection and data analysis processes are occurring simultaneously. As new data evolve, new questions emerge. This evolution of data collection is part of the reason for the lack of structure in interview guides. Although many qualitative researchers prefer to analyze data by hand, many software programs are available to assist in the organization and coding of data. Data collection to saturation implies a level of data analysis as data collection occurs.

From the brief descriptions of data analysis in the methods previously described, one can see that qualitative data analysis can be quite complex. While quantitative data analysis usually involves numbers and statistics, qualitative data analysis involves deep examination of large volumes of written data.

The qualitative research methods of grounded theory, phenomenology, and ethnography require specific steps in data analysis. Other qualitative methods have no specific "rules" for the analysis of data. In such cases, a researcher might simply state that content analysis was conducted. Content analysis is a generic term for the process of data being analyzed and categories of data being created by experts.

Methodological Rigor in Qualitative Research

Both qualitative and quantitative research methods require the researcher to strive for **rigor**, or the criteria for trustworthiness of data and interpretation of data. The major methods for ensuring rigor are intricately linked with reliability and validity checks. Lincoln and Guba (1985) provided pioneering work in the area of qualitative research, particularly in the area of methodological rigor. The criteria frequently used to ensure qualitative rigor include (1) credibility, (2) transferability, (3) dependability, (4) confirmability, and (5) authenticity (Cope, 2014). A discussion follows on how each criterion can be achieved to establish the trustworthiness of a study.

Credibility, or the truth value of data and data analysis, can be achieved in a proposed study through several methods. First, when possible, the data should be taken back to subjects to ensure accuracy. Upon coding of data, the coded data can be checked with available participants. Additionally, coded data can be reviewed by experts in both the area of research and in the method used for the study. These checks usually consist of validation of data, validation of findings, and checking of interpretations.

Transferability refers to the applicability of findings to other populations in different contexts. Often, this process is accomplished by providing a thorough description of the sample, setting, and data in the report to allow the reader to determine the transferability of the study's findings. The process requires that those aspects that can be effectively transferred are readily denoted for the readers to understand and consider. The aspect within rigor provides understanding concerning the applicability of the findings to other settings.

Dependability in qualitative research can also be described as auditability. If other researchers can follow the investigator's decisions throughout the study and come to similar conclusions, the study is auditable (Lincoln & Guba, 1985). Thus, an audit trail also provides an element of rigor to any study. The audit trail documents the development of the project and provides an adequate amount of evidence for interested parties to reconstruct the process by which the investigators reached their conclusions (Morse, 1998). Audit trails can be documented in a variety of ways. Documenting where the information was collected, how it was stored, and how it was analyzed provides a picture of the movement of information toward the final outcome of the study.

Confirmability represents freedom from bias, or neutrality (Lincoln & Guba, 1985). It is important to analyze data in a way that keeps researcher biases, assumptions, and perspectives separate. These elements should be clearly identified early in the proposal process. Reviewing the analyzed data with informants or study participants and review by experts also serves to mitigate the effects of researcher bias.

Although many ways are available to establish the quality of qualitative data, researchers can select the appropriate criteria for the topic under investigation. It is not necessary for all of these criteria to be incorporated into each study project. Application of any research results to practice, whether qualitative or quantitative, must be considered in light of the study's reliability, validity, and generalizability. Further, qualitative researchers themselves may face a number of challenges as they approach qualitative research. Inherent in qualitative research is the recognition of multiple realities. This concern about challenges is also true when interpreting qualitative findings; however, when reasonable methodological rigor is applied to qualitative methods, one can have assurance regarding the authenticity of the results (Snelgrove, 2014). Care must be taken by the research team to clearly and effectively address how the results were determined.

Understanding and Using Qualitative Study Results

Virtually all areas within nursing lend themselves to qualitative study. Nursing practice should be guided by nursing theory that is solidly grounded in research data. Qualitative studies are often the first step in the development of a theoretical framework for a phenomenon that has not been fully explored. Andrews and Waterman (2005) collected interview and observation data using the grounded theory approach in their study about how hospital-based staff used vital signs and the Early Warning Score to predict physiologic deterioration in clients. The authors reported that quantifiable evidence is the most effective means of referring patients to doctors and improving communication between professionals. The authors concluded that the Early Warning Score leads to successful referral of patients by providing an agreed-upon framework for assessment, increasing confidence in the use of medical language, and empowering nurses.

Qualitative research affords an opportunity to explore human issues that have previously been understood by way of assumption or simply not understood. For example, the high turnover and burnout rate of nursing staff has historically been assumed to be a function of long hours, physically strenuous work, and lack of power. The combined qualitative and quantitative studies of Cohen-Katz, Wiley, Capuano, Baker, and Shapiro (2004) have illuminated the causes of nursing burnout and led to system-wide changes to help nurses manage stress and burnout.

Qualitative studies often offer immediate clinical applicability. These studies are a source of rich descriptions of a wide range of physical and psychosocial experiences of healthcare consumers. By gaining a deeper understanding of those experiences, nurses can counsel, plan interventions, and develop programs to meet the needs of clients in similar conditions.

A study exploring adapting qualitative research strategies to technology-savvy adolescents provides an example of how to determine which communication method was preferred by youth (Mason & Ide, 2014). A grounded theory methodology was used to explore how 23 adolescents were interviewed by email rather than traditional face-to-face interviews. Participants indicated email communication was slow and that they preferred instant messaging instead. The adolescents in this study preferred text-based communication, suggesting the need to modify the traditional qualitative approach of in-person interviews (Mason & Ide, 2014). Each step within the study was clearly presented to allow the readers to understand the path taken to arrive at the conclusions presented.

Qualitative research brings increased knowledge to the evidence-based practice of nursing. Qualitative research methods are often used to develop theories and research questions needed to guide future quantitative studies. Qualitative studies can illuminate issues that are poorly or inaccurately understood. Finally, qualitative studies often offer immediate clinical applicability and can guide teaching and practice.

■ Mixed Methods Research

Broadly defined, **mixed methods research** is a combination of quantitative and qualitative research methods and techniques for collecting and analyzing data that together make possible an increase in the understanding to be gained from the research data (Creswell, Klassen, Plano Clark, & Klegg Smith, 2010). This form of research is also referred to in the literature by several other names—multimethod, triangulated, and integrated designs. Mixed methods research is growing in use in the health sciences. A "best practices" guideline has been developed for use by healthcare professionals who are developing and evaluating mixed methods studies (Office of Behavioral and Social Sciences, 2011). The use of mixed methods requires a strong research team to effectively integrate both qualitative and quantitative into one research project.

Mixed methods research is often possible within the clinical arena. For example, nurses may believe that the dryness of quantitative research needs to be tempered with the "touchy-feely" aspects of qualitative research. Within the realm of evidence-based nursing practice, a nurse might realize that the time spent in the surgical holding area causes increased stress to the patients. A study could collect physiologic data related to stress, such as blood pressures and time in the surgical holding area, as well as observed signs of stress and emotional data (e.g., verbal comments about the experience while in the surgical holding area awaiting the surgical procedure). The conclusions resulting from the collection of both types of data would reveal each aspect of the individual's experiences while in the surgical holding area. This mixed methods study would provide needed data to facilitate the provision of evidence-based nursing practice within the institution.

Quantitative research, which is considered the foundational method, permits the researcher to make inferences only about the data that are being examined. These studies, however, are not designed to detect contextual nuances, which may produce a biased understanding of the variables being studied. By comparison, qualitative research spreads a much broader net, allowing for in-depth examination of elements of a phenomenon not considered when research is conducted using quantitative methods. Because both quantitative and qualitative methods have strengths and weaknesses, neither can perfectly establish the full truth about phenomena of interest to nursing (Polit & Beck, 2011). Joining methods is done to reduce the biases associated with one design alone, provide insight into the complexity of the problem under study, and introduce rigor into the study design (Creswell et al., 2010). This form of research entails more than just the combination of two or more methods in a single study. Multimethod (mixed methods) research implies the integration of both numbers and narrative, pragmatically offering enhanced results in terms of quality and span (Shaw, Connelly, & Zecevic, 2010).

An example of what is meant by multimethod research can be seen when a questionnaire includes both closed-ended questions (numbers) to provide quantitative data and open-ended questions (narrative) that require qualitative analysis.

Simply stated, mixed methods design views both quantitative and qualitative research as useful and important, while avoiding the constraints that might hamper a study carried out using a single research methodology (Chow, Quine, & Li, 2010). Researchers must carefully consider each of the different pieces to determine the optimal method for addressing the research problem identified.

As the field of research has advanced, the use of mixed methods has sometimes been referred to as "**action research**" and/or "participatory research." It is seen as a research technique that may be useful in the implementation of evidence-based practice (Munten, van den Bogaard, Cox, Garretsen, & Bongers, 2010). This form of research may be employed to facilitate a change in strategy based on feedback about what is being observed in real time (Goodnough, 2008; Ponic, Reid, & Frisby, 2010). With the advancement of mixed methods research, attention must be given to the optimal avenue to get at the information being sought to address the identified problem and/or challenge.

Components of Mixed Method Procedures

In using mixed method procedures, the researcher attempts to blend a combination of methods (qualitative and quantitative) that have complementary strong points, while defusing the non-overlapping weaknesses. Bliss (2001) has stated, "A common misconception about mixed method research is that it requires a blending of contradictory or competing research paradigms" (p. 331). This view is also supported by Johnson and Onwuegbuzie (2004): "Mixed methods research is an attempt to legitimate the use of multiple approaches in answering research questions, rather than restricting or constraining researchers' choices (i.e., it rejects dogmatism)" (p. 17). Allowing researchers to use multiple techniques to answer the questions posed provides clarity within the research project.

Although quantitative and qualitative methods each have an established focus, the two are neither contradictory nor competing. Within the delivery of the methodology, the two research designs are frequently

---

? THINK OUTSIDE THE BOX

Carefully consider the idea of mixed methods studies. Which elements would need to be present to reflect effective use of quantitative methods in a qualitative research project? Explain your answer.

meshed within the sampling, data collection, and analysis aspects of the research project. Although these aspects are the current levels, the process does not restrict the versatility or variety of the potential combinations within the two methodologies. As Bliss (2001) has noted, "mixed method research seems to offer an opportunity to deepen our insights, sharpen our thinking, develop sensitive methods, and accelerate our advances" (p. 331). By allowing the researcher to identify a combination of methods, this process merges the best of both worlds of research to address the identified healthcare problem in the optimal manner available to the profession. The primary restriction on the joining of the methodologies is the obstruction occurring through lack of vision and risk-taking on the part of the researcher.

According to Creswell, Fetters, and Ivankova (2004), mixed methods (multimethod) research possesses the potential for rigor, methodologic effectiveness, and investigation within the primary care setting. Even though rigidity is not a problem within this kind of research, the aspects of each methodology employed must still be carefully considered and weighted by the researcher. Within any of the research designs, each method has identified strengths and limitations. As a researcher tries to maximize the complementary points while modifying the limitations, certain concerns emerge to be considered.

The ability to merge quantitative and qualitative data is one of the main advantages of using the mixed methods approach to research and may be referred to as triangulation. This principle states that the validity of the results from the use of various research approaches determines the appropriateness of the resulting outcomes of the analysis. A mixed methods design allows for the utilization of words, pictures, and narrative within the data collection process. Each of these qualitative aspects of the study augments the data provided via the statistical process. Numbers provide the precision, while the words, pictures, and narrative supply the textural aspects of the experience (Office of Behavioral and Social Sciences Research, 2011). Each part provides a view of the uniqueness of the experience being investigated.

As a result of having this intensity of data available for data analysis of the event, an extensive and more comprehensive array of research questions and/or hypotheses can be answered. Put simply, the researcher is not limited regarding the breadth of the questions to be searched within the study. Because both quantitative and qualitative aspects of the issue are being addressed through the mixed methods, the research team can draw from the different designs to develop the optimal research project to address the identified problem.

An example of how the use of mixed methodologies uncovers perceptions that might otherwise be missed is illustrated in the work published by Chen and Goodson (2009), who studied barriers to adopting genomics into public health education. On the one hand, qualitative data were collected from a small number (n = 24) of public health educators through personal interviews. Quantitative data, on the other hand, were collected using a large (n = 1,607), web-based survey method. The combined data gathered via the two methods highlighted barriers that extended beyond a lack of knowledge to more nuanced and complex issues of incompatibility of the individual's personal ethics and beliefs about genomics as factors in the adoption of genomics into public health education.

An additional strength visualized by the use of a mixed methodology for a research project relates to the enthusiasm of the evidence. This resulting power from the in-depth evidence comes about from the triangulation (convergence and corroboration) of the results identified (Johnson, n.d.). Because the evidence is managed through several different processes, the truth of the results may be strengthened.

A further strength associated with use of mixed methods strategies can be seen when complementary insights and perceptions arise that might have been missed if only one research methodology were employed. The use of both quantitative and qualitative methodologies allows the researcher to pull together a wider and deeper understanding about the identified research problem, as it is considered from multiple viewpoints.

Mixed methods strategies are not without limitations, however. When both quantitative and qualitative methods are employed, the researcher must be well versed in both methodologies, especially if the two methods are managed concurrently. If the researcher does not feel competent to implement both methods, a research team may be required to complete the process effectively. The combination of the two methods should not be engaged in haphazardly. When this strategy is selected for implementation, care must be given to learning about the various methods and tactics to allow for the successful incorporation of the necessary approaches. Mixed methodology research can also be especially expensive to complete due to the use of teams, and it can result in additional time-consuming steps.

When an investigator elects to use this methodology, rationales for the decisions made must be documented and supported. These rationales need to be based on a thorough understanding of the relevant characteristics of both the quantitative and qualitative methodologies. Clear justification for the selection of a mixed methods approach to the research problem must be provided to ensure that the research community comprehends the reasons for the decisions. These rationales are most often cited in the introduction section of the study report, the study aims discussion, or the overview of the section on methods to be used. As a researcher initiates this discussion concerning the rationales, the priority of the data collection process must be one key aspect that is presented clearly and concisely. This dialogue addresses the question of whether the quantitative and qualitative data are both emphasized equally. Regardless of the direction a researcher elects to go with the prioritization of the data, understandable and succinct logic for the choice should be carefully and thoroughly documented within the project.

Creswell and colleagues (2004) have elaborated on the labor-intensive process needed for the involvement of multiple points of data collection and analysis. This process should not be seen as an easier way of arriving at results but rather as a process for obtaining richer and more thorough information about the phenomenon under investigation. Johnson and Onwuegbuzie (2004) contend that the fundamental piece driving this process should be the research question or identified problem. From the identified research problem, a researcher ought to be free to select those research methods that best address the research questions, thereby taking the best opportunity to obtain meaningful answers. If a single research design is considered the best option, then a researcher should utilize that design methodology. When the research problem is viewed as progressively complex, however, all avenues of research methodology should be contemplated to identify the best manner to successfully gain a thorough understanding of the phenomenon.

■ Types of Mixed Method Strategies

As researchers conceptualize using both quantitative and qualitative methodologies, at least three aspects of this process need to be considered: implementation, prioritization, and integration. Each of these three aspects results in one of two subtypes of mixed methods models—within-stage or across-stage methods. Within-stage methods reflect the use of quantitative and qualitative approaches within one or more stages of the research process. An example of this method would be the inclusion of both open-ended questions and closed-ended questions on the same tool for administration at the same time. Across-stage mixed method approaches involve mixing the two research designs transversely between at least two of the stages within the research endeavor. Returning to the example given earlier concerning the surgical holding room, the use of physiologic data collected while the individual is in the holding area, followed by development of a narrative regarding how the experience was perceived after the surgical process, is an example of the use of across-stage mixed methods. With this approach, the data are not collected at the same time, but rather data collection at each stage builds on data collection from the other stages.

In addressing the implementation question, the principal decision relates to whether the two methods—quantitative and qualitative—will be executed at the same time or sequentially. The research question aids in this choice. At times, the information discovered within one of the methods is perceived as a valuable foundation for the gathering of the data within the following method. For example, to determine the extent of research used within an acute care facility, researchers could conduct focus groups with a select group of nurses to determine perceived barriers to the use of research. Based on the data collected via the focus groups, a questionnaire could be developed and given to all staff nurses to determine their level of agreement with the information identified by the focus group members. In this scenario, the qualitative data results and analysis are seen as critical forces determining the data to be collected within the quantitative piece of the project. When neither type of data is needed to drive the data collection, quantitative and qualitative data can be collected concurrently. The surgical holding area example could be considered from this viewpoint. If the nurse collected physiologic data of blood pressures, observation of stressed behaviors, and time in the surgical holding area, while also questioning the individual about his or her perceptions of being in the holding area, the data would be collected concurrently. The determination of the appropriateness of this implementation comes directly from the identified research problem and resulting research questions and hypothesis.

If the decision is to conduct both the quantitative and qualitative data collection aspects at the same time, the process tends to be used to confirm, cross-validate, or corroborate findings within a single study (Creswell, 2003). Even when the two methods are conducted simultaneously, the question concerning how the information will be delivered must still be answered. If one method is embedded into the other method, then the process is termed **nesting**, where the less predominant method is implanted into the other method.

An example of nesting would be the inclusion of open-ended questions at the conclusion of a previously validated quantitative tool. An advantage of using concurrent design for the mixed methods process is the shortened data collection time period. Because all of the data are collected at one phase, the expense and time allocation can be reduced.

Within the concurrent implementation of the methodology, each piece of data is weighted equally within the data analysis phase. That is, for concurrent implementation, neither quantitative nor qualitative data are awarded a higher priority relative to the other; each aspect is judged on its own merits. Within this approach to mixed methods research, data integration begins during the data collection phase and continues through the data analysis phase and into the data interpretation phase. The data are interconnected for the initiation of the research process. When concurrent processing is selected for the research project, the investigator must be competent in both methodologies. This proficiency in both methods is imperative, because the researcher must ensure that the protocols for the quantitative and qualitative processes are appropriately carried out at each juncture of the research process.

Data Collection Procedures

In research methods of all types, the collection of data refers to information collected and organized by the researcher. Research data are collected in an effort to measure specific variables that are relevant to the study (Macnee, 2004).

One often thinks first of data taking the form of numbers or statistics. Many preliminary steps must occur prior to the collection of such data in quantitative research. Polit and Beck (2008) describe the data collection plan in quantitative research as including the following steps:

1. Determine the data that need to be gathered.
2. Consider the type of measurement to be used for each variable.
3. Identify the instruments available to capture each variable.
4. Develop data collection forms/protocols.
5. Collect and manage the data.

In mixed methods research, data collection may also take non-quantitative forms. Narratives, verbal feedback from focus groups, transcripts, and videotapes are examples of sources of non-quantitative data (Vogt, 2005). The purpose of qualitative data collection in mixed record research may vary. For example, qualitative data may be collected for the purpose of developing questions for a quantitative survey or instrument. This step assists in developing a more comprehensive understanding of the dimensions of a construct under study or in generating hypotheses.

The rationale for the data collection process used in mixed methods research studies should be stated clearly: Why and how did using one or more methods of collecting and integrating data contribute to the purpose of the study? The specific data that are collected by quantitative and qualitative methods and the priority and emphasis given to each type of data are determined by the researchers and driven by the research problem and goals of the study (Creswell et al., 2004). Johnson and Onwuegbuzie (2004) describe their mixed method process as having eight distinct steps:

1. Determine the research question.
2. Determine whether a mixed design is appropriate.
3. Select the mixed methods or mixed model research design.
4. Collect the data.
5. Analyze the data.
6. Interpret the data.
7. Legitimate the data.
8. Draw conclusions (if warranted), and write the final report.

Johnson and Onwuegbuzie's (2004) mixed methods process focuses on data collection. Data collection in multimethod studies is frequently carried out such that quantitative and qualitative components of the study are kept separate during the actual conduct of the study and are combined only later in the interpretation and reporting of results (Creswell et al., 2004; Polit & Beck, 2011). Careful thought concerning the timing and flow of the data collection process is required.

To illustrate this idea, consider the research reported by Long and colleagues (2013), in which quantitative methods were used to measure the differences among fruit, vegetable, and fat consumption in college students. Participants used digital pictures recorded on personal cell phones as a memory prompt prior to entering their diet information online and then crossed over to record their diet information online without the use of cell phone pictures for memory recall. Qualitative methods were employed to understand participant perceptions, satisfaction, and usability of personal cell phones for this purpose. In this study, the researchers identified statistical analysis and significance testing to evaluate the difference in diet recording with and without digital pictures for memory prompt. Focus group interviews and structured short answers were used to evaluate how participants felt about using personal cell phones for this purpose. In this study, both quantitative and qualitative mixed methods suggested the use of digital pictures of diet on cell phones as an acceptable and effective way to prompt short-term memory of what had been eaten (Long et al., 2013). Allowing the participants' voices to be heard within the process strengthened the outcomes found within the research project.

■ Data Analysis and Validation Procedures

How data are analyzed is inextricably tied to the type of information that has been collected. Quantitative data will, at minimum, be counted and described. Inferential statistical analysis will be applied depending on the type and level of data available to the researcher. Qualitative data analysis also takes multiple forms, but it generally involves the coding of narrative themes for depth of understanding. It is not surprising, therefore, that analysis of mixed methods research mirrors the variety seen in analyses of both quantitative and qualitative methodologies.

To illuminate this point, consider the subset of data analysis in the study conducted by Long and colleagues (2006), which compared the results from two quantitative measurements of fruit, vegetable, and fat intake for **convergent validity**. Quantitative data from a computer-based self-report and from a structured interview were compared statistically (triangulated) and determined to have a small to medium correlation (Long et al., 2006). This form of mixed methodology is generative. It assisted the researcher in determining the need for further development of the measurement methods used to determine fruit, vegetable, and fat consumption in an adolescent population. In the same study, the qualitative feedback obtained from observations of student enjoyment with using the web-based educational intervention and verbal feedback from focus groups was analyzed and coded thematically to capture observed variances among learners, raising new questions about the population and about how to best provide meaningful health education to this group.

In summary, both quantitative and qualitative research designs can be combined through the use of a mixed methods approach to data collection and analysis. The specific data collected by both methods and the emphasis given to each should be determined based on the research problem and the goals of the study. A research team whose members are experienced with use of both types of methods is important to the success of mixed methods research. While each of the methods has its own strengths and weaknesses, mixed methods research offers the opportunity for a more complete investigation into the problem being studied (Creswell et al., 2004; Elliott, 2004; Ramprogus, 2005). Given the complexities and the nature of the problems of interest to nursing, mixed methods research holds promise for advancing evidence-based understanding that might lead to enhanced quality patient care.

■ Evidence-Based Practice Considerations

Problems of interest to nursing are characteristically complex in nature. Nurses in clinical practice need to know how to find, evaluate, and use research so that they can implement best practices at the bedside (Spruce, 2015). Understanding mixed methods research is important because it holds the potential for promoting methodologically sound studies that capture complexities which might otherwise be over-

---

❓ THINK OUTSIDE THE BOX

1. Debate the benefits and restrictions involved in using a mixed methodology for a research project.
2. How would you handle a PICOT (population, intervention, comparison, outcome, time) question format when using a mixed methodology?
3. Consider a clinical situation that you have confronted. How could you address the clinical problem using both a quantitative method and a qualitative method?
4. Debate which types of rationales are necessary when a mixed methods approach is used.

looked. According to Rolston-Blenman (2009), "Clinical stakeholders must participate in planning and championing the changes taking place. Staff must feel they have a voice in making decisions" (p. 21). Through the use of mixed methods (action research), the staff at the bedside can actively participate in different aspects of research, resulting in better management of the problems so identified. According to Myers and Meccariello (2006), "It's critical to help nurses understand how crucial their role is in the research process and how they can improve patient care by validating their own trial and error experiences" (p. 24). Each day, individuals must realize the importance of connecting the research process to key activities that occur within the workplace—one patient at a time. This permeation of the workplace with a critical thinking mindset allows for the deep consideration of multiple problems at the ground-zero level. Taking advantage of the strengths of qualitative and quantitative research design methods, while planning for ways to overcome the limitations of the research designs, allows the discipline of nursing to advance the body of knowledge toward clinical practice confirmed by evidence.

■ Conclusion

Qualitative research lends itself well to the study of complex human issues. Qualitative research is the study of the quality of something rather than the quantity, amount, or frequency of something. Subjectivity is an expected trait of a qualitative study. Qualitative and quantitative research methods differ in many ways. As described previously, qualitative studies approach phenomena from the emic perspective—the perspective of the participant provides the meaning rather than the perspective of the researcher. Qualitative methods are inductive, as opposed to the deductive approach of quantitative methods. Although quantitative methods seek to minimize differences among subjects, qualitative methods embrace differences among participants. Sample size in qualitative research is often small compared with the requisite larger sample sizes in quantitative research.

Case studies, ethnography, grounded theory, and phenomenology are methods used within qualitative research to seek the essences of the situation being investigated. In data collection and analysis, saturation occurs when no new themes or codes emerge or the data analysis becomes redundant. The reliability and validity of qualitative research can be ensured by verifying credibility, transferability, dependability, confirmability, and authenticity of data.

Mixed methods design (called multimethod, triangulated, and integrated design) is an amalgamation of quantitative and qualitative research methods and techniques used to collect and analyze data. In mixed methods studies, two research patterns are regularly interlocked within the sampling, data collection, or analysis aspects of the project. The use of both methods permits the researcher to develop a wider and deeper understanding of the identified research problem as a result of the consideration of the problem from multiple viewpoints.

The fundamental force driving the use of mixed methods research continues to be the clear and concise identification of the research problem.

---

❷ THINK OUTSIDE THE BOX

1. Look at the table, which compares emic and etic research designs. Which other aspects can you identify that might be added to this table to further delineate the differences and similarities between these two research design methods?

Differences Between Quantitative and Qualitative Research Methods

	Point of View	Attachment to Participant	Process of Inquiry	Sample
Outsider view	Etic—analyzed without considering their role as a unit within a system	Seeks to minimize the differences among subjects	Deductive	Large sample size required
Insider view	Emic—analyzed with consideration of their role as a unit within the system	Embraces different perspectives of each participant	Inductive	Individuals; sample size is typical

2. Discuss how sample sizes for qualitative versus quantitative research projects differ. How do researchers determine optimal sample size for qualitative studies as opposed to quantitative studies?

3. Think for a moment about your current workplace. Identify one problem, process, or policy in your work area whose improvement by the healthcare team would favorably affect patient outcomes. Once you have identified a problem, list ideas about which quantitative data would assist you and your colleagues in solving the problem. Further consider those aspects of the issue in which your understanding would be enhanced through collection of qualitative data. How could you apply best practices to solve the problem you identified using aspects of both research methods? Now consider an unmet educational need of new staff members on your unit. How might an "action research" mixed methods approach assist you in understanding and meeting the changing educational needs of new staff members?

The investigator must rigorously examine the issue of whether the two research designs should be conducted concurrently or sequentially.

Triangulation allows the researcher to fully understand a phenomenon of interest through validation or supplementation of data. The term *triangulation* is used to describe the situation in which data are analyzed for the purpose of corroborating data from multiple methods. Justification for the ordering and prioritization of the different methods must be documented, with rationales being presented for each of the decisions made concerning the research process. During collection and analysis of data in mixed methods research, quantitative and qualitative data are often treated as independent components in the research design.

Summary Points

1. Qualitative research is the study of the quality of something rather than the quantity, amount, or frequency of something. Subjectivity is an expected trait of a qualitative study.
2. Qualitative research is conducted from the emic perspective; quantitative research is conducted from the etic perspective.
3. Sample size in qualitative research is often small compared with the requisite larger sample sizes in quantitative research.
4. The criteria for reliability and validity of a qualitative study include credibility, transferability, dependability, confirmability, and authenticity of data.
5. Mixed research methods—combinations of qualitative and quantitative methods—are used to supplement or validate data.
6. Saturation occurs in data collection or analysis when there is repetition or redundancy in the themes or patterns in the data.
7. Mixed methods design (called multimethod, triangulated, and integrated design) is an amalgamation of quantitative and qualitative research methods and techniques used to collect and analyze data.
8. In mixed methods studies, two research patterns are regularly interlocked within the sampling, data collection, or analysis aspects of the project.
9. The use of both methods permits the researcher to develop a wider and deeper understanding of the identified research problem as a result of the consideration of the problem from multiple viewpoints.
10. The fundamental force driving the use of mixed methods research continues to be the clear and concise identification of the research problem.
11. The criteria used when choosing the combination of methods for inclusion in a mixed methods study are related to implementation, prioritization, and integration needs.

12. The investigator must rigorously examine the issue of whether the two research designs should be conducted concurrently or sequentially.
13. Justification for the ordering and prioritization of the different methods must be documented, with rationales being presented for each of the decisions made concerning the research process.
14. During collection and analysis of data in mixed methods research, quantitative and qualitative data are often treated as independent components in the research design.
15. The term *triangulation* is used to describe the situation in which data are analyzed for the purpose of corroborating data from multiple methods.

RED FLAGS

- Care must be given to explaining how different research methodologies are entwined as a single project.
- A lack of a rationale for using mixed methods is problematic.
- Any indication that quantitative and qualitative methods are competing with each other reflects lack of planning.
- When the rationale for weighting of the methods is not provided, then concerns must be raised about the results of the data analysis.
- The data collection process for each of the two research methodologies should be kept distinctive.
- If data collection methods are improperly conducted for the identified research methodology, then the validity of the results must be questioned.
- Attention must be given to the auditability of the data collected via a qualitative methodology.
- Within a qualitative research report, the reader should be able to pick out aspects that demonstrate credibility, transferability, dependability, confirmability, and authenticity of the research.
- Qualitative research designs use an inductive reasoning process.
- Patterns and/or themes coming from the data should be documented and supported by the discussion.
- Given that qualitative research deals with volumes of written data, the documentation of statistic results would cause concern when evaluating a project.

Multiple-Choice Questions

1. Qualitative research examines which of the following characteristics of a phenomenon?
   A. Frequency
   B. Quantity
   C. Quality
   D. Distribution

2. Which of the following best illustrates the emic perspective in research?
   A. Finding a quality of a phenomenon and looking for examples of the quality
   B. Taking an outsider's view of a phenomenon
   C. Exploring the way members of a group view themselves
   D. Validating perspectives about a group through discussion

3. Which of the following types of studies is considered qualitative research?
   A. Delphi technique
   B. Cross-sectional design
   C. Phenomenology
   D. Survey

4. Mixed methods research combines elements of which two methods?
   A. Quantitative and qualitative
   B. Transferability and trustworthiness
   C. Prospective and retrospective
   D. Phenomenology and ethnography

5. A researcher explores the phenomenon of how nurses make decisions about when to discuss end-of-life issues with clients. From this research, a model is developed to explain the decision-making process. Which type of research does this represent?
   A. Grounded theory
   B. Ethnography
   C. Phenomenology
   D. Case study

6. The extent to which a researcher is able to accurately express the feelings and emotions of the study participants in a faithful manner is a measure of which of the following concepts?
   A. Credibility
   B. Transferability
   C. Authenticity
   D. Dependability

7. A researcher conducts a study in which participants are asked to describe the lived experience of being a caregiver of a parent with Parkinson's disease. Which type of qualitative study does this represent?

   A. Constant comparison
   B. Ethnography
   C. Phenomenology
   D. Case study

8. Which of the following statements is true with regard to comparing qualitative and quantitative research methods?

   A. Qualitative studies seek to generalize findings.
   B. Qualitative studies don't require evidence of reliability and validity.
   C. Qualitative studies don't allow for the use of computerized data analysis.
   D. Qualitative research is often inductive in nature, whereas quantitative research is deductive in nature.

9. When writing up a research project, the researcher describes in detail the audit trail used as conclusions about data were drawn. Which criterion for reliability and validity was met?

   A. Credibility
   B. Transferability
   C. Dependability
   D. Confirmability

10. When writing up a research project, the researcher describes in detail the sample, setting, and data. Which criterion for reliability and validity was met?

    A. Credibility
    B. Transferability
    C. Dependability
    D. Confirmability

11. When writing up a research project, the researcher describes in detail how biases, assumptions, and personal perspectives were identified and set aside, or bracketed. Which criterion for reliability and validity was met?

    A. Credibility
    B. Transferability
    C. Dependability
    D. Confirmability

12. The researcher collecting data notices that she is beginning to hear the same things repeatedly and that no new themes are emerging. The researcher recognizes that what has occurred?

    A. Triangulation
    B. Saturation
    C. Quantizing
    D. Redundancy

13. Another term used within the literature for mixed methods design is:
    A. Quantitative design.
    B. Qualitative design.
    C. Multimethod design.
    D. Experimental design.

14. When a researcher endeavors to use mixed methods design to answer an identi-fied research problem, the blending of the methods is based on:
    A. Combining the methods to capitalize on their strong points while negating their flaws.
    B. Combining the methods to blend both their strengths and their weaknesses.
    C. Separating the strengths from the weaknesses within the different designs.
    D. Separating the weaker method from the stronger method.

15. The research designs are merged within which sections of the report on the research project?
    A. Introduction, sampling, and problem identification
    B. Problem identification, data collection, and analysis
    C. Sampling, data collection, and analysis
    D. Introduction, data collection, and analysis

16. What is a primary reason the researcher might consider the use of mixed methods research?
    A. The need to examine a problem that calls for real-life and contextual understanding of multilevel perspectives
    B. Willingness to engage in the use of, and confidence in, one research method
    C. Willingness for risk taking
    D. Lack of confidence in qualitative methods

17. A nurse identifies individuals who seem to comply better with a treatment plan when several different teaching methods are used within the discharge planning process. In developing a mixed methods design for researching which educational methods work best, a question concerning the type of data to be collected is confronted. Which of the following groups of data collection methods represents a mixed methods format?
    A. Likert scale tool with a demographic component
    B. Observation of teaching sessions with videotaping
    C. Focus group discussion with audiotaping
    D. Likert scale tool with focus group discussion

18. The determination of the mixed methods design approach must address the meshing of the qualitative and quantitative methodologies through the use of which of the following criteria?
    A. Implementation, prioritization, and integration
    B. Implementation, analysis, and investigation
    C. Analysis, prioritization, and integration
    D. Collection, prioritization, and analysis

19. A researcher has elected to conduct a mixed methods research project. Within this project, the decision has been made to conduct the two types of data collection concurrently, with each type of data having equal weight within the analysis process. Based on these decisions, what must the researcher make sure is done for the reporting of the process?
    A. Establish a team to aid in the management of the study.
    B. Reevaluate the decision, because quantitative research is the stronger method.
    C. Ensure that confidentiality is maintained within the process.
    D. Document the rationale for the decisions made within the process.

20. Triangulation in mixed methods research is utilized for the purposes of supporting _____ validity.
    A. Criterion
    B. Convergent
    C. Construct
    D. Variable

21. The data collected in mixed methods research and the emphasis given to each type of data should be determined by the _____ and goals of the study.
    A. Source of funding
    B. Preference of the research team
    C. Research problem
    D. Literature

22. Qualitative data analysis seeks _____ in understanding a phenomenon.
    A. Rigor
    B. Depth
    C. Numbers
    D. Statistical significance

23. A primary reason for using mixed research methodologies is the opportunity to _____ that might otherwise be overlooked.
    A. Catch complexities
    B. Define concepts
    C. Describe new research problems
    D. Uncover opportunities

24. In mixed methods research, how is the collection of quantitative and qualitative data often treated?

   A.   Synchronously
   B.   Stringently
   C.   Independently
   D.   Statistically

25. An advantage of using a mixed methods design for a research study is to:

   A.   Increase the biases associated with the use of two designs.
   B.   Provide insight into the complexity of the problem under study.
   C.   Impart generalizability to the findings of the study.
   D.   Decrease the impartiality associated with the use of one design.

26. Limitations related to the use of mixed method strategies include the:

   A.   Cost and additional time required.
   B.   Extensive and comprehensive research questions involved.
   C.   Vivacity of the evidence provided.
   D.   Complementary insights and perceptions provided.

Discussion Questions

1. You are the nurse manager of a perinatal care unit. You have read a phenomenology research report on the positive effects of music on the labor and delivery process for mothers. Consider the following: The study is one of many of this type with similar findings, there were five informants in the study, and the researcher did not provide a discussion of reliability and validity in the write-up. Will you use this study to support the practice of ensuring that all labor and delivery rooms are equipped to play music throughout the labor and delivery process? Support your answer.

2. You are the charge nurse on a medical–surgical floor. After reading several qualitative research reports on pet therapy, you approach your nurse manager about the possibility of implementing a pet therapy program on your floor. Your nurse manager states that no changes should be made based on qualitative research, because the sample sizes are always too small. What is your best response?

3. You are reading a research report about a long-term care facility. The researcher describes in detail the demographics of administration, staff, and clients. There is a lengthy discussion about how problems are solved in the facility, how various departments communicate, and how the facility values family involvement in client care. Which type of qualitative study does this represent? Support your answer.

4. A nurse on the labor and delivery unit wants to study the effects of having small children participate with the family in the delivery process on the bonding process between mother and child. For this study, the nurse has determined that a questionnaire will be mailed out to families who elect to have their toddlers in the delivery room during the delivery of a sibling. The questionnaire will include both open-ended questions and closed-ended (Likert-type) questions. Which aspects of the study should be considered to provide a rationale for selecting this mixed methods strategy?

5. A researcher working within a hospital striving to gain Magnet status wants to study the barriers to use of research at the bedside. For the design of this study, the individual is considering using a mixed methods format. Which pieces of the design should be considered as the researcher prepares the study?

6. A group of researchers has developed a new instrument to assess the degree of destruction noted within decubitus ulcers (pressure ulcers). As part of their study, the researchers are planning to compare the new instrument with instruments currently used within their acute care setting. Which components of the mixed methods strategies need to be carefully considered as the researchers develop the study design?

Suggested Readings

Bader, M. K., Palmer, S., Stalcup, C., & Shaver, T. (2002). Using a FOCUS-PDCA quality improvement model for applying the severe traumatic brain injury guidelines to practice: Process and outcomes. *Reflections on Nursing Leadership, 28*(2), 34–35.

Balas, E. A., & Boren, S. A. (2000). Managing clinical knowledge for health care improvements. In V. Schattauer, J. Bemmel, & A. T. McCray (Eds.), *Yearbook of medical informatics* (pp. 65–70). Stuttgart, Germany: Schattauer.

Borkan, J. M. (2004). Mixed methods studies: A foundation for primary care research [Editorial]. *Annals of Family Medicine, 2*(1), 4–6.

Classen, S., & Lopez, E. (2006). Mixed methods approach explaining process of an older driver safety systematic literature review. *Topics in Geriatric Rehabilitation, 22*(2), 99–112.

Foss, C., & Ellefsen, B. (2002). The value of combining qualitative and quantitative approaches in nursing research by means of method triangulation. *Journal of Advanced Nursing, 40*(2), 242–248.

Freshwater, D. (2005). Book review: Integrating qualitative and quantitative research methods: Trend or foe? *Journal of Research in Nursing, 10*(3), 337–338.

Freshwater, D., Walsh, L., & Storey, L. (2002, February). Prison health care part 2: Developing leadership through clinical supervision. *Nursing Management, 8*(9),16–20.

Grassley, J. S., & Nelms, T. P. (2008). The breast feeding conversation: A philosophic exploration of support. *Advances in Nursing Science, 31*(4), E55–E66.

Halcomb, E., & Andrew, S. (2005). Triangulation as a method for contemporary nursing research. *Nurse Researcher, 13*(2), 71–82.

Hanson, W. E., Creswell, J. W., Clark, V. L., Petska, K. S., & Creswell, J. D. (2005). Mixed methods research designs in counseling psychology. *Journal of Counseling Psychology, 52*(2), 224–235.

Happ, M. B. (2009). Mixed methods in gerontological research. *Research in Gerontological Nursing, 2*(2), 122–127.

Happ, M. B., Dabbs, A. D., Tate, J., Hricik, A., & Erlen, J. (2006, March/April). Exemplars of mixed methods data combination and analysis. *Nursing Research, 55*(2 Suppl.), S43–S49.

Harland, N., & Holey, E. (2011). Including open-ended questions in quantitative questionnaires—theory and practice. *International Journal of Therapy and Rehabilitation, 18(*9), 482–486.

Kinn, S., & Curzio, J. (2005). Integrating qualitative and quantitative research methods. *Journal of Research in Nursing, 10*(3), 317–336.

Kreutzer, J. S., Stejskal, T. M., Godwin, E. E., Powell, V. D., & Arango-Lasprilla, J. C. (2010). A mixed methods evaluation of the Brain Injury Family Intervention. *NeuroRehabilitation, 27*(1), 19–29.

Law, M., Stewart, D., Letts, L., Pollock, N., Bosch, J., & Westmoreland, M. (1998). *Guidelines for critical review of qualitative studies*. Retrieved from http://www.usc.edu/hsc/ebnet/res/Guidelines.pdf

Melnyk, B. M., & Fineout-Overholt, E. (2006, Second Quarter). Advancing knowledge through collaboration. *Reflections on Nursing Leadership, 32*(2), 1–5.

Melnyk, B. M., Fineout-Overholt, E., Stetler, C., & Allen, J. (2005). Outcomes and implementation strategies from the first U.S. evidence-based leadership summit. *Worldviews on Evidence-Based Nursing, 2*(3), 113–121.

Miller, S. I., & Fredericks, M. (2006). Mixed-methods and evaluation research: Trends and issues. *Qualitative Health Research, 16*(4), 567–579.

O'Neill, R. (2006). Advantages and disadvantages of qualitative and quantitative research methods. Retrieved from http://www.learnhigher.ac.uk/analysethis/main/quantitative1.html

Onwuegbuzie, A. J., & Leech, N. L. (2005). Taking the "Q" out of research: Teaching research methodology courses without the divide between quantitative and qualitative paradigms. *Quality & Quantity, 39*(3), 267–295.

Paton, B., Martin, S., McClunie-Trust, P., & Weir, N. (2004). Doing phenomenological research collaboratively. *Journal of Continuing Education in Nursing, 35*(4), 176–181.

Priest, H., Roberts, P., & Woods, L. (2002). An overview of three different approaches to the interpretation of qualitative data. Part 1: Theoretical issues. *Nurse Researcher, 10*(1), 30–42.

Rapport, F., & Wainwright, P. (2006). Phenomenology as a paradigm of movement. *Nursing Inquiry, 13*(3), 228–236.

Sale, J. E. M., Lohfeld, L. H., & Brazil, K. (2002). Revisiting the quantitative–qualitative debate: Implications for mixed-methods research. *Quality & Quantity, 36*(1), 43–53.

Schifferdecker, K. E., & Reed, V. A. (2009). Using mixed methods research in medical education: Basic guidelines for researchers. *Medical Education, 43*(7), 637–644.

Shih, F. J. (1998). Triangulation in nursing research: Issues of conceptual clarity and purpose. *Journal of Advanced Nursing, 28*(3), 631–641.

Silverstein, L. B., Auerbach, C. F., & Levant, R. R. (2006). Using qualitative research to strengthen clinical practice. *Professional Psychology: Research & Practice, 37*(4), 351–358.

Vishnevsky, T., & Beanlands, H. (2004). Qualitative research. *Nephrology Nursing Journal, 31*(2), 234–238.

Williamson, G. R. (2005). Illustrating triangulation in mixed-methods nursing research. *Nurse Researcher, 12*(4), 7–18.

References

Andrews, T., & Waterman, H. (2005). Packaging: A grounded theory of how to report physiological deterioration effectively. *Journal of Advanced Nursing, 52*(5), 473–481. doi:10.1111/j.1365-2648.2005.03615.x

Bliss, D. Z. (2001). Mixed or mixed up methods? *Nursing Research, 50*(6), 331.

Carnegie Foundation Report. (n.d.) Educating nurses: A call for radical transformation. Retrieved from http://www.carnegiefoundation.org/elibrary/educating-nurses -highlights

Chen, L. S., & Goodson, P. (2009). Barriers to adopting genomics into public health education: A mixed methods study. *Genetics in Medicine, 11*(2), 104–110.

Chow, M. Y., Quine, S., & Li, M. (2010). The benefits of using a mixed methods approach—quantitative and qualitative—to identify client satisfaction and unmet needs in an HIV healthcare centre. *AIDS Care, 22*(4), 491–498.

Cohen-Katz, J., Wiley, S. D., Capuano, T., Baker, D. M., & Shapiro, S. (2004). The effects of mindfulness-based stress reduction on nurse stress and burnout: A quantitative and qualitative study. *Holistic Nursing Practice, 18*(6), 302–308.

Cope, D. G. (2014). Methods and meanings: Credibility and trustworthiness of qualitative research. *Oncology Nursing Forum, 41*(1), 89–91.

Creswell, J. W. (2003). *Research design: Qualitative, quantitative, and mixed method approaches* (2nd ed.). Thousand Oaks, CA: Sage.

Creswell, J. W., Fetters, M. D., & Ivankova, N. V. (2004). Designing a mixed methods study in primary care. *Annals of Family Medicine, 2*(1), 7–12.

Creswell, J. W., Klassen, A. C., Plano Clark, V. L., & Klegg Smith, C. (2010). Best practices for mixed methods in the health sciences. Retrieved from http://obssr.od.nih.gov/scientific_areas/methodology/mixed_methods_research/pdf/Best_Practices _for_Mixed_Methods_Research.pdf

Denzin, N. K., & Lincoln, Y. S. (Eds.). (1998). *Collecting and interpreting qualitative materials.* Thousand Oaks, CA: Sage.

Denzin, N. K., & Lincoln, Y. S. (2011). *The SAGE handbook of qualitative research* (4th ed.). Thousand Oaks, CA: Sage.

Dictionary.com. (n.d.). Boolean algebra. Retrieved from http://dictionary.reference .com/browse/Boolean+algebra

Donnelly, F., & Wiechula, D. F. (2013). An example of qualitative comparative analysis in nursing research. *Nurse Researcher, 20*(6), 6–11.

Elliott, J. (2004). Multimethod approaches in educational research. *International Journal of Disability, Development and Education, 51*(2), 135–149.

Glaser, B. G., & Strauss, A. L. (1967). *The discovery of grounded theory: Strategies for qualitative research.* Chicago, IL: Aldine De Gruyter

Goodnough, K. (2008). Moving science off the "back burner": Meaning making within an action research community of practice. *Journal of Science and Teacher Education, 19*(1), 15–39.

Holloway, I., & Wheeler, S. (2010). *Qualitative research in nursing and healthcare* (3rd ed.). Ames, IA: Wiley-Blackwell.

Iverson, K. M., Huang, K., Wells, S., Wright, J. D., Gerber, M. R., & Wiltsey-Stirman, S. (2014). Women veterans' preferences for intimate partner violence screening and response procedures within the Veterans Health Administration. *Research in Nursing & Health, 37*(4), 302–311.

Joanna Briggs Institute. (2015). Retrieved from www.Joannabriggs.org

Johnson, R. B. (n.d.). Mixed research: Mixed method and mixed model research [Online lecture]. Retrieved from http://www.southalabama.edu/coe/bset /johnson/dr_johnson/lectures/lec14.htm

Johnson, R. B., & Onwuegbuzie, A. J. (2004). Mixed methods research: A research paradigm whose time has come. *Educational Researcher, 33*(7), 14–26.

Lincoln, Y. S., & Guba, E. G. (1985). *Naturalistic inquiry.* Beverly Hills, CA: Sage.

Long, J. D., Armstrong, M. L., Amos, E., Shriver, B., Roman-Shriver, C., Feng, D., ... Blevins, M. W. (2006). Pilot using World Wide Web to prevent diabetes in adolescents. *Clinical Nursing Research, 15*(1), 67–79.

Long, J. D., Boswell, C., Rogers, T., Littlefield, L. A., Estep, G., Shriver, B., ... Song, H. (2013). Effectiveness of cell phones and mypyramidtracker.gov to estimate fruit and vegetable intake. *Applied Nursing Research, 26*(1), 17–23.

Macnee, C. L. (2004). *Understanding nursing research: Reading and using research in practice.* Philadelphia, PA: Lippincott Williams & Wilkins.

Malinowski, B. (1922). *Argonauts of the western Pacific: An account of native enterprise and adventure in the archipelagos of Melanesian New Guinea.* New York, NY: E. P. Dutton & Co.

Mason, D. M., & Ide, B. (2014). Adapting qualitative research strategies to technology savvy adolescents. *Nurse Researcher, 21*(5), 40–45.

Mead, M. (1935). *Sex and temperament in three primitive societies.* New York, NY: Morrow.

Morse, J. M. (1991). *Qualitative nursing research: A contemporary dialogue.* Newbury Park, CA: Sage.

Morse, J. (1998). Designing funded qualitative research. In N. K. Denzin & Y. S. Lincoln (Eds.), *Strategies of qualitative inquiry* (pp. 56–85). Thousand Oaks, CA: Sage.

Munten, G., van den Bogaard, J., Cox, K., Garretsen, H., & Bongers, I. (2010). Implementation of evidence-based practice in nursing using action research: A review. *Worldviews on Evidence-Based Nursing, 7*(3), 135–157.

Myers, G., & Meccariello, M. (2006). From pet rock to rock-solid: Implementing unit-based research. *Nursing Management, 37*(1), 24–29.

Office of Behavioral and Social Sciences Research. (2011). Best practices for mixed methods research in the health sciences. Retrieved from http://obssr.od.nih .gov/mixed_methods_research/

Polit, D. F., & Beck, C. T. (2008). *Nursing research: Generating and assessing evidence for nursing practice* (8th ed.). Philadelphia, PA: Lippincott Williams & Wilkins.

Polit, D. F., & Beck, C. T. (2011). *Nursing research: Generating and assessing evidence for nursing practice* (9th ed.). Philadelphia, PA: Lippincott Williams & Wilkins.

Ponic, P., Reid, C., & Frisby, W. (2010). Cultivating the power of partnerships in feminist participatory action research in women's health. *Nursing Inquiry, 17*(4), 324–335.

Ramprogus, V. (2005). Triangulation. *Nurse Researcher, 12*(4), 4–6.

Rolston-Blenman, B. (2009). Nurses roll up their sleeves at the bedside to improve patient care. *Nurse Leader, 7*(1), 20–25.

Rosenberg, J. P., & Yates, P. M. (2007). Schematic representation of case study research designs. *Journal of Advanced Nursing, 60*(4), 447–452.

Scott Tilley, D., Rugari, S. M., & Walker, C. A. (2008). Development of violence in men who batter intimate partners: A case study. *The Journal of Theory Construction & Testing, 12*(1), 28–32.

Shaw, J. A., Connelly, D. M., & Zecevic, A. A. (2010). Pragmatism in practice: Mixed methods research in physiotherapy. *Physiotherapy Theory and Practice, 26*(8), 510–518.

Siddiqui, N., & Fitzgerald, J. A. (2014). Elaborated integration of qualitative and quantitative perspectives in mixed methods research: A profound enquiry into the nursing practice environment. *International Journal of Multiple Research Approaches, 8*(2), 137–147.

Smythe, L. (2012). Discerning which qualitative approach fits best. *New Zealand College of Midwives Journal, 46,* 5–12.

Snelgrove, S. R. (2014). Conducting qualitative longitudinal research using interpretive phenomenological analysis. *Nurse Researcher, 22*(1), 20–25.

Spruce, L. (2015). Back to basics: Implementing evidence-based practice. *AORN Journal, 101*(1), 106–112.

Stake, R. (1998). Case studies. In N. K. Denzin & Y. S. Lincoln (Eds.), *Strategies of qualitative inquiry* (pp. 86–109). Thousand Oaks, CA: Sage.

Strauss, A., & Corbin, J. (1998). *Basics of qualitative research: Techniques and procedures for developing grounded theory* (2nd ed.). Thousand Oaks, CA: Sage.

Vogt, W. P. (2005). *Dictionary of statistics and methodology: A nontechnical guide for the social sciences* (3rd ed.). Thousand Oaks, CA: Sage.

Chapter 7

Ethics for Nursing Research and Evidence-Based Practice

Sharon Cannon, Theresa Delahoyde, and Jane Sumner

Chapter Objectives

At the conclusion of this chapter, the learner will be able to:

1. Explain why ethical theories used in nursing practice are important for nursing research.
2. Acknowledge how international and national ethical principles have influenced ethical nursing research.
3. Discuss the impact of the history of human experimentation on nursing research today.
4. Delineate the ethical implications in each step of the research process.
5. Identify specific ethical issues when various research methodologies are utilized.

Key Terms

Autonomy	Ethics
Beneficence	Fidelity
Code of ethics	Honesty
Deontology	Human experimentation
Ethical theories	Informed consent

Institutional review board (IRB)

Justice

Morality

Nonmaleficence

Respect

Teleology

Trustworthiness

Scientific misconduct

Veracity

Vulnerable subjects

■ Introduction

This chapter focuses on ethics in two areas: research and evidence-based practice. The literature for ethics in research is plentiful. However, literature regarding ethics in evidence-based practice is just emerging. Similarities and differences in ethics exist in both research and evidence-based practice (EBP). Because ethics in research is abundantly found in the literature, ethics in research is examined first.

Nurses practice within a unique social world with norms, controls, rules, and regulations. Nurses embody the art of caring and are required to do no harm to patients. Nurse researchers are further constrained by this principle. The following statement encapsulates all the principles important for ethical nursing research; the most important and critical principle is the protection of the rights of all and any individuals participating in biomedical research:

> No one shall be subjected to torture or to cruel, inhuman or degrading treatment or punishment. In particular, no one shall be subjected without his/her free consent to medical or scientific experimentation. (United Nations, 1976, p. 175)[*]

Nurse researchers, acting as social scientists, examine the human condition in relation to health and illness. They, too, are governed by all the ethical principles encompassed within biomedical research. The International Council of Nurses (ICN) and the American Nurses Association (ANA) have developed ethical codes that control the practice of the nursing profession. Whether providing nursing care or doing EBP projects or research, nurses must engage in moral, ethical activities. Each ethical code specifies that a nurse researcher needs to be qualified to conduct research, regardless of the particular role (e.g., principal investigator, clinical research coordinator, or member of an institutional review board). This clarification means the researcher must understand all the elements required to maintain the highest ethical standards.

---

[*]From International covenant on civil and political rights, article 7. Universal declaration of human rights. In Council for International Organizations of Medical Sciences (CIOMS), International ethics guidelines for biomedical research involving human subjects, © 2002 United Nations. Reprinted with the permission of the United Nations.

The nurse researcher must understand what is morally and ethically appropriate to study and disseminate so as to protect the vulnerable—a group that includes everyone who participates as a subject and who trusts the nurse researcher will be ethical. "All research has ethical dimensions, and all research must be ethical" (Cipriano Silva, 2006, p. 178).

Nursing research, which lies within the domain of social science, is critical for the development of nursing knowledge. As a social science, nursing research is concerned with the human condition and, as such, is directed and controlled by all international ethical codes. The pursuit of nursing research requires participants to respect the specific ethical constraints and standards that are discussed in the sections that follow. This chapter discusses the ethical issues in each step of the research process. Universal ethical theories and their relevance to nursing research are presented, as well as theories that underpin all the health disciplines. A brief review of the history of human experimentation and the need for ethical practice is also provided.

Ethical Theories

To appreciate **ethical theories**, it is important to first understand the definitions of morality and ethics. **Morality** refers to "traditions or beliefs about right and wrong conduct" and is influenced by social and cultural practices, whereas **ethics** is "the study of social morality" (Burkhardt & Nathaniel, 2014, p. 35). Morality is what a person believes to be right and wrong and is shaped by what a person has been taught within society and their own culture. Cipriano (2015) suggests a moral person possesses integrity, respect, moderation, and industry, which are characteristics expected of nurses. Ethics is how a person makes judgments between right and wrong. Not infrequently, little distinction is made between the two, however, both morality and ethics are important in making decisions.

Ethical theories provide society with general guidelines for making decisions, but it is a person's moral philosophy that ultimately factors into the decision. According to Burkhardt and Nathaniel (2014), moral philosophy is "the philosophical discussion of what is considered good or bad, right or wrong, in terms of moral issues" (p. 35). Individuals have their own personal moral philosophies that guide ethical decision making. Tschudin (1992) points out that ethics are identified as either normative or descriptive. Normative ethics are prescriptive ethics; they relate to the standards that have been laid down and are generally accepted in any society as the guidelines for what one should do. From normative ethics emerges the code by which a profession lives, which is particularly true in nursing. In contrast, descriptive (or scientific) ethics arise from what people do.

Most occupations have a professional **code of ethics** to provide a more formal process for applying moral philosophy and to "govern professional behavior" (Burkhardt & Nathaniel, 2014, p. 35). In nursing, the ANA has a "Code of Ethics for Nurses," which was revised in 2015. This code of ethics guides the practice of nursing and is "the promise that nurses are doing their best to provide care for their patients and their communities and are supporting each other in the process so that all nurses can fulfill their ethical and professional obligations" (ANA, 2015). In recognizing the importance of ethics to nursing practice, the ANA declared the 2015 National Nurses' Week theme to be "Ethical practice, Quality care" (The American Nurse, 2015, p. 1). In addition, the ANA promoted 2015 as the year of ethics. In health care, professional codes of ethics incorporate several basic principles to help guide healthcare professionals in determining right from wrong and in making ethical decisions. These basic principles include autonomy, beneficence, nonmaleficence, veracity, justice, and fidelity.

The first basic ethical principle is **autonomy**. Autonomy, which comes from the Greek language, means self (*autos*) and governance (*nomos*). Autonomy incorporates three basic elements, "the ability to decide; the power to act on your decision, and a respect for the individual" (Edge & Groves, 2005, p. 60). From autonomy comes informed consent, which is an essential component in the research process and includes "understanding, voluntariness, competence, and permission given" by the individual (Edge & Groves, 2005, pp. 60–61). In health care, informed consent means the patient has been "given the opportunity to autonomously choose a course of action" related to their medical care (Burkhardt & Nathaniel, 2014, p. 64).

A second basic ethical principle is **beneficence**, which means to prevent harm or to promote good. This principle ensures that the healthcare worker will act to protect the patient. In research, beneficence "implies the protection from harm and discomfort" and includes a "balance between the benefits and risks of a study" (Burkhardt & Nathaniel, 2014, p. 525).

Along with beneficence comes the ethical principle **nonmaleficence**. This is commonly known as "do no harm." Specifically, nonmaleficence, means "avoid causing harm to another," including "deliberate harm, risk of harm, and harm that occurs during the performance of beneficial acts" (Burkhardt & Nathaniel, 2014, p. 529). In health care, the principles of beneficence and nonmaleficence can conflict and become an ethical dilemma as some forms of treatment may cause harm in order to provide for the greater benefit of care for the patient.

Another basic ethical principle is **veracity**, which refers to "the practice of telling the truth" (Burkhardt & Nathaniel, 2014, p. 73). Veracity encompasses mutual truth by the healthcare provider and the patient. Both parties have the right to know the truth and to be told the truth. Veracity is a fundamental principle in health care. Veracity also encompasses confidentiality, which refers to the individual's basic right to privacy. Confidentiality is "an important aspect of the trust the patients place in healthcare professionals" (Burkhardt & Nathaniel, 2014, p. 68). In 1996, the Health Insurance

---

❓ THINK OUTSIDE THE BOX

Consider the basic principles of ethics and morality. What basic principle shapes your decisions? How will your morals shape ethical decisions related to your nursing practice?

Portability and Accountability Act (HIPAA) was created to protect patients' rights and confidentiality by requiring and enforcing strict laws with regard to patient information. According to the U.S. Department of Health and Human Services (HHS; n.d.a, para 1), HIPAA "provides federal protections for individually identifiable health information" and "gives patients an array of rights with respect to that information."

A fifth basic ethical principle is **justice**. Justice is also known as fairness and equality to another. It encompasses a general guideline of "what is due or owed to persons" and "implies the rights of fair treatment and privacy, including anonymity and confidentiality" (Burkhardt & Nathaniel, 2014, p. 528).

A final ethical principle is **fidelity**. Fidelity refers to "faithfulness in the practice of keeping promises" (Burkhardt & Nathaniel, 2014, p. 84). Nurses are called to uphold "the profession's code of ethics, to practice within the established scope of practice and definition of nursing" (Burkhardt & Nathaniel, 2014, p. 84). All healthcare providers need to uphold ethical principles in their profession. This is equally important in the area of research.

Utilitarianism (Teleology)

Aristotle is regarded as a teleologist, although he does not necessarily take a wholly utilitarian perspective (utilitarianism is identified somewhat more narrowly than teleology). The theory of **teleology** is closely associated with Jeremy Bentham and John Stuart Mill (Mill, 1863/1967), two English philosophers. Simply put, it relates to the means justifying the ends and consequences of actions, which may be either good or bad. Bentham and Mill (Mill, 1863/1967) emphasized the duty of "good action" on the basis of happiness, or the greatest happiness that required the right action.

Three propositions form the basis of utilitarianism:

1. Actions are judged right or wrong based on the "virtue" of their consequences.
2. In assessing the consequences, all that is of concern is the amount of happiness that results.
3. When calculating happiness or unhappiness, no one person's reaction is more important than the reaction of anyone else (Rachels, 1995).

According to the views espoused by advocates of utilitarianism, the only thing that matters in the final analysis is the consequences. Rachels (1995) states that utilitarianism, with its adherence to the principle of utility, is the standard for judging right and wrong and firmly "rejects corruption" (p. 115). This perspective reduces—if not eliminates—feelings, desires, and "intuition" (p. 115) from rational and moral decision making.

While this ethical theory is used in healthcare delivery, it is perhaps somewhat difficult to apply and of limited use, except in weighing all the consequences of an action before it occurs and in making the decision whether the end truly justifies the means. In many instances, teleology would not be correctly applied if one is to do no harm to the patient. However, if adherence to the principle of utility is applied, then it can be assumed that reason will trump feelings and emotions.

The implication for nursing is that all nursing actions should be focused on doing the right thing or good (beneficence), rather than on doing harm (maleficence). In relation to nursing research, Edwards and Mauthner (2002) describe ethical theory as applied to research as follows: Doing the "right thing" is to perform research that produces new knowledge, provided that the human subject is not put at increased risk during the process of conducting the research.

Deontology

Deontology is a theory that focuses on the intrinsic nature or "rightness" of the action itself, with some actions seen as right and others as wrong. With "right" action, the individual is obligated to act regardless of the consequences. Immanuel Kant is believed to be the first to put duty at the forefront of moral behavior (Norman, 1998). In particular, Kant believed that because humans are "rational" entities, they are entitled to be treated with dignity, they always have value, and they must never be used as means—they are always ends. With this thinking comes responsibility, and Kant made clear his position that individuals must take responsibility for their actions.

Kant (1785) also defined "oughts" of reasoned behavior as "act[ing] only according to that maxim by which you can at the same time will that it should become a universal law" (cited by Rachels, 1995, p. 110). The limitation of this perspective is that a universal law should be upheld without exception, which makes it difficult or impossible to take into account the context for the behavior. The obligated duties of deontology are as follows:

- Fidelity
- Reparation
- Gratitude
- Justice

- Beneficence
- Self-improvement
- Nonmaleficence (Ross, 1954, as cited by Norman, 1998)

If one understands the meanings of these duties, then it is not difficult to accept why deontology is more easily accepted within the healthcare delivery system, and particularly in the nursing profession, which has a strong sense of duty and obligation to the patient.

Embedded in this ethical theory is the freedom of the individual but also consideration for the common good: "A right action is only right if it is done out of a sense of duty, and the only good thing without any qualification is a person's goodwill: the will to do what one knows to be right" (Tschudin, 1992, p. 51). Nursing has the obligation to protect the vulnerable patient—and therein lies the cause for justice. Edwards and Mauthner (2002) describe this theory as "actions governed by principles" (p. 20), including **honesty**, respect, and justice. For the nurse researcher, the obligation is to protect the human subject through demonstration of respect and honesty.

Values Theories

Principles of ethics not uncommonly used in health care include (1) respect, (2) autonomy, (3) beneficence (or nonmaleficence), and (4) justice. All ethics codes related to **human experimentation** stress **respect** for persons, both from the perspective of individual autonomy and by emphasizing the rights of those with diminished autonomy to the same protections. Autonomy refers to the ability to make careful choices. In relation to research, a potential subject should receive all the information required to make an informed decision.

Beneficence refers to the practice of maximizing benefits while minimizing risks. In relation to research, as stated by the Council for International Organizations of Medical Sciences (CIOMS),

> this principle gives rise to norms requiring that the risks of research be reasonable in light of the expected benefits…the research design be sound … investigators competent to perform the research and to safeguard the welfare of the research subjects. (2002)

Another term for beneficence is nonmaleficence, or the doing of no harm to the individual. Beneficence is identified as an obligation, and every effort must be made to ensure the wellbeing of the research subject. The Belmont Report (National Institutes of Health [NIH], 1979) indicated that the principle of beneficence applies to society at large as well as to specific investigators. Thus, obligations are inherent in all human research projects that have implications measured in terms of long-term effects for society at large.

Finally, the principle of justice is particularly applicable to the "vulnerable," but is more widely viewed as the "ethical obligation to treat each person in accordance with what is morally right and proper, to give each person what is due to him or her" (CIOMS, 2002, p. 11). The Belmont Report (NIH, 1979) describes what is due as "(a) to each person an equal share, (b) to each person according to individual need, (c) to each person according to individual efforts, (d) to each person according to societal contribution, and (e) to each person according to merit." "Equal" in this instance implies equity, although clearly at times not everyone will be equal. Nevertheless, there should be equity or justice in distribution of whatever is distributed. The implication of "distributive justice," to which both CIOMS and The Belmont Report refer, is that the issue of vulnerability of human subjects must be addressed as the same for everyone.

In human studies, nursing and medical practitioners are tending to **vulnerable subjects** simply by virtue of the illnesses that brought patients to the attention of healthcare providers. CIOMS (2002) describes vulnerability as:

> substantial incapacity to protect one's own interests owing to such impediments as lack of capability to give informed consent, lack of alternative means of obtaining medical care or other expensive necessities, or being a junior or subordinate member in a hierarchical group. (p. 11)

Human subjects are therefore vulnerable before they are invited to participate in research projects, and this imposes further ethical obligations on the researcher to protect them.

Virtues Theory

Virtues are regarded as character traits. Norman (1998) cites David Hume's (1751) list of virtues, which gives insight into these traits:

- Qualities useful to others: benevolence, justice, and fidelity
- Qualities useful to their possessor: discretion, industry, frugality, strength of mind, and good sense
- Qualities agreeable to their possessor: cheerfulness, magnanimity, courage, and tranquility
- Qualities agreeable to others: modesty and decency (p. 55)

Rachels (1995) adds "courage, self-control, generosity, and truthfulness" (p. 159) to this list, and suggests that moral philosophers can frame these virtues within the larger question of "what is the right thing to do" (p. 160) for the moral agent in "habitual action" (p. 163). Nevertheless, these characteristics, while important, do not offer a complete ethical theory. They assist in explaining how they can influence moral reasoning and behaviors. Rachels indicates that they may provide moral motivation,

THINK OUTSIDE THE BOX

Consider the various ethical theories. Which one seems to align with your nursing practice and why?

but it is important to realize that emotion may be an influence and that care is required to maintain impartiality. The virtue characteristics clearly play a role in determining how ethical theories are interpreted and utilized, but the theory itself does not depend on virtues themselves.

Historical Overview

The 20th century saw an explosive increase in human research, with a need for ethical oversight and controls. Significant medical breakthroughs, however, have occurred throughout history as a result of experimenting upon other human beings. For example, in 1789 in England, Edward Jenner first inoculated his son at 1 year of age with swinepox against smallpox, a lethal disease. This vaccination method proved to be ineffective, and later Jenner used cowpox on other human subjects. This approach was successful and led the way for effective inoculation against smallpox (Reich, 1995). Despite his undoubted achievement, Jenner's work raises a number of key ethical issues:

- No consent was obtained from the subject.
- No understanding was established as to whether the agents used (i.e., swinepox and cowpox) were safe for human use.
- Research was performed on a minor who would have had no understanding of what was happening, although the argument could be made that because the researcher was the father of the child, it was a nonissue. However, this practice would be deemed unacceptable today.

Nevertheless, throughout Western European history, there is evidence of the relevance of ethical behaviors in human research. Moses Maimonides (1135–1204), a physician and philosopher, "instructed colleagues always to treat patients as ends in themselves, not as means for learning new truths" (Reich, 1995, p. 2248). Claude Bernard, writing in France in 1865, stated

> Morals do not forbid making experiments on one's neighbor or one's self ... the principle of medical and surgical morality consists in never performing on man an experiment which might be harmful to him to any extent, even though the result might be highly advantageous to science, i.e., to the health of others. (Reich, 1995, p. 2249)

However, recognition of the need for regulated ethical constraints emerged as a result of horrific episodes during the 20th century. The worst documented atrocities were probably the Nazi experiments that were conducted mainly on prisoners during World War II. These experiments included "putting subjects to death by long immersion in subfreezing water, deprivation of oxygen to learn the limits of bodily endurance, or deliberate infection by lethal organisms in order to study the effect of drugs and vaccines" (Reich, 1995, p. 2253). In addition, "Nazi experimental atrocities included investigation of quicker and more effective means of inducing sexual sterilization (including clandestine radiation dosing and unanesthetized male and female castration and death)" (Reich, 1995, p. 2258).

In addition to these appalling events, highly unethical human research studies were performed in the United States. The most infamous was the Tuskegee Syphilis Study (Centers for Disease Control and Prevention [CDC], 2011), which involved African American males suffering from secondary syphilis; the treatment of penicillin (the recommended and available medication) was deliberately withheld from these patients so that the progression of the disease could be studied. The Tuskegee study, which was initiated in the mid-1930s, was not halted until 1972, when a newspaper published an account of it. At no time were the human subjects fully informed about the study, and in some instances they appear to have been deliberately misinformed. Among the many sad aspects of the study was the fact that subjects more than likely, in all innocence, infected others, because their syphilis was not being treated. Therefore, maleficence was directed not only toward the study subjects, but also toward their families, which compounded the researchers' ethical lapses.

Instances of human drug testing or usage with inadequate ethical oversight have also occurred. Thalidomide, a widely used sedative in the 1950s (though not in the United States), was given to some pregnant women to control morning sickness. When the tragic malformations of their fetuses were made public, thalidomide was removed from the market for this particular use. Thalidomide was one of a group of drugs for which it is evident that there was already knowledge about the potential for teratogenicity (malformation of fetuses). Yet, because this drug had been "widely praised, advertised, and prescribed on the grounds that it was unusually safe" (Dally, 1998, p. 1197), it was never properly tested for safety before human use. Instead, because of the highly effective advertising campaign conducted by the drug's manufacturer, the medical community ignored the evidence and went on using thalidomide. This case highlights another aspect of the relevance of stringent ethical controls in human research studies.

More recently, the inadequate design of a medical research study at Johns Hopkins School of Medicine led to the death of one of the subjects. In this instance, prior to the initiation of the study on the inhalation of

> **? THINK OUTSIDE THE BOX**
>
> Consider several examples of human experimentation that have occurred during the history of medical research. Have these projects resulted in beneficial outcomes for society? Can human experimentation be justified when the greater good of society is at stake? Defend your thoughts.

the drug hexamethonium, a limited and sketchy review of the literature was performed using only a medical index website. Such reviews are limited in terms of how far back they can search. The failure to explore the full history of the drug resulted in a healthy 24-year-old female losing her life: A review of the literature from an earlier period would have revealed potential hazards in association with this drug and its proposed route of administration. This case points to the importance of the careful design and organization of a study before it is initiated. Fault lay at many levels, not the least of which was the researcher, but also perhaps with Johns Hopkins' research review board (Perkins, 2001).

Interestingly, the World Medical Association in 1964 first made ethical principles for medical research involving human subjects public in the Declaration of Helsinki. Specifically, in section B, Basic Principles for All Medical Research, item #11 states, "Medical research involving human subjects must conform to generally accepted scientific principles, be based on a thorough knowledge of the scientific literature, [and] other relevant information" (World Medical Association, 1964–2004). Clearly, in the Johns Hopkins study, the study design did not adhere to international standards.

◼ Research Ethics: Progress in the 20th Century

The core ethical issue in medical research is the need for voluntary consent of the potential research subject so that a fully informed individual participates. Many efforts have been made to address this issue, but perhaps the most significant progress came from the Nuremberg Trials, in which the Nazi war crimes were investigated. The result was the Nuremberg Code of 1946, in which it is stated, "the voluntary consent of the human subject is absolutely essential … This means that the person involved should have legal capacity to give consent … the research subject should be so situated as to be able to exercise free power of choice" and human subjects "should have sufficient knowledge and comprehension of the elements of the subject matter involved as to make an understanding and enlightened decision" (Reich, 1995, p. 2253).

In the United States during the 1960s, different agencies within the federal government began more stringently regulating funded research on human subjects. On July 1, 1966, the NIH, through the Public Health Service, assigned "responsibility to the institution receiving the grant for obtaining and keeping documentary evidence of informed patient consent" (Reich, 1995, p. 2254). It also mandated "review of the judgment of the investigator by a committee of institutional associates not directly associated with the project" (Reich, 1995, p. 2254). Finally, the "review must address itself to the rights and welfare of the individual, the methods used to obtain informed consent, and risks and potential benefits of the investigation" (Reich, 1995, p. 2254).

In 1973, Congress formally recognized the importance of ethical standards in human research when it created the National Commission for the Protection of Human Subjects of Biomedical and Behavioral Research, whose mission was to protect the rights and welfare of research human subjects. Research oversight by the federal government continues with a constant updating of regulations, which can be found in the Code of Federal Regulations, Title 45 and 21—specifically in the Protection of Human Subjects Rule (HHS, 2005). Federal efforts to improve the safeguards to human subjects in research continue apace, culminating most recently with HIPAA.

ICN (2012) has followed suit, making the need for protection of human rights very clear in its own code of ethics, which focuses on four principal elements: (1) nurses and people, (2) nurses and practice, (3) nurses and the profession, and (4) nurses and coworkers. Ethical behaviors within these relationships are expected at all times, not just in areas of research. The second statement in the "nurses and people" element of the "ICN Code of Ethics for Nurses" (2012) reads as follows: "In providing care, the nurse promotes an environment in which the human rights, values, customs and spiritual beliefs of the individual, family and community are respected" (p. 2). As a social science, nursing research must demonstrate ethical values that reflect the values of the profession at any one time (Jeffers, 2005). Human rights, equity, and justice are stressed specifically in relation to educators and researchers. The "nurses and the profession" element of the ICN's code of ethics states that the researcher must "conduct, disseminate and utilise research to advance the nursing profession" (p. 8). Although ethics is not named directly here, its importance is inherent in the entire document.

As mentioned earlier, the ANA (2015) also has a "Code of Ethics for Nurses," in which specific vulnerable populations are identified. These populations include children, the elderly, prisoners, students, and the poor. The code was published in 1994, copyrighted in 1997, updated and republished in 2001, and revised in 2015. It also indicates that the nurse clinician identifies clinical problems that need examining and the researcher designs the study in association with the clinician. What is clear in this statement is that research topics in nursing should be focused on practice, which in itself should provide an ethical underpinning for nursing research.

Environment for Ethical Research

Most nurse researchers are associated with institutions that already have ethical regulations in place that the researcher is required to follow. This offers protection to the institution, the researcher, and the human subjects. The research institution housing the project typically has an office for reviewing all research proposals, usually called the **institutional review board (IRB)**. The main purpose of an IRB is to protect human subjects, especially vulnerable populations such as children, prisoners, pregnant women, handicapped or mentally disabled persons, or economically/educationally disadvantaged persons. The issues that receive the most intense IRB scrutiny relate to thorough evaluation by the research team of the risks and benefits of the project, the provision of sufficient protection for human subjects, and the implementation of sufficient monitoring of the project once approval is given to proceed (Rothstein & Phuong, 2007). In addition, this office is most helpful in ensuring that the researcher submits all the required paperwork, including the proposal for the study, the consent form that study participants will sign, the budget, and whatever tools the researcher will be using in data gathering (e.g., surveys or instruments, or interview guides in the case of qualitative studies).

The HHS Code of Federal Regulations controls the IRB offices of various types of healthcare organizations. The membership of the IRB must include at least five members of different backgrounds who also have the competence to review research proposals. It is expected that the membership will have cultural and gender diversity, as well as an awareness of local community mores. Thus, not only will there be healthcare professionals on the board, but there will also be members who are "unaffiliated" with the institution; at least one member must have scientific interests, and one may not (Rothstein & Phuong, 2007). The members are expected to be knowledgeable about all federal guidelines and regulations. When reviewing a proposal, an IRB member may not have involvement with the project (HHS, 2009). Unfortunately, there have been instances when IRB members have had some sort of conflict of interest or lack of objectivity that renders the board less capable of being just, fair, and protective of human subjects (Rothstein & Phuong, 2007).

The IRB members meet once a month to review all proposals, which they have already carefully scrutinized, and they may request further information to make informed decisions. When the IRB is satisfied that the researcher will provide full protection of the human subjects, the researcher is given permission to proceed and the project is given an identifying number. The researcher must report progress back to the IRB every 12 months. The IRB members expect the researcher to follow the protocol exactly as laid out in the proposal. If the project has more than one researcher, all must be listed on the protocol and, if requested by the institution, the curriculum vitae (CV) of each must also be attached. The issues of specific concern for ensuring ethical research are that the risks to the subjects are minimized (or are at least reasonable, providing the expected outcomes or benefits can be attained); subject selection is equitable; informed consent is sought from participants; and issues relating to data collection and storage, privacy, and confidentiality are managed according to regulations (HHS, 2005).

HHS (2009) outlines regulations specific to the IRB and the subjects being researched; the current version of the regulations includes five subparts:

- Subpart A is the basic set of protections for all human subjects of research conducted or supported by HHS, and was revised in 1981 and 1991, with technical amendments made in 2005. Three of the other subparts provide added protections for specific vulnerable groups of subjects.
- Subpart B, issued in 1975 and most recently revised in 2001, provides additional protections for pregnant women, human fetuses, and neonates involved in research.
- Subpart C, issued in 1978, provides additional protections pertaining to biomedical and behavioral research involving prisoners as subjects.
- Subpart D, issued in 1983, provides additional protections for children involved as subjects in research.
- Subpart E, issued in 2009, requires registration of institutional review boards (IRBs) which conduct review of human research studies conducted or supported by HHS.[†]

The researcher is expected to be competent to perform the research. Lenz and Ketefian (1995) indicate that in 1989, the Institute of Medicine's Committee on the Responsible Conduct of Research was concerned that there was "a lack of formal training in scientific ethics and the responsible conduct of science as a deficit in the training of scientists and clinicians" (p. 217). Although baccalaureate degree programs and higher levels of nursing education include courses on research, it is oftentimes not until a student is writing either a master's thesis or a doctoral dissertation that he or she begins to understand the process that ensures that the research is ethical and legal.

[†] Reproduced from U. S. Department of Health and Human Services (HHS). (n.d.b). Regulations. http://www.hhs.gov/ohrp/humansubjects/

According to Ketefian and Lenz (1995), "Scientists have traditionally valued their independence in the conduct of their research. In the main, society and academic institutions have to be willing to give certain freedoms and latitude ... in return, increased accountability is ... demanded" (p. 268). However, an institution does not want its reputation sullied by unprofessional, illegal, or unethical research. Research **trustworthiness**, reliability, and usefulness are utterly dependent on the credibility of the researcher, the work, and the institution. The rules and regulations are generally the most rigorous when an institution receives federal funding. In such cases, the IRB office is insistent on all requirements being met. Ultimately, the research has to be honest.

Although multiple brakes are now applied in an attempt to prevent unethical research from occurring, some continue to have concerns that there is still the potential for inadequate protection of human subjects. Wood, Grady, and Emanuel (2002) believe that the review process is "bureaucratic and inefficient" (p. 2) and suggest that IRB members are overworked, frightened by the possibility of federal audits, and do not always understand "ambiguous regulations" (p. 2). They continue: "Federal regulators are aggravated by the limited scope of their authority and variable adherence to regulations" (p. 2), and their concerns are not limited to these particulars. For the nurse researcher, however, adherence to the ethical standards for human subject protection applied by the organization for which the researcher works and the codes of ethics developed by ICN and ANA is crucial, regardless of external concerns.

Developing a Researchable Topic

Although nurse researchers may have curiosity about and interest in many topics they believe have the potential for expanding the body of nursing knowledge, some topics may not be realistically researchable for a number of reasons. The critical factor relates to protection of the vulnerable subject. As nurses, we are deeply and intimately involved with human beings at their most vulnerable, and the research topic may well pose a further increase in those individuals' vulnerability. When developing a researchable topic, the nurse researcher is called upon to utilize "ethical sensitivity" to decide what is appropriate, to have the "ability to perceive rightness and wrongness" (Weaver, 2007, p. 142), and to know what one is doing that affects the welfare of another person either directly or indirectly. Iverson and colleagues (2014) discuss the importance of sensitivity in their study of female veterans who were victims of intimate partner violence (IVP).

Issues related to the researcher also determine whether a topic is researchable. Volker (2004) indicates that attempting to research certain topics could put the researcher at risk "for loss of professional license, legal actions, imprisonment and peer ostracism" (p. 119). The types of topics that pose a threat to the researcher, according to Volker (2004), include those examining "social deviance, [those impinging] on powerful social interests, or [those examining] a deeply personal sacred value held by study participants" (p. 117). Nurses should not be studying illegal activities as a general rule, of course. Volker uses the example of a patient requesting assistance with suicide—an issue that nurses confront in their practice. A topic such as this presents problems when considering a research project: According to the ANA's 1994 statement on assisted suicide, "Nursing has a social contract with society that is based on trust, and therefore patients must be able to trust that nurses will not actively take human life" (p. 4). Volker does not state that the topic of assisted suicide cannot be examined in a research project, but rather that careful vigilance must be exercised to ensure the study design is meticulously developed to protect both the researcher and the research subject. Cipriano (2015) indicates nurses must speak up regarding decisions and actions that are questionable.

In legally sensitive research projects, further measures can be sought that protect the researcher against "compelled disclosure" (Anderson & Hatton, 2000, p. 249) or breaking confidentiality covenants (Volker, 2004) and that offer additional protection for the study subjects. In particular, a Certificate of Confidentiality may be issued by the HHS in such cases. Federal law states that a Certificate of Confidentiality:

> may authorize persons engaged in biomedical, behavioral, clinical, or other research (including research on the use and effect of alcohol and other psychotic drugs) to protect the privacy of individuals who are the subject of such research by withholding from all persons not connected with the conduct of such research the names or other identifying characteristics of such individuals. Persons so authorized to protect the privacy of such individuals may not be compelled in any Federal, State, or local civil, criminal, administrative, legislative, or other proceedings that identify such individuals. (Public Health Service Act, 42 USC 163, 1988)

Volker (2004) makes it clear that "researchers who engage in socially sensitive research must be prepared for scrutiny by diverse professional and lay parties who have varying agendas and interests" (p. 123). Research projects are usually undertaken in institutions that have a well-developed ethical structure and that are highly conscientious in following federal guidelines and regulations to protect the vulnerable patients under their care. As a consequence, the researcher, while developing the project, has resources immediately available for advice and consultation, including the IRB, professional colleagues, attorneys, and an ethics committee.

> **? THINK OUTSIDE THE BOX**
>
> Vulnerable populations are always with us. Can you think of some additional ones that are emerging in the current healthcare environment? Explain why you see these groups as vulnerable. Which issues need to be considered when determining the vulnerability of a group of people? Of the two articles regarding diabetes and IVP, which involves a vulnerable population? Give a rationale for your choice.

The topic that the nurse researcher chooses should be one of real interest to him or her. The researcher should be willing to allocate the preparatory time and effort to ensure that the project meets all of the institution's ethical guidelines. Ethical behavior requires intellectual honesty of the researcher—giving credit due to others, not using ideas from others without acknowledgment, and not initiating data collection before institutional approval has been given. Plans for seeking funding for the study, the study design, methodology, data collection, and the dissemination of results (even if insignificant) at the conclusion of the study are also critical parts of developing the topic for research.

Pilkington (2002) makes it clear that if a research project is not scientifically valid, then it is unethical to involve human subjects. It is the responsibility of the IRB (known as a "research ethics board" in Canada) to ensure that a study is scientifically valid. In defining whether a research project is scientifically valid, Pilkington (2002) states bluntly, "If a study does not hold substantial promise of answering a significant question(s), thereby generating valuable knowledge, then there is no justification for exposing persons to the actual or potential risks and inconvenience of participation" (p. 197). Scientific validity, therefore, influences how a researchable topic is developed to be an ethical research study.

■ Developing Researchable Questions

Although the nurse researcher may have a burning interest in a particular topic, developing the question(s) appropriately is most important when gearing up for a formal study. This development is necessary to narrow down the topic to a specific focus, clarify the methodology, determine whether the topic has embedded in it useful questions that will give shape to the study, and ensure that significant research results will emerge and add to the body of nursing knowledge. The questions should be broad enough to obtain results, yet not so broad as to yield diffuse and possibly meaningless results.

Thorough reading on the subject can assist in developing questions that meet these criteria. This preliminary investigation can help identify the gaps in the literature and hone the researcher's thinking about what it is specifically that he or she wants to investigate. Communication with both clinician colleagues and fellow nurse researchers can also assist in refining the questions.

The ethical component of this endeavor derives from ANA's demand for effective and efficient care of the patient. If the research design is faulty at any level—and specifically the question development level—then one must ask if the results will improve the efficiency and effectiveness of patient care.

■ Participant Recruitment and Informed Consent

Vulnerable populations are always a concern for all research regulatory bodies, but there are some populations who are particularly vulnerable—the very young, the frail elderly, prisoners, the mentally incompetent, and women. In addition, issues related to socioeconomic status, education, and language may contribute to a specific population's vulnerability (Anderson & Hatton, 2000; Rogers, 2005). The researcher must be sensitive to these issues and to the points specifically outlined in federal regulations. This can make recruitment more difficult and the need for true **informed consent** crucial. Very specific regulations can be found in the Belmont Report (NIH, 1979), the International Ethics Guidelines for Biomedical Research Involving Human Subjects (CIOMS, 2002), and the HHS's Protection of Human Subjects document (2009), including sections relating to the protections needed for specific vulnerable populations.

The key ethical issue embedded in informed consent is that the individual always has the freedom of choice to participate or not participate, and may withdraw from the study at any time. Another term used in conjunction with informed consent is valid consent. Valid consent is thought to be more informative of the process. This freedom of choice is built on a series of components:

- The language is simple enough to be clearly understood.
- The potential subject adequately comprehends the project.
- The subject has had time to think about the study and its potential risks and benefits and to discuss it with family members.
- The consent is not coerced.
- The written consent is documented.

CIOMS (2002) discusses "inducements" to participation, which can be identified as coercion and, therefore, are not appropriate. Several authors have expressed concern over how to achieve the consent and indicate that, in fact, obtaining consent should be a continuous process throughout a research project. In other words, the researcher should regularly check in with the subject to ensure that he or she is still a willing and informed participant (Edwards & Mauthner, 2002; Miller & Bell, 2002). The only payment or compensation allowed includes the costs of transportation or loss of earnings due to participation in the research project. It is unethical to offer more financial incentives, as they may encourage a potential subject to consent against his or her better judgment. It is also unethical for the researcher to receive compensation from a pharmaceutical company to conduct a study.

Research using child participants encompasses all the usual ethical issues relating to informed consent, privacy, and confidentiality, but includes several other factors that may compound these issues: Children exist in a natural power hierarchy with adults, but are able to communicate and understand according to their interpretation of the world around them (Kirk, 2007). Children must believe they are part of the project, but researchers must be alert to the specific child's "agenda" and continually check back with the child to ensure that he or she wants to continue to participate. Parents are also involved with providing informed consent, but researchers must ensure that children do understand what they are getting into and that their consent is given freely. Hanna, Weaver, Slaven, Fortenberry, and DiMeglio (2014) obtained informed consent of parents and youths 18 years old or older. In some instances, only one parent's consent is required, although two parents' consent is preferable. On occasion, a child and parents may not agree on continued participation; in general, it is the child's decision that is accepted in such cases.

The success of the study may depend on the warmth, interest in the child, and rapport established by the researcher, so that the child trusts the researcher. These characteristics have been demonstrated to be critical in longitudinal studies with children (Ely & Coleman, 2007), particularly when ill children are subjected to discomforting treatments. A slightly different issue arises with teenagers who, while still legally minors, have the right to give informed consent without parental consent (Roberson, 2007). Parents still have legal responsibility "to ensure the child [receives] appropriate medical care, [but] there is also the ethical need to 'respect the rights and autonomy of every individual, regardless of age'" (Kunin, 1997, cited by Roberson, 2007, p. 191).

Recruiting the desired composition and number of participants may require establishing multiple research sites, which can create some problems for the researcher, even as it confers some distinct advantages to the study: Such studies are "likely to produce generalizable, high quality results ... [increase the] likelihood of attracting funding ... [provide access to] a broader range of practice settings and patients with a wider range of diagnoses … [and] expedite data collection" (Twycross & Corlett, 2007, p. 35). Multisite research enables experts to work together and perhaps close the theory–practice gap. Of course, some notable difficulties in conducting multisite studies are noted, including those related to establishing and maintaining collaborative, trusting relationships with one's colleagues; meeting face to face; overcoming organizational cultural differences; and having to gain IRB approval at each site.

Data Collection and Data Analysis

Protection of vulnerable human subjects remains the critical ethical issue with data collection and analysis. First and foremost, the privacy and confidentiality of the subjects must be protected, which means that the data must be locked securely in a safe place at all times. Data may include audiotapes, podcasts, digital recordings, surveys, or videotapes, among other media.

Video recording is becoming more popular for data collection because of "its inherent accuracy and reliability as a record of events and detailed, nuanced levels of observation and analysis permitted" (Broyles, Tate, & Happ, 2008, p. 59). Additional ethical issues must be addressed when such data collection methods are used, however—namely, privacy; participant burden and safety; storage, location, and condition of storage of recordings; maintenance of the recordings in storage; access to recordings; use of the recordings as part of a presentation; and whether the actual taping will interfere with clinical care. The IRB will make decisions on all these issues and may require that faces be blurred and/ or eyes are covered with a black box in the final recording.

Each institution has specific guidelines about how long data files must be kept. Lutz (1999) has raised the issue of premature destruction of original data, predominantly in studies on particularly vulnerable populations (e.g., battered women). According to this author, such destruction could occur if the researcher were concerned about court subpoenas that could compromise the participants' safety. However, premature destruction could lead to institutional accusations of scientific misconduct, which suggests that the researcher has a fine line to walk between ethical and unethical actions.

Ethical analysis and interpretation depend on the honesty and trustworthiness of the researchers. Although healthcare organizations make every effort to ensure ethical behaviors within their research environments, ultimately it rests with the researchers to ensure that the project is indeed conducted ethically in all areas, including analysis, interpretation, and dissemination of results. The opposite of ethical behavior is scientific misconduct, which brings dishonor to both the individual and the institution, and renders the research project

THINK OUTSIDE THE BOX

Determine if your school or hospital has an institutional review board (IRB). Which criteria do the board members use when approving a research project?

meaningless. In addition, concern for the welfare of the vulnerable human subjects is negated when misconduct occurs. **Scientific misconduct**, an extremely serious issue, is defined by HHS as follows:

> Fabrication, falsification, plagiarism or other practices that seriously deviate from those that are commonly accepted within the scientific community for proposing, conducting or reporting research. It does not include an honest error or honest differences in interpretations or judgments of data. (Commission on Research Integrity, 1995, p. 1)

Lutz (1999) has cited Macrina (1995), who states that falsification involves results being manipulated or tampered with, fabrication refers to "totally unfounded results" (p. 90) being produced, and plagiarism is "theft of another person's ideas" (p. 90). History makes evident that falsification, fabrication, and plagiarism are unconscionable and utterly unethical.

Issues in Quantitative and Qualitative Research

There is concern in qualitative research about the increased risk for ethical lapses inherent with this research methodology. As Birch and Miller (2002) state, this "type of research relationship may involve acts of self-disclosure, where personal, private experiences are revealed" (p. 92) and is never value free or "value neutral" (Christians, 2003, p. 213). The researcher must be aware of this potential and approach this type of research by making every attempt to acknowledge any personal biases.

In qualitative research, interviews are commonly used to gather data, resulting in face-to-face exposure for both the researcher and the researched as was the case in the study of IVP. The dialogue serves as the research data that are then analyzed and interpreted. The vulnerable patient immediately becomes more vulnerable as the researcher delves into his or her lived experience. Anonymity and confidentiality are inevitably compromised in the interaction between researcher and human subject, which means there is an even greater need for data security and constant awareness on the part of the researcher of these issues. Honesty and trustworthiness of the research are even more important in such cases. Firby (1995) has stated, in relation to an IRB giving permission for a qualitative research project, "We should not simply assume that because research has been accepted by a committee it is morally justifiable in its methods" (p. 41). The moral obligation of nursing is to do good and to do no harm. Therefore, qualitative nursing research must meet that obligation.

In contrast to qualitative research, quantitative research, which initially arose from the objective methodology of the Enlightenment's scientific paradigm, is more apt to be value neutral. The quantitative researcher is less likely to engage in face-to-face self-disclosure, which protects him or her and the subject. The facts should speak for themselves. However, the researcher must be alert to the potential for his or her biases to influence the interpretation of data. Nevertheless, there remains the ethical principle of justice and the need for informed consent for human participants in such studies.

■ External Pressures

Conducting research studies is never easy, but various pressures making it more difficult may push the researcher toward unethical behaviors. According to Lutz (1999), these pressures include limited funding, the competition for achieving tenure for faculty, and "increasing emphasis on producing research reports" (p. 92). New technology and seeking cures also place pressure on healthcare providers (Cipriano, 2015).

HIPAA is designed to protect patients against unauthorized disclosure of their health and medical records. At the same time, it adds another source of pressure for nurse researchers, as passage of HIPAA has led to some new concerns related to health research. According to Erlen (2005), these regulations were written for healthcare delivery organizations, and not for universities per se; nevertheless, the latter organizations have had to develop their own policies and procedures that meet the requirements of HIPAA. At times it has proven difficult to draw "clear boundaries," and universities have tended to err on the side of caution by providing for additional protection of human subjects, privacy, confidentiality, and informed consent. HIPAA compliance has meant additional training for anyone who wishes to engage in research. The institution's IRB office sets the policy for how the researchers of that institution can proceed while adhering to HIPAA regulations.

HIPAA and its ramifications are key ethical considerations for the nurse researcher. With the drive for evidence-based research to underpin practice, the nurse researcher needs to be aware that study data and their interpretation must be shared, but within the constraints of HIPAA.

To meet these criteria, data must contain no identifiers of an individual in a sample. Thus, subjects may be given a code number or letter. Only the researcher maintains a list linking the sample identifiers with their associated codes, and this document must be kept secure at all times.

Evidence-Based Practice and Ethical Implications

Now that we have explored ethics in the research process, let's examine ethics and EBP. In the clinical environment, considerable effort is being made to implement evidence-based nursing practice. Such practice is derived from several elements, including experiential knowledge on the part of the nurse (i.e., knowing what works in practice and why), having clinical judgment and skills of critical inquiry, knowing the individual patient both as a human being and in terms of his or her pattern of responses to what is occurring, and knowledge of current scientific research findings (Borsay, 2009; Redman, 2007; Tanner, 2006). EBP is designed to reduce unthinking, ritualistic practices in nursing care (Siedlecki, 2008). Nurses are uniquely placed to establish an ethical practice environment that protects the patient (Cipriano, 2015).

Quality improvement (QI) is constantly performed in healthcare organizations: Data are gathered in order to improve patient outcomes through "local innovations in and assessment of the processes and systems of care delivery" (Redman, 2007, p. 217). This process is designed for rapid implementation of change. It is different from the slower rigorous, empirical research approach, which is more deliberative and follows a "fixed protocol with a clearly defined method and ... a period of analysis after completed data collection" (Lynn et al., 2007, p. 668). QI is not empirical research. There is some concern, however, related to the ethics of human subject protection in QI practices (Grady, 2007; Lynn et al., 2007). To date, there has been no standard established regarding whether there should be a separate IRB process for QI.

Changes that are derived from QI are not regarded as the strongest evidence in EBP. Rather, EBP is dependent on generalizable scientific evidence (Batalden & Davidoff, 2007). The research utilized in evidence-based nursing practice uses well-tested scientific study data from studies that have undergone the required ethical scrutiny.

Developing an Evidence-Based Project

Similar to some nurses interested in researchable topics, other nurses may want to pursue EBP projects. Much interest has been generated in QI, patient autonomy, quality of life, and end-of-life issues. The specific process of developing an EBP project is discussed elsewhere; however, ethical issues need to be addressed prior to, during, and after the completion of EBP projects that parallel ethical issues in research projects.

EBP is a broad area that encompasses more than scientific research. In fact, research is considered to be one aspect of EBP. Not all nurses have the knowledge and skill to conduct research but that does not mean they don't encounter clinical situations that arouse their curiosity. As a result, they may wish to pursue information to improve nursing care. Developing an EBP topic also requires sensitivity to vulnerable populations, confidentiality, and existing federal and state guidelines, as well as professional regulations to practice nursing. Keeping all this in mind, the nurse should choose an EBP topic that is of specific interest to him or her to improve nursing practice. EBP projects also require the nurse to meet the institution's ethical guidelines.

The PICOT (population, intervention, comparison, outcome, time) format can be used as a starting point for developing an EBP question. Nurses must consider the ethics of asking an EBP question. The topic selected must be narrow enough to produce results that will improve patient care. At the same time, the design must be carefully planned to eliminate the potential of harm to participants.

Protection of human subjects is as important to EBP projects as it is to research. Thus, vulnerable populations are a concern for EBP projects. For example, if you want to collect data about fall rates in your institution, the population might include the elderly and/or children. Ethically, you must ensure that patient privacy and confidentiality are protected. Even if you are only conducting a retrospective chart review of patients who have fallen, you must still keep all patient information in confidence and not reveal any patient identification information.

It is also necessary to ensure that participants in an EBP project will be honest in their responses. If a nurse is investigating nurses' medication errors in his or her institution, nurses in the institution must report that a medication error is made. If the nurses making the errors do not report them for fear of reprisal, the information about the number, type, or reasons for the error(s) will not be accurate, and recommendations to decrease medication errors will not be effective. The EBP project must also be ethical in all areas, including design, implementation, and evaluation. EBP projects require the same ethical rigor required in research.

Data collection for EBP generally focuses on institutional benchmarks to improve patient outcomes, patient satisfaction, communication techniques, hospital readmissions, and staff/physician satisfaction, to name just a few potential areas of investigation. An example might be a hospital that wants to decrease the occurrence of pressure ulcers. To accomplish this, the hospital wound care nurse obtains permission to adapt the Braden Scale as part of the nursing assessment of skill. The wound care nurse then educates the staff regarding the use of the Braden Scale and how it is mandatory to chart this assessment so that pressure ulcers can be prevented by early detection. After 1 month, the wound care nurse performs a chart review to determine if nurses used the Braden Scale, charted the skin assessment results, and if the number of new pressure ulcers decreased. The wound care nurse may also compare the results with other hospitals in the same geographic area or with other hospitals of the same size and same general population. Thus, data analysis does not necessarily involve statistical tests/methods as seen in research projects.

Data collection and data analysis for EBP projects, such as the wound care example, require the same ethical considerations for protection of human subjects. Many hospitals request patients to allow their information to be used to promote better outcomes and/or for teaching purposes. To be ethical in the example given, the wound care nurse must protect patient confidentiality, remove patient identifying information, and report results in the aggregate (group) and not as individuals.

Issues in Evidence-Based Projects

As in research projects, anonymity and confidentiality in EBP projects are paramount. The person(s) responsible for EBP projects must protect the human subjects and must do no harm. In addition, they must be alert to any bias that may influence how the data are interpreted.

Because EBP projects are often specific to an institution, care must be taken to avoid pressure from individuals within the organization who want to show positive results. The EBP project must ensure that policies and procedures are followed and that data are accurately represented. Training regarding such things as HIPAA is necessary to ensure no violations occur.

A further ethical dimension is encountered when, at the end of the research or EBP project, it is time to publish the results: Journals accept only peer-reviewed manuscripts (Ketefian & Lenz, 1995). Peer referees are required to evaluate the scientific merit of the research study as well as the manuscript's acceptability for a particular journal. To warrant publication, the findings are expected to contribute new knowledge to the practice of nursing (Driever & Pranulis, 2003). Without that expectation, the research is inappropriate, if not unethical. Those who review manuscripts for publication must have the knowledge and expertise to evaluate the work appropriately (Pilkington, 2002).

---

❷ THINK OUTSIDE THE BOX

Should it be a requirement that EBP projects be approved by an IRB? List the reasons why or why not IRB approval is necessary.

An emerging segment of the literature is focusing on issues related to publication. Conn (2008) discusses how pressure may be put on the author to change results because the manuscript reviewers resist "unexpected outcomes" (p. 161) and want revisions that are not consistent with the results. The authors may need to make changes, but those changes should not come at the expense of reliable data results. Freda and Kearney (2005) discuss how editors can face ethical issues when articles have been published in more than one journal; when data are published in more than one journal with no changes; or when there is evidence of author misconduct, demand for credit for someone "undeserving" of credit, lack of IRB approval, or misconduct related to lack of informed consent or an undeclared conflict of interest.

A study by Henley and Dougherty (2009) revealed another potential problem related to publication of research results: discrepancies in the quality of the reviews submitted by many persons who serve as peer reviewers. According to these authors, "Peer review is the mainstay of the editorial process" (p. 18). The key issues of concern within a paper were poor reviews related to the study's theoretical framework (47.2%), literature review (35.15%), discussion and interpretation of results (22%), and data analysis/presentation (21.9%). In terms of usefulness of the written comments to the author, 14.4% of peer reviews were deemed poor (Henley & Dougherty, 2009). Finally, in terms of usefulness to the editor, 12.2% of peer reviews were poor or inadequate (Henley & Dougherty, 2009). These authors recommended formal training and a probationary period for all potential reviewers.

A further ethical issue relates to who should be listed as first author when multiple researchers participated in the study. Generally, the principal investigator is listed as first author. However, in the case of multiple authors, negotiation determines the first author named on various publications. Ketefian and Lenz (1995) point out that listing authors in order of the extent of effort they made is the most ethical way of recognizing authorship. These authors also suggest that it is unethical to publish the same manuscript or article in multiple journals. It is appropriate to publish several articles on the same study, provided that each manuscript is written with a different focus. In addition, all contributions and funding sources for an article must be acknowledged.

Emerging Issues in Research and EBP

The prevalence of EBP projects has caused much controversy about whether EBP and research are separate. One school of thought is that research is not a component of EBP; the other side of course is that research is one aspect of EBP. Much depends on the definition of each. Proponents of research argue that EBP is specific to an institution, has no theoretical framework, and data are not able to be statistically tested and analyzed. Proponents of EBP state that EBP is broader, includes research where appropriate, and that data collected from specific institutions can be compiled and added to national data banks providing information that has broad implications. Ethical considerations for both will continue to be required regarding protection of human subjects, regardless of the prevailing school of thought.

Although nurses generally have not been involved in animal, genetic, or biological material research in the past, this situation is changing and is likely to continue to do so as more transdisciplinary, translational research occurs. The issues of concern with animals include ensuring that the least harm and suffering are inflicted, using animals only when absolutely necessary, using the fewest animals possible, and, when seeking IRB permission, ensuring that someone on the board understands the implications of animal research. In relation to genetic and biological materials research, the same moral and ethical obligations apply as when dealing with any human subjects (Cipriano Silva, 2006).

An environment that has been neglected as a site for study in the past, but is likely to draw increasing attention from researchers in the future because of the aging of the U.S. population, is the community-based care facility (i.e., nursing home). All of the usual ethical research issues apply in this setting, but some additional concerns may arise relating to ensuring the quality of life, safety, and satisfaction of those residing in nursing homes, and ensuring that the study will not impose an undue burden on the participants. Proxies may be required to give consent for resident participation if the resident is mentally incompetent or extremely frail; however, use of proxies requires that the proxy holder have the authority to give this type of consent, and he or she must be adequately informed of the study's focus. In a study by Cartwright and Hickman (2007), it was discovered that community-based facility administrators had limited understanding of the protections established by an IRB that gives consent to a study, although most seemed aware of federal and state statutory requirements in terms of informed consent. In an attempt to overcome these deficits, Cartwright and Hickman developed a Bill of Rights for Community-Based Research Partners that could prove valuable for similar institutions.

■ Conclusion

The lessons learned from the history of human experimentation have led to the development of ethical codes, both nationally and internationally. These controls are crucial for the protection of vulnerable human subjects. Indeed, ensuring adequate protection of human subjects requires that particular care be taken in each step of the research or EBP process.

The obligations inherent within nursing demand the "moral deliberation, choice and accountability" (Edwards & Mauthner, 2002, p. 14) of the nurse researcher. Nurses in their practice are tending to humans at their most vulnerable, and this level of understanding adds to the responsibility of the nurse as researcher or EBP project director. Achieving valid research and EBP that enhances nursing knowledge is dependent on adherence to the highest ethical standards. The key components necessary to ensure that these ethical standards are met, as described in this chapter, should provide a useful guide for all nurses embarking on a research or EBP project.

Summary Points

1. History provides many lessons on the importance of protection of vulnerable human subjects. These history lessons have led to the development of national and international ethical codes of conduct.
2. Both the International Council of Nurses (ICN) and the American Nurses Association (ANA) acknowledge the obligations of the nursing profession to the vulnerable human and, as such, stress ethical standards in nursing research.
3. Ethical theories guide the standards of nursing research.
4. Some populations (e.g., children) are more vulnerable than others; as such, they must be provided with the utmost protection during the research or EBP project.
5. Each step of the research process involves meeting ethical standards.
6. The privacy and confidentiality of the human subject must always be guaranteed.
7. Informed consent must be given by a human subject participant who truly understands to what he or she is consenting.
8. The honesty and trustworthiness of the nurse researcher or EBP project directors are crucial in ensuring valid—and valuable—results are derived from any study.

RED FLAGS

- Every study must address the ethical aspects of that study. Documentation of this focus may be demonstrated through a statement reflecting IRB approval of the study.
- Every study must speak to how the subjects will be protected from harm—physical and/or psychological—during the research process.

Critical Discussion: Ethical Issues in Nursing Research and EBP Projects

1. A research study of incarcerated women who are human immunodeficiency virus (HIV) positive or have acquired immunodeficiency syndrome (AIDS) is being conducted. You are not the principal investigator, but you are one of the researchers who have received permission to interview some of the women who volunteered to participate. One woman gives you inappropriate information about another prisoner, whom she states propositioned her for sex; the interviewee claims this prisoner has AIDS. As you leave the prison, the warden asks you to relate what happened during this interview. Discuss your responsibilities as a researcher in this sensitive study. A number of critical elements must be taken into account: the interviewee divulging information about another prisoner's possible HIV/AIDS status and behaviors, confidentiality and protection of human subjects, the warden's request, and your ethical responsibility to the study and to your institution.

2. You are the principal investigator studying young teenagers (10–14 years old) who are receiving aggressive treatment for life-threatening cancers. One 11-year-old boy has had many bouts of chemotherapy, which have made him acutely ill. His parents would like the child to participate in the study, but he refuses. What he shares could potentially be of use in treating other young teenagers. Clearly, there are some issues of consent here. Discuss what you should do.

3. You are one of a group of nurse researchers who are participating in a multinational study. The sample will include people of many different ethnic groups, all of whom speak different languages, and will include women and children. You understand the process of IRB review in your own institution, but many other issues arise when one is participating in international studies. Among the issues of concern here are the need for an interpreter, confidentiality, local permission requirements, management of the study in the foreign country, recruitment of persons into the study, and protection of human subjects in a different country. How can these issues be resolved so that the study may be conducted?

4. Your hospital wants to decrease the rate of falls in patients older than 65 years of age. You have been asked to conduct an EBP project regarding these patient outcomes. What are some ethical considerations you must incorporate into this project?

Multiple-Choice Questions

1. When developing a nursing research project, why is it important to remember the ethical constraints?

    A. The study will not be approved by the institutional review board without these constraints.

    B. The protection of human subjects underlies all human research projects.

    C. The results will not be trustworthy and replicable.

    D. The nurse researcher will not be able to get funding for the project and, therefore, will not be able to complete the project.

2. The atrocities performed on prisoners in Nazi Germany violated which ethical principles?

    A. Value of life, justice, and respect

    B. Beneficence, nonmaleficence, and value of life

    C. Autonomy, nonmaleficence, and respect

    D. Justice, autonomy, and nonmaleficence

3. Protection of vulnerable individuals is a critical ethical component in human research studies. How did Edward Jenner fail to meet this standard when he tested swinepox on his 1-year-old son?

    A. He thought the new knowledge overrode any concern he should have for the rights of his son.

    B. He did not know any better.

    C. He ignored the point that he could not get informed consent from his son, who was particularly vulnerable.

    D. He did not fail: Given that smallpox was such a lethal disease at that time, it was better for Jenner to ignore his son's vulnerability in order to gain new knowledge.

4. The Tuskegee Syphilis Study lasted many years, and none of the human subjects were properly informed about the study's conduct. Which ethical principle was egregiously ignored in this study?

    A. Autonomy

    B. Respect

    C. Nonmaleficence

    D. Justice

5. Why does an ethical research environment assist with ensuring scientific integrity?

   A. Within this environment, expectations for scientific integrity are laid out.
   B. Federal regulations related to ethical standards are adhered to, increasing the likelihood of integrity.
   C. The researcher always works within an ethical environment, which encourages the practice of ethical research behaviors.
   D. Scientific integrity ensures funding, which means that the study will be completed.

6. Why do federal regulations specify that the makeup of the institutional review board should reflect cultural and gender diversity and an awareness of local mores?

   A. This practice ensures that all research projects presented to the IRB will receive fair examination and will not be denied without discussion.
   B. Gender studies have not been common until recently and females react differently to different treatments.
   C. Awareness of local customs and culture means that both IRB members and researchers understand issues of concern in a non-American population.
   D. There is now great interest in researching healthcare issues in persons of different cultures.

7. Why is it important that the researcher be competent to conduct research?

   A. It is not ethically appropriate for an incompetent person to conduct research.
   B. An incompetent researcher will not be able to get informed consent from the vulnerable subject, which is unethical.
   C. An incompetent researcher should always work with someone who is competent, so that he or she can learn the process.
   D. Research is a complicated process that has to be learned.

8. What is the issue of greatest concern when developing a research project?

   A. The competence of the researcher to do the research
   B. The availability of funding
   C. The protection of the vulnerable subject
   D. Informed consent

9. A Certificate of Confidentiality may be required to protect both the researched and the researcher. Why?

    A. The nurse researcher will not lose his or her license to practice and do research because of the sensitive topic being researched.

    B. If the research topic is particularly sensitive, this certificate protects patients from divulging issues uncomfortable to them.

    C. The certificate protects the researcher and the researched from being coerced by governmental authorities to reveal sensitive information.

    D. The certificate means that no information is shared with those who should not be informed.

10. Why do research questions have to be developed carefully?

    A. The wrong question for the study means the wrong answer.

    B. Carefully developed and refined questions focus the research project.

    C. Without careful development of the questions, the research results will be meaningless.

    D. It is unethical not to develop questions carefully.

11. Why is informed consent a crucial issue in research projects?

    A. Research results will be more meaningful.

    B. The researcher will be adhering to international codes of ethics from which federal regulations are drawn.

    C. The project will be rejected by the IRB, because the subject is not informed about the study.

    D. The consenting subject will understand what the research is about and will have the choice to participate (or not).

12. Scientific misconduct on the part of the researcher is very serious. What constitutes scientific misconduct?

    A. Lying about the project to subjects when seeking informed consent

    B. Fabrication, falsification of data, and plagiarism

    C. Attributing only partial authorship to other contributors when they have done most of the work

    D. Making false claims about a project being funded when the researcher is talking about his or her work

13. HIPAA, which was designed to protect all humans and their medical records in this era of electronic paperless records, has imposed another restraint on conducting research. Why?

   A. It is more difficult to obtain IRB permission to conduct a research project.
   B. With paperless medical records, there are no data to analyze, even when interview data and surveys are involved.
   C. The regulations protect against unauthorized disclosure; although IRB permission includes this protection, additional care is taken under HIPAA.
   D. HIPAA ensures that highly sensitive data (e.g., HIV/AIDS status) are not disclosed.

14. Privacy and confidentiality are always issues in human subject research. What are the important steps to ensure that they are protected?

   A. The researcher does not talk about what the subject shares until the project's results are published in a peer-reviewed journal.
   B. All data are kept securely locked in a safe place and destroyed when the study is completed.
   C. Care with replication studies must be taken so that original data are not shared in the second study.
   D. All data are kept securely locked in a safe place and may be destroyed only according to IRB instructions.

15. Both the International Council of Nurses and the American Nurses Association make it clear that the ethical standards of the profession require the same obligations from the nurse researcher. Why?

   A. For the protection of vulnerable clients and patients
   B. For the protection of the nurse researcher
   C. Because of an obligation inherent within the nursing profession
   D. Because practice on which these ethical standards are built focuses nursing research

16. The nurse is developing a question for an EBP project involving the fall rate of patients 65 years of age and older. What should the initial ethical consideration be?

   A. The age of the researcher
   B. The number of falls
   C. The age of the population
   D. The sample size of the population

17. EBP projects in your institution are not required to obtain IRB approval. What must the nurse in charge of the EBP project still do?

   A. Maintain anonymity and confidentiality of patient information
   B. Maintain professionalism in gathering patient information
   C. Provide all staff access to the patient information
   D. Provide patient information obtained to the hospital board of directors

Discussion Questions

1. Several nurses are working together to develop a research project. Only one is doctorally prepared; the others have either a master's degree or a baccalaureate degree. The preparatory work is to be shared equally among all the nurses. As the project evolves, it turns out that those who do not have a doctorate do all the work. At a meeting, the doctorally prepared nurse insists that she be listed as the principal investigator for the grant to be submitted and as the first author on all publications. She bases her request on a belief that the reviewers of the grant would "pay more attention to the application" if the principal investigator has a doctoral degree. Discuss the ethical issues embedded in this situation.

2. The protection of human subjects lies at the heart of any research project. Part of this protection entails the need to obtain informed consent. A female nurse wants to do a qualitative study investigating what it means for males to live with diabetes mellitus and the resultant impotence. Qualitative research usually involves interviewing the human subject, and sexual impotence is a particularly sensitive subject. How should the nurse explain the study to her potential sample to ensure that the consent is truly informed and that the subjects will not drop out of the study because of extreme discomfort during the interview? What are the ethical issues involved?

3. Codes of ethics in human research, developed partly as a result of the atrocities of the mid-20th century, continue to be refined. The dictionary definitions of "moral" and "ethics" suggest that the meanings of these terms can and will change, and the evolving codes support this idea. Yet codes of ethics are based on some universal theories and values theories. Discuss why, despite the universality of these theories, the codes continue to evolve.

4. You have an idea for an EBP project that your hospital has approved regarding the fall rates of pediatric patients on your unit. Discuss the ethics involved with this particular population. How would you incorporate ethics in the data collection, analysis, and report of the project?

Suggested Readings

American Association of Critical-Care Nurses (AACN). (2015). Ethics in critical care nursing research. Retrieved from http://www.aacn.org/wd/practice/content/research/ethics-in-critical-care-nursing-research.pcms

Im, E.-O., & Chee, W. (2002, July/August). Issues in protection of human subjects in Internet research. *Nursing Research, 51*(4), 266–269.

International Council of Nurses (ICN). (2012). *The ICN code of ethics for nurses.* Retrieved from http://www.icn.ch/images/stories/documents/about/icncode_english.pdf

Lanter, J. (2006). Clinical research with cognitively impaired subjects. *Dimensions of Critical Care Nursing, 25*(2), 89–92.

Levine, C., Faden, R., Grady, C., Hammerschmidt, D., Eckenwiler, L., & Sugarman, J. (2004). The limitations of "vulnerability" as a protection for human research participants. *American Journal of Bioethics, 4*(3), 44–49.

National Institutes of Health (NIH). (1979). The Belmont report: Ethical principles and guidelines for the protection of human subjects of research. Retrieved from http://www.hhs.gov/ohrp/humansubjects/guidance/belmont.html

Rogers, B. (2005). Research with protected populations: Vulnerable participants. *AAOHN Journal, 53*(4), 156–157.

Smith, L. (2001, May/June). Ethics and the research realist. *Nurse Educator, 26*(3), 108–110.

United Nations. (2002). International covenant on civil and political rights, article 7. Universal declaration of human rights. Retrieved from https://treaties.un.org/doc/Publication/UNTS/Volume%20999/volume-999-I-14668-English.pdf

U.S. Department of Health and Human Services (HHS). (1998). Sponsor–investigator–IRB interrelationship—information sheet. Retrieved from http://www.fda.gov/RegulatoryInformation/Guidances/ucm126425.htm

U.S. Department of Health and Human Services (HHS). (2005). Protection of human subjects rule, 45 C.F.R. 46. Retrieved from http://www.hhs.gov/ohrp/humansubjects/guidance/45cfr46.html

World Medical Association (WMA). (1964–2004). World Medical Association: Declaration of Helsinki: Ethical principles for medical research involving human subjects. Retrieved from http://www.wma.net/en/30publications/10policies/b3/17c.pdf

References

American Nurses Association (ANA). (1994). *Position statement: Assisted suicide.* Washington, DC: Author.

American Nurses Association (ANA). (2015). *Code of ethics for nurses.* Retrieved from http://www.nursingworld.org/codeofethics

Anderson, D. G., & Hatton, D. C. (2000). Accessing vulnerable populations for research. *Western Journal of Nursing Research, 22*(2), 244–251.

Batalden, P. B., & Davidoff, F. (2007). What is "quality improvement" and how can it transform healthcare? *Quality and Safety in Health Care, 16*(1), 2–3.

Birch, M., & Miller, T. (2002). Encouraging participation: Ethics and responsibilities. In M. Mauthner, M. Burch, J. Jessop, & T. Miller (Eds.), *Ethics in qualitative research* (pp. 91–106). London, UK: Sage.

Borsay, A. (2009). Nursing history: An irrelevance for nursing practice? *Nursing History Review, 17*(1), 14–27.

Broyles, L. M., Tate, J. A., & Happ, M. B. (2008). Videorecording in clinical research: Mapping the ethical terrain. *Nursing Research, 57*(1), 59–63.

Burkhardt, M. A., & Nathaniel, A. K. (2014). *Ethics and issues in contemporary nursing* (4th ed.). Stanford, CT: Cengage Learning.

Cartwright, J. C., & Hickman, S. E. (2007, October). Conducting research in community-based care facilities: Ethical and regulatory implications. *Journal of Gerontological Nursing, 33*(10), 5–11.

Centers for Disease Control and Prevention (CDC). (2011). *The Tuskegee timeline.* Retrieved from http://www.cdc.gov/tuskegee/timeline.htm

Christians, C. G. (2003). Ethics and politics in qualitative research. In N. K. Denzin & Y. S. Lincoln (Eds.), *The landscape of qualitative research: Theories and issues* (2nd ed., pp. 208–244). Thousand Oaks, CA: Sage.

Cipriano, P. F. (2015). Ethical practice environments, empowered nurses. *The American Nurse, 47*(2), 3.

Cipriano Silva, M. (2006). Ethics of research. In J. Fitzpatrick & M. Wallace (Eds.), *Encyclopedia of nursing research* (2nd ed., pp. 177–180). New York, NY: Springer.

Commission on Research Integrity. (1995). *Integrity and misconduct in research* (U.S. Department of Health and Human Services, Publication No. 1996–746–425). Washington, DC: U.S. Government Printing Office.

Conn, V. S. (2008). Staying true to the results. *Western Journal of Nursing Research, 30*(2), 161–162.

Council for International Organizations of Medical Sciences (CIOMS). (2002). *International ethics guidelines for biomedical research involving human subjects.* Retrieved from http://www.cioms.ch/publications/guidelines/guidelines _nov_2002_blurb.htm

Dally, A. (1998). Thalidomide: Was the tragedy preventable? *Lancet, 351*(9110), 1197–1199.

Driever, M. J., & Pranulis, M. F. (2003). New challenges for issues in clinical nursing research. *Western Journal of Nursing Research, 25*(8), 937–947.

Edge, R. S., & Groves, J. R. (2005). *Ethics of healthcare: A guide for clinical practice.* Clifton Park, NY: Thomas Delmar Learning.

Edwards, R., & Mauthner, M. (2002). Ethics and feminist research: Theory and practice. In M. Mauthner, M. Burch, J. Jessop, & T. Miller (Eds.), *Ethics in qualitative research* (pp. 14–31). London, UK: Sage.

Ely, B., & Coleman, C. (2007). Recruitment and retention of children in longitudinal research. *Journal for Specialists in Pediatric Nursing, 12*(3), 199–202.

Erlen, J. A. (2005). HIPAA: Implications for research. *Orthopedic Nursing, 23*(2), 139–142.

Firby, P. (1995). Critiquing the ethical aspects of a study. *Nurse Researcher, 3*(1), 35–41.

Freda, M. C., & Kearney, M. H. (2005). Ethical issues faced by nursing editors. *Western Journal of Nursing Research, 27*(4), 487–499.

Grady, C. (2007). Quality improvement and ethical oversight. *Annals of Internal Medicine, 146*(9), 680–681.

Hanna, K. M., Weaver, M. T., Slaven, J. E., Fortenberry, J. D., & DiMeglio, L. A. (2014). Diabetes-related quality of life and the demands and burdens of diabetes care among emerging adults with Type I diabetes in the year after high school graduation. *Research in Nursing & Health, 37*(5), 399–408.

Henley, S. J., & Dougherty, M. C. (2009). Quality of manuscript reviews in nursing research. *Nursing Outlook, 57*(1), 18–26.

Hume, D. (1751). *An enquiry concerning the principles of morals.* Oxford, UK: Oxford University Press.

Iverson, K. M., Huang, K., Wells, S. Y., Wright, J. D., Gerger, M. R., & Wiltsey-Stirman, S. (2014). Women veterans' preferences of intimate partner violence screening and response procedures within Veterans Health Administration. *Research in Nursing & Health, 37*(4), 302–311.

International Council of Nurses (ICN). (2012). *The ICN code of ethics for nurses.* Retrieved from http://www.icn.ch/images/stories/documents/about/icncode_english .pdf

Jeffers, B. R. (2005). Research environments that promote integrity. *Nursing Research, 54*(91), 63–70.

Kant, I. (1785). Fundamental principles of the metaphysics of morals. In J. Rachels (1995), *The elements of moral philosophy* (2nd ed., pp. 107–131). New York, NY: McGraw-Hill.

Ketefian, S., & Lenz, E. R. (1995). Promoting scientific integrity in nursing research. Part II: Strategies. *Journal of Professional Nursing, 11*(5), 263–269.

Kirk, S. (2007). Methodological and ethical issues in conducting qualitative research with children and young people: A literature review. *International Journal of Nursing Studies, 44*(7), 1250–1260.

Kunin, T. F. (1997). Ethical issues in longitudinal research with at-risk children and adolescents. Cited in A. J. Roberson. (2007). Adolescent informed consent: Ethics, law, and theory to guide policy and nursing research. *Journal of Nursing Law, 11*(4), 191–196.

Lenz, E. R., & Ketefian, S. (1995). Promoting scientific integrity in nursing research. Part I: Current approaches in doctoral programs. *Journal of Professional Nursing, 11*(5), 213–219.

Lutz, K. F. (1999). Maintaining client safety and scientific integrity in research with battered women. *Image: Journal of Nursing Scholarship, 31*(1), 89–93.

Lynn, J., Baily, M. A., Bottrell, M., Jennings, B., Levine, R., Davidoff, F., … James, B. (2007). The ethics of using quality improvement methods in health care. *Annals of Internal Medicine, 146*(9), 666–673.

Macrina, F. L. (1995). *Scientific integrity: An introductory text with cases.* Washington, DC: ASM Press.

Mill, J. S. (1967). *Utilitarianism*. London, UK: Longmans. (Original work published 1863)

Miller, T., & Bell, L. (2002). Consenting to what? Issues of access, gate-keeping and informed consent. In M. Mauthner, M. Burch, J. Jessop, & T. Miller (Eds.), *Ethics in qualitative research* (pp. 53–69). London, UK: Sage.

National Institutes of Health (NIH). (1979). The Belmont report: Ethical principles and guidelines for the protection of human subjects of research. Retrieved from http://www.hhs.gov/ohrp/humansubjects/guidance/belmont.html

Norman, R. (1998). *The moral philosophers: An introduction to ethics* (2nd ed.). Oxford, UK: Oxford University Press.

Perkins, E. (2001). Johns Hopkins tragedy: Could librarians have prevented a death? *Information Today*, *18*(8), 51, 54. Retrieved http://newsbreaks.infotoday.com/nbreader.asp?ArticleID=17534

Pilkington, F. B. (2002). Scientific merit and research ethics. *Nursing Science Quarterly*, *15*(3), 196–200.

Public Health Service Act, 42 USC~163. (1988). Cited in D. L. Volker (2004). Methodological issues associated with studying an illegal act: Assisted dying. *Advances in Nursing Science*, *27*(2), 117–128.

Rachels, J. (1995). *The elements of moral philosophy* (2nd ed.). New York, NY: McGraw-Hill.

Redman, R. W. (2007). Knowledge development, quality improvement, and research ethics. *Research and Theory for Nursing Practice: An International Journal*, *21*(4), 217–219.

Reich, W. T. (Ed.). (1995). *Encyclopedia of bioethics*. New York, NY: Simon & Schuster Macmillan, pp. 2248–2259.

Roberson, A. J. (2007). Adolescent informed consent: Ethics, law, and theory to guide policy and nursing research. *Journal of Nursing Law*, *11*(4), 191–196.

Rogers, B. (2005). Research with protected populations: Vulnerable participants. *AAOHN Journal*, *53*(4), 156–157.

Ross, W. D. (1954). *Kant's ethical theory*. Oxford, UK: Oxford University Press.

Rothstein, W. G., & Phuong, L. H. (2007). Ethical attitudes of nurse, physician and unaffiliated members of institutional review boards. *Journal of Nursing Scholarship*, *39*(1), 75–811.

Siedlecki, S. L. (2008). Making a difference through research. *AORN Journal*, *88*(5), 716–729.

Tanner, C. A. (2006). Thinking like a nurse: A research-based model of clinical judgment in nursing. *Journal of Nursing Education*, *45*(6), 204–211.

The American Nurse. (2015). Welcoming in the "year of ethics." *The American Nurse*, *47*(1), 1.

Tschudin, V. (1992). *Ethics in nursing: The caring relationship*. Oxford, UK: Butterworth Heinemann.

Twycross, A., & Corlett, J. (2007). Challenges of setting up a multi-centered research study. *Nursing Standard*, *21*(49), 35–38.

United Nations. (1976). International covenant on civil and political rights, article 7. Universal declaration of human rights. Retrieved from https://treaties.un.org/doc/Publication/UNTS/Volume%20999/volume-999-I-14668-English.pdf

U.S. Department of Health and Human Services (HHS). (2005). Protection of human subjects rule, 45 C.F.R. 46. Retrieved from http://www.hhs.gov/ohrp/humansubjects/guidance/45cfr46.html

U.S. Department of Health and Human Services (HHS). (2009). Protection of human subjects, title 45, code of regulations, part 46. Retrieved from http://www.hhs .gov/ohrp/humansubjects/regbook2013.pdf.pdf

U. S. Department of Health and Human Services (HHS). (n.d.a). Health information privacy: Understanding health information privacy. Retrieved from http://www .hhs.gov/ocr/privacy/hipaa/understanding/

U. S. Department of Health and Human Services (HHS). (n.d.b). Regulations. Retrieved from http://www.hhs.gov/ohrp/humansubjects/

Volker, D. L. (2004). Methodological issues associated with studying an illegal act: Assisted dying. *Advances in Nursing Science, 27*(2), 117–128.

Weaver, K. (2007). Ethical sensitivity: State of knowledge and needs for further research. *Nursing Ethics, 2*(4), 141–155.

Wood, A., Grady, C., & Emanuel, E. J. (2002). The crisis in human participants research: Identifying the problems and proposing solutions. Retrieved from http://bioethics.georgetown.edu/pcbe/background/emanuelpaper.html

World Medical Association (WMA). (1964–2004). World Medical Association Declaration of Helsinki: Ethical principles for medical research involving human subjects. Retrieved from http://www.wma.net/en/30publications/10policies /b3/17c.pdf

Chapter **8**

Asking the Right Question

Lucy B. Trice and Kathaleen C. Bloom

Chapter Objectives

At the conclusion of this chapter, the learner will be able to:

1. Discuss processes involved in identifying a researchable problem in nursing practice.
2. Write an effective problem statement.
3. Discuss essential characteristics needed to pose a research question.
4. Identify the criteria for establishing research variables.
5. Contrast the various types of hypotheses.
6. Explain the differences between conceptual and operational definitions.
7. Critically evaluate research questions and hypotheses found in research reports for their contribution to the strength of evidence for nursing practice.

Key Terms

Associative hypothesis	Complex hypothesis
Categorical variable	Confounding variable
Causal hypothesis	Continuous variable

Demographic variable	Nondirectional hypothesis
Dependent variable	Null hypothesis
Dichotomous variable	Problem statement
Directional hypothesis	Research hypothesis
Discrete variable	Research question
Extraneous variable	Simple hypothesis
Hypothesis	Variable
Independent variable	

■ Introduction

Every research study begins with a problem the researcher would like to solve. For such a problem to be researchable, it must be one that can be studied through collecting and analyzing data. Some problems, although interesting, are by their nature not appropriate research problems because they are not researchable. Problems involving moral or ethical issues are not researchable, because the solutions to these problems are based on an individual's values. For example, one could not research a question such as, "Should physician-assisted suicide be legalized?" because the answer to the question depends on one's values rather than on a clearly right or wrong answer. This is not to say that physician-assisted suicide cannot be studied. One could study people's opinions regarding physician-assisted suicide. For example, one might ask the question, "Do cancer patients hold more favorable opinions regarding legalization of physician-assisted suicide than the general public?" The need to avoid moral/ethical questions as a research topic applies to both quantitative and qualitative studies.

Other factors influence whether a problem is researchable using quantitative methods. For a problem to be considered researchable by quantitative methods, the **variable** to be studied must be clearly defined and measurable. This clarity is necessary to apply statistical measures that will identify relationships among the variables. Qualitative studies are not subject to the same restriction, as the purpose of these studies is to describe in detail the phenomenon of interest as it is perceived by the study subjects. In other words, qualitative studies are descriptive in nature and are not concerned with relationships among variables.

■ Identifying Researchable Problems

There are a number of sources from which researchable problems can arise. Personal experience, whether as a healthcare professional or as a consumer of health care, is a rich source. For example, reviewing procedure manuals might raise the question, "Does one procedure for giving mouth care apply to all patients?" In considering diverse groups of patients such as those with endotracheal or nasogastric tubes in place, those with acquired immuno-deficiency syndrome (AIDS)—often accompanied by buccal mucosal lesions, and cancer patients on chemotherapy, one might ask, "Does one size fit all, or should separate procedures be established for each case?" Thus, as many authors point out (Macnee & McCabe, 2008; Norwood, 2010; Polit & Beck, 2014; Schmidt & Brown, 2015), practice experience is a major source for identifying gaps in knowledge that would benefit from research.

The nursing literature can also be a valuable source for researchable problems, particularly for the novice researcher (Burns & Grove, 2007; Norwood, 2010; Polit & Beck, 2014). For example, the researcher might identify a topic of interest and then review the nursing research literature to determine which kinds of studies have been done in that area. Seeing how other researchers have approached a problem can often spark new ideas or perhaps point to studies that would benefit from replication. In addition to offering such indirect assistance in the development of a problem statement, the research literature, including unpublished dissertations and theses as well as published research articles, provides direct assistance through specific suggestions for future research in the area. These suggestions may be offered under a special heading for future research, or they may be part of the discussion of the findings.

Social issues often give rise to topics relevant to healthcare research (Norwood, 2010; Polit & Beck, 2008, 2014). For example, the feminist movement raised questions about gender equity in health care and in healthcare research. The civil rights movement led to research on minority health problems in general and to explorations of the differences in effectiveness of medical treatment in different ethnic groups.

Shifts in the U.S. population including increasing numbers of elderly, and increasing numbers of individuals with one or more chronic diseases, also provide impetus for healthcare research. For example, the emergence of conditions such as Alzheimer's disease has led to research dealing with the nursing care of these patients, as well as research in how best to give "care for the caregiver" (Elliott, Burgio, & DeCoster, 2010). The rising

---

 THINK OUTSIDE THE BOX

Using the following examples, develop problem statements, research questions, and/or hypotheses for each:

1. Which information has been used to determine the method of catheterizing a laboring mother?
2. Which information serves as the basis for the range of blood sugars used within newly diagnosed elderly diabetics?
3. Which items need to be included into the formation of a problem statement, research question, and hypothesis?

Box 8-1

Funding Priorities of NINR

1. Health Promotion and Disease Prevention
2. Advancing the Quality of Life: Symptom Management and Self-Management
3. End-of-Life and Palliative Care
4. Innovation
5. Developing Nurse Scientists

Key Themes:

1. Symptom Science: Promoting Personalized Health Strategies
2. Wellness: Promoting Health and Preventing Illness
3. Self-Management: Improving Quality of Life for Individuals with Chronic Illness
4. End-of-Life and Palliative Care: The Science of Compassion

---

Source: National Institute of Nursing Research (NINR). (n.d.). Implementing NINR's Strategic Plan: Key Themes. Retrieved from http://www.ninr.nih.gov/aboutninr/keythemes. Further elaboration within each priority is provided at this source.

---

epidemic of obesity at all ages of the population, and especially in childhood, highlights the need for research into methods to promote skill building with regard to healthy lifestyles (Melnyk, 2008). The Institute of Medicine's report on professional education suggests that these shifts in population and the changing face of our society also demand a revamping of professional education to better deal with these issues (Institute of Medicine Board on Health Care Services, 2003).

The research priorities of the profession, and particularly of the funding bodies interested in healthcare research, are also a primary source for generating researchable problems (Burns & Grove, 2011; Norwood, 2010). For example, the National Institute of Nursing Research (NINR, n.d.) is the largest federal funding body dedicated specifically to nursing research. The NINR has as its mission "to promote and improve the health of individuals, families, communities, and populations" (p. 4). The NINR supports clinical and basic research and also provides funding for researcher training. The ongoing funding priorities of the NINR are listed in **Box 8-1**.

◼ Determining Significance of the Problem

Once the problem of interest has been identified, and before going any further, the researcher must determine the significance of the problem to nursing and the feasibility of studying the problem. Significance refers to whether a problem is worth studying. A number of authors agree on the criteria that can be used to determine the significance of a problem to nursing (Burns & Grove, 2011; LoBiondo-Wood & Haber, 2010; Polit & Beck, 2008):

- Will nursing's stakeholders (patients, nurses, healthcare community) benefit from the findings of the study?

- Will the findings be applicable to practice, education, or administration?
- Will the findings extend or support current theory or generate new theory?
- Will the findings support current nursing practice or provide evidence for changing current practice and/or policies?

Some authorities recommend that two additional criteria be considered when determining the significance of a problem:

- Will the findings address nursing research priorities? (Burns & Grove, 2007; Polit & Beck, 2014)
- Will the results of the proposed study build on previous findings? (Burns & Grove, 2011; Polit & Beck, 2008, 2014)

If the research problem does not meet the majority of these criteria, it should be reworked or, if that is not possible, simply abandoned. The single most important of these criteria is perhaps the first one: Will nursing's stakeholders (patients, nurses, healthcare community) benefit from the findings of the study? If this question cannot be answered with a resounding "yes," then the problem is probably not worth studying. Nursing is a discipline that takes pride in research aimed at benefitting patients and changing practice for the better. In the move to evidence-based practice (EBP), benefit to patients and applicability to practice—and especially support for current practice or evidence for changing current practice—are paramount in assessing the significance of a research problem. According to Farrell (2010), "Practices are sorely needed that are based on sound evidence" (p. 113).

▪ Examining Feasibility of the Problem

Feasibility refers to whether the study can be done. It includes considerations such as cost of the study, availability of study subjects, time constraints, availability of facilities and equipment, cooperation of others, interest of the researcher, and expertise of the researcher (Burns & Grove, 2009, 2011; LoBiondo-Wood & Haber, 2010; Norwood, 2010; Polit & Beck, 2008).

Cost

EBP has emerged from the desire of the majority of healthcare providers (both institutions and individuals) to do what is right for the patient and what will result in more good than harm (Craig & Smyth, 2002). The evidence for EBP is gathered through research (DiCenso, Guyatt, & Ciliska, 2005; Schmidt & Brown, 2015), and all research studies cost money to some degree. It is the researcher's task to obtain support for the research from the institution in which it will be conducted as well as from potential funding bodies, both within the institution itself and in outside agencies. When seeking this support, the researcher must present a clear picture of the value of the research in terms of patient outcomes versus the costs involved. The current economic climate, which emphasizes the link between outcomes value and resources expenditure, demands nothing less (Malloch & Porter-O'Grady, 2010). In the final analysis, the deciding factor with regard to feasibility of a particular study may be how much the study will cost versus the funds and other necessary support that are available to the researcher.

Availability of Subjects

The type and number of study subjects will vary depending on the purpose and design of the study. Larger numbers of participants are generally needed for quantitative studies if the findings are to be considered significant, whereas smaller numbers of subjects are appropriate for studies using a qualitative design. Clearly, a sufficient number of subjects must be available for the study to be feasible.

Time Constraints

Studies done in connection with the pursuit of academic degrees (e.g., research projects, theses, dissertations), of necessity, have a timeframe for their completion. The same is true for studies supported by grant monies, as well as studies for which grant monies are being sought. For a study to be considered feasible, it must have the possibility of being completed within the applicable time constraints.

Availability of Facilities and Equipment

The need for special facilities and equipment can add greatly to the cost of a study. Although not all studies require specialized equipment or facilities, for those that do, both the cost and the availability of these items must be taken into consideration when determining the feasibility of the study.

Cooperation of Others

All studies require a certain amount of cooperation from others. The researcher may need referrals from others to obtain research subjects, for example, or to arrange for use of laboratories or other kinds of facilities. Student researchers in particular often need assistance with data entry in quantitative studies, data transcription in qualitative studies, and statistical analysis. These types of assistance are frequently offered to student researchers without a fee; however, obtaining the assistance requires cooperation from those providing these services. The study subjects themselves must also cooperate in a sense, if the data are to be collected in a timely manner. Thus, the cooperation of these important others is an essential ingredient of a feasible study. Securing that cooperation falls squarely on the shoulders of the researcher. In their discussion of obtaining cooperation from various others, Burns and Grove (2001) contend that researchers need to maintain objectivity throughout the course of the study, avoiding a tendency to take themselves too seriously; "a sense of humor is invaluable" (p. 426).

Interest of the Researcher

Conducting research, although often rewarding when the final results are in, is nevertheless hard work. To embark on a study that is not of fairly profound interest to the researcher is foolhardy at best, and at worst it can lead to failure to complete the study. If the researcher is not interested in doing the research, then carrying out the study is not generally feasible.

Expertise of the Researcher

Ideally, the researcher should have prior knowledge and experience in the field of study in question. This is not to say that a study would be considered not possible solely because it is a new area of study for the researcher. Certainly, seasoned researchers frequently "branch out" into new areas of study. When less experienced researchers are involved, however, Polit and Beck (2008) caution that difficulties may arise in developing and carrying out a study on a topic that is totally new and/ or unfamiliar.

■ Addressing Nursing Research Priorities

If the body of knowledge that deals with the practice of nursing is to be expanded, the major focus of nursing research should be on issues that influence patient outcomes. Further, it is through this type of research that we will gather the evidence to document the quality and effectiveness of nursing care (Moorhead, Johnson, Maas, & Swanson, 2008). The specific areas of focus, in terms of patient outcomes, vary widely. As noted earlier, doing research can be costly, so it behooves the researcher to attempt to match his or her research interests not only with those of the institution where the individual works, but also with the priorities established by funding agencies. The major federal funding agency dedicated to nursing is NINR. Other funding bodies with research priorities relevant to nursing include the Agency for Healthcare Research and Quality, private organizations such as the W.K. Kellogg Foundation and the Helene Fuld Health Trust, professional organizations such as the American Nurses Foundation and Sigma Theta Tau International, and nursing specialty organizations such as the Association of periOperative Registered Nurses and the American Association of Critical-Care Nurses, to name a few. Taking care to address the funding priorities of a particular organization enhances the possibility of obtaining from that organization the funding needed to complete the research project.

Problem Statement

The **problem statement** presents the idea, issue, or situation that the researcher intends to examine in the study. The statement should be broad enough to cover the concern prompting the study, yet narrow enough to provide direction for designing the study. It can be conceptualized in the form of a declarative sentence or a question. In some cases, the term *research question* is used interchangeably with *problem statement*.

The problem statement is the foundation of the study, and as such is usually preceded by several paragraphs of background information that set the stage for the proposed study. These paragraphs identify the significance of the problem, present justification that the problem is researchable, and provide supporting documentation from the literature. This general discussion of the problem culminates in the problem statement. The problem statement is often further clarified by including the purpose and goal(s) of the study, which are derived from the problem statement.

Research Question

Although the terms **research question** and *problem statement* are sometimes used interchangeably, the research question is often more specific than the problem statement. Additionally, research questions (rather than hypotheses) are frequently used to guide studies that are exploratory in

---

? THINK OUTSIDE THE BOX

Formulate conceptual and operational definitions for *catheterization, laboring mother, blood sugar,* and *newly diagnosed elderly diabetic.*

nature and aimed at describing variables or perhaps identifying differences between groups in relation to these variables. Research questions also guide studies that examine relationships among the variables being studied but do not test the nature of these relationships. Studies designed to test the nature of the relationships among variables are generally guided by hypotheses rather than research questions (Burns & Grove, 2009; Fain, 2009).

Research questions can be used to guide both quantitative and qualitative studies. Quantitative studies are often initiated to answer several questions derived from the problem of interest, each focused on a specific variable to be measured in the population. For example, West and colleagues (2011) were interested in obesity prevention—specifically, how to prevent regaining weight initially lost during a weight-loss regimen. Most weight-loss methods focus on behavioral skill refinement, that is, changing food choice and/or eating patterns. These same methods are used in maintenance programs, but with disappointing results (Wing et al., 2008). West and colleagues (2011) devised a study to compare the efficacy of a motivation-focused treatment versus a skill-based treatment in maintaining weight loss. The following research questions might be used to guide this study:

1. Does a motivation-focused intervention affect weight maintenance in individuals who have recently lost weight?
2. Does a skill-based intervention affect weight maintenance in individuals who have recently lost weight?
3. Do individuals who follow a motivation-focused intervention maintain their weight loss for a longer time period than those who follow a skill-based intervention?

Questions 1 and 2 are narrowly focused, dealing with one **independent variable** (participation in a motivation-focused intervention and participation in a skill-based intervention, respectively) and the **dependent variable** (weight maintenance). The third question, while more complex, gets at the heart of the matter: Does one intervention work better than the other?

In another example, Hanna, Weaver, Slaven, Fortenberry, and DiMeglio (2014) were interested in diabetes-related quality of life (DQOL) experienced by young adults. They were specifically concerned with the effect of the demands and burdens of diabetes on quality of life during the year following high school graduation. This is a time of fairly dramatic change for young adults as they move toward independent living, physically, psychologically, and emotionally. Those with type 1 diabetes must also assume independence in managing their diabetes during this time. The authors wished to study the effect assuming responsibility for their own diabetes management had on DQOL among these young adults. They designed a study to examine the association of

DQOL and, among others, various aspects of diabetes care, including glycemic control and assuming primary responsibility for diabetes. The following research questions might be among those used to guide this study:

1. Does glycemic control affect DQOL?
2. Does assuming primary responsibility for diabetes care affect glycemic control?
3. Do those with consistent glycemic control have a higher perceived DQOL than those who do not have consistent glycemic control?

Questions 1 and 2 are again fairly narrow and contain one independent variable (glycemic control and assuming responsibility for diabetes care, respectively) and one dependent variable (DQOL and glycemic control, respectively). Question 3, while seemingly more complex, still contains one independent variable (consistent glycemic control) and one dependent variable (perceived DQOL).

Qualitative studies, by their nature, explore phenomena about which little is known (Polit & Beck, 2014). Burns and Grove (2007) point out that the research questions guiding these types of studies are limited in number and generally broad in scope, and they include variables or concepts that are more complex than those guiding quantitative studies.

For example, Karlsson, Bergbom, and Forsberg (2012) investigated the lived experiences of adult intensive care patients who were conscious while undergoing mechanical ventilation. Using a qualitative approach (namely phenomenology), they conducted in-depth interviews with 12 patients who were determined to be conscious while they were being mechanically ventilated. The interviews took place approximately 1 week following their discharge from the intensive care unit. The research question guiding this study might be stated as follows: What are the essential themes common to the experience of being conscious while undergoing mechanical ventilation? The concepts in this question are much broader than those cited for the earlier quantitative example.

In a second example, Iverson and colleagues (2014) explored women veterans' preferences for intimate partner violence (IPV) screening and response procedures within the Veterans Health Administration. While all women are at risk for IPV, research suggests that women veterans are at a higher risk than other women (Dichter, Cerulli, & Bossarte, 2011). Data were gathered through focus groups, with separate groups for women who had experienced IPV during their lifetime and those who had not. A total of five focus groups were conducted over a 1-year period. The data obtained were analyzed using conventional content analysis, and common themes were identified. A research question guiding this study might be stated in this manner: What are women veterans' preferences for IPV screening and response procedures within the Veterans

Health Administration? Again, the concepts in this question are broad and more complex than those for the earlier examples of questions guiding quantitative studies. Qualitative studies, because they are designed to get at understanding behavior and the values/perceptions that underlie it, are particularly important as a starting point for designing and implementing nursing interventions (Ketefian & Redman, 2013).

Components of the Problem Statement

A well-written problem statement for a quantitative study, whether written as a declarative statement or a question, has at a minimum, two components: the population of concern and the variable(s) to be studied. The PICOT (population, intervention, comparison, outcome, time) format described elsewhere has the advantage of clarifying more fully the population of the study, the intervention/comparison of interest, the outcome desired, and the timeframe involved. For example, a researcher might be interested in investigating the use of pet therapy to increase morale in hospitalized patients. As stated, the population (hospitalized patients) is fairly broad and does not provide a lot of direction for the literature search or for the study design. Depending on the specific concern and age group under investigation, the researcher could narrow the population by age (e.g., hospitalized patients between the ages of 6 and 10 years) or other characteristics, such as disease and/or treatment (e.g., hospitalized patients between the ages of 6 and 10 years undergoing treatment for cancer). The variables of interest would be pet therapy and morale. Following the PICOT format, the population of interest (P) would be hospitalized patients between the ages of 6 and 10 years undergoing treatment for cancer, the intervention of interest (I) would be pet therapy, the comparison of interest (C) would be no pet therapy, the outcome of interest (O) would be increased morale, and the time (T) would refer to time of hospitalization.

Strictly speaking, the term *variable* refers to measurable qualities or characteristics of people, things, or situations that can change, vary, or fluctuate. For example, blood pressure, pulse rate, anxiety level, and degree of pain are all characteristics of people that can vary from one person to another. A child's reaction to the presence (or absence) of a parent in the hospitalized child's room during painful procedures can vary from one hospitalized child to another. Variables are the foundation of quantitative studies; they constitute what is being studied in the designated population.

Researchers often want to know what causes or influences a particular phenomenon or, in some cases, what alleviates or diminishes that phenomenon. For example, one might want to know if a hospitalized child's anxiety level during a painful procedure would be lessened if a parent were present during the procedure. In this case, there are two variables of interest: the child's anxiety level and the presence of a parent during the painful procedure. The researcher is investigating the effect that the presence of a parent has on the child's anxiety level during a painful procedure. Because the variable "presence of a parent" is having an effect on the variable "child's anxiety level," it is termed the independent variable. By the same token, the variable being affected (i.e., child's anxiety level) is termed the dependent variable. In a study investigating more than one variable, the variable(s) that is (are) acting on, influencing, or causing an effect on the other variable(s) is (are) called the independent variable(s), and the variable(s) being acted on is (are) called the dependent variable(s) (Burns & Grove, 2011; LoBiondo-Wood & Haber, 2010; Norwood, 2010; Polit & Beck, 2014).

Another types of variable that can affect the outcome of the study but is not the variable the researcher is investigating is referred to as an **extraneous variable**. In the example cited in the preceding paragraph, the age of the child could affect his or her anxiety level, regardless of whether a parent is present in the room, and therefore would be considered an extraneous variable. The researcher could control for the variable of age by limiting the study population to a particular age group. Another variable that might affect the child's anxiety level, regardless of whether a parent is present in the room, is the nature of the painful procedure. The procedure could be specified to control for this variable. With any study, it is important to identify and control for extraneous variables; otherwise, the study results may be confusing and inaccurate. Most studies have extraneous variables of one sort or another. It is important for the researcher to recognize and control for these variables, either in the study design or through statistical procedures, to preserve the validity of the study results. If a study cannot control for an extraneous variable, the variable is then termed a **confounding variable**.

The term **demographic variable** refers to characteristics of the subjects in the study. Data on these characteristics are usually collected during the study and are then used to describe the study group. Many different kinds of demographic information can be collected, including details about age, gender, ethnicity, educational level, marital status, and number of children. The types of demographic data collected depend on the purpose of the study; however, at a minimum, data on age, gender, and ethnicity should be gathered.

 THINK OUTSIDE THE BOX

Why is it necessary to have a problem statement, research question, or hypothesis? What benefit does it provide? Is one better than others? What restrictions arise related to the use of the problem statement, research question, or hypothesis?

If a variable can take on a wide range of values (from 0 to 100 or larger), it is often referred to as a **continuous variable**. A continuous variable is not limited to whole-number values. Examples of continuous variables include age, weight, salary, and blood pressure. In contrast, a variable that can take on only a finite number of values, usually restricted to whole numbers, is referred to as a **discrete variable**. For example, respiratory rate would be considered a discrete variable, as it can take on only whole-number equivalents; although variation in respiratory rate can occur from person to person, a finite number of these variations are compatible with life.

Categorical and dichotomous variables are similar because they represent characteristics that can be measured only in the sense that they are either present or not present. These kinds of variables are often assigned a number for identification, but the number does not represent a quantity. For example, ethnicity might be divided into white, African American, Hispanic, Native American, Pacific Islander, and Asian American, with each classification assigned an identifying number. The assigned number, however, would have no meaning other than identifying the occurrence of each race, perhaps to facilitate counting the number of occurrences of that particular race in the study. In this case, race would be considered a **categorical variable**, with each race included in the study representing a category. If only two categories are possible for a categorical variable, it may be referred to as a **dichotomous variable**. For example, sex is considered a dichotomous variable, as two categories are possible—male and female.

Writing the Problem Statement

As noted previously, problem statements for quantitative studies may be written in the form of a declarative statement or a question (**Table 8-1**). The two components that must be included in every problem statement are the population of interest and the variable(s) to be measured. For example, if we were interested in studying the effect of presence of a parent on anxiety level in children undergoing painful procedures, we might construct a problem statement in the form of a question: "Does the presence of a parent affect the anxiety level in children ages 3–5 years undergoing initiation of intravenous therapy?" Alternatively, the same problem could be stated as a declarative statement: "The presence of a parent affects the anxiety level in children ages 3–5 years undergoing initiation of intravenous therapy." Both statements contain a population of interest (children ages 3–5 years undergoing initiation of intravenous therapy) and two variables (presence of a parent—independent variable; anxiety level of the child—dependent variable). The only difference between the two is the form of the statement—one is presented as a question and the other as a declarative statement. Note also that the elements of the PICOT format are readily apparent in each of these examples.

Table 8-1	
Problem Statements	
Declarative Statement Format	**Question Format**
Music therapy decreases the level of maternal anxiety during cesarean section.	Does music therapy decrease the level of maternal anxiety during cesarean section?
Nursing home residents who participate in regular exercise have fewer falls than those who do not.	Do nursing home residents who participate in regular exercise have fewer falls than those who do not?
Participation in a support group improves morale in family caregivers of Alzheimer's patients.	Does participation in a support group improve morale in family caregivers of Alzheimer's patients?
Diabetic patients who perceive themselves as obese will participate in a weight management program.	Will diabetic patients who perceive themselves as obese participate in a weight management program?
The number of medication errors made by nurses increases when the number of medications per patient is greater than three (3).	Does the number of medication errors made by nurses increase when the number of medications per patient is greater than three (3)?

❓ THINK OUTSIDE THE BOX

Identify the elements of the PICOT format for each of the problem statements in Table 8-1.

■ Hypotheses

A research question asks whether a relationship exists between variables in a particular population. In contrast, a **hypothesis** stipulates or predicts the relationship that exists. For example, if the research question is "Does the presence of a parent in the room affect the anxiety level in children ages 3–5 years undergoing initiation of intravenous therapy?", then we might develop several hypotheses:

1. The presence of a parent in the room affects the anxiety level in children ages 3–5 years who undergo initiation of intravenous therapy.
2. The presence of a parent in the room reduces the anxiety level in children ages 3–5 years who undergo initiation of intravenous therapy.
3. The presence of a parent in the room has no effect on the anxiety level in children ages 3–5 years who undergo initiation of intravenous therapy.
4. The presence of a parent in the room increases the anxiety level in children ages 3–5 years who undergo initiation of intravenous therapy.

The advantage of a hypothesis over a research question is that the hypothesis puts the question into a form that can be tested. It is the nature of hypotheses to predict relationships among or between variables. For a hypothesis to be testable, it must stipulate a relationship between at least two variables in a given population.

Within EBP, the research question format incorporates the population of interest, the intervention, a comparison of interest, outcomes, and timing to ensure clarity of the subject (note that these are the components of the PICOT format). This process can also be applied to developing one or more hypotheses for a research study. Each hypothesis should contain the population of interest, the independent variable(s), the dependent variable(s), and the comparison of interest, all of which should lead to the outcome of the study.

Hypotheses and Qualitative Studies

Hypotheses are used in quantitative studies but are not appropriate for qualitative studies. By their nature, they present the researcher's opinion in the form of a prediction about the outcome of the study. In qualitative studies, however, researchers focus on the viewpoints of the subjects participating in the study rather than on their own. Thus, the participants' viewpoints, rather than the researcher's hypothesis, guide the qualitative study. Generally, the purpose of qualitative studies is to explore new concepts and ideas about which little is known or to discover new meanings for concepts. In keeping with this purpose, researchers using qualitative methods take great care to set aside their preconceived notions about the phenomena under investigation. A hypothesis would be a disadvantage in a qualitative study, because it would predict the outcome of the study and potentially bias the results. Thus, while qualitative studies may generate hypotheses that can then be tested using quantitative methods, they are not themselves guided by research hypotheses.

Types of Hypotheses

A testable hypothesis, also called the **research hypothesis**, predicts the relationship between two or more variables in a population of interest. All four of the hypotheses in the previous example could be considered testable.

Hypotheses may be directional, nondirectional, or null:

- A **directional hypothesis** predicts the path or direction the relationship will take. In the preceding example, both hypothesis 2 and hypothesis 4 are directional hypotheses. Hypothesis 2 predicts a decrease in anxiety with the presence of a parent, and hypothesis 4 predicts an increase in anxiety with the presence of a parent.

THINK OUTSIDE THE BOX

Describe a problem in which a null hypothesis would be used, and state the null hypothesis.

- A **nondirectional hypothesis** predicts a relationship but not the path or direction of the relationship. Hypothesis 1 in the previous example is a nondirectional hypothesis; it states that the presence of a parent affects the anxiety level in children ages 3–5 years but does not stipulate the direction of the effect.
- A **null hypothesis**, also called a statistical hypothesis, predicts that no relationship exists among or between the variables in the study. When inferential statistics are used to analyze data, the assumption is that the null hypothesis is actually being tested. Because this is understood, many researchers do not state the null hypothesis when reporting their findings in the literature. In the previous example, hypothesis 3 is stated in the null form.

Hypotheses may also be classified as simple or complex: A **simple hypothesis** specifies the relationship between two variables, whereas a **complex hypothesis** specifies the relationships between and among more than two variables. In the previous example, all four of the hypotheses could be classified as simple hypotheses. In each case, there are only two variables—the presence of a parent and the anxiety level in children ages 3–5 years. An example of a complex hypothesis might be "Religious beliefs, presence of social support, and ethnic background affect the perception of pain in patients who are terminally ill with cancer." Here there are four variables—religious beliefs, the presence of social support, ethnic background, and perception of pain. Complex hypotheses may also be termed *multivariate hypotheses* for the simple reason that they contain more than two variables.

In addition, hypotheses may be categorized as associative or causal. These terms reflect the relationship between or among the variables in the hypothesis. For example, in an **associative hypothesis**, the hypothesis is stated in a way indicating that the variables exist side by side, and that a change in one variable is accompanied by a change in another. However, there is no suggestion that a change in one variable causes a change in another—merely that the variables change in association with each other (Reynolds, 1971).

In contrast, a **causal hypothesis** is stated in a way indicating that one variable causes or brings about a change in one or more other variables (Burns & Grove, 2011). As one might expect, the variable inducing the change is referred to as the independent variable, and the variable being changed is the dependent variable. Causal hypotheses may also be called directional hypotheses. Continuing with the example of the presence of a parent in the room with a child during a painful procedure and its effect on the child's anxiety level, two of the hypotheses can be termed causal—hypothesis 2 and hypothesis 4. Hypothesis 2 predicts a decrease in anxiety (dependent variable) with the presence of a parent in the room (independent variable), and hypothesis 4 predicts an increase in anxiety (dependent variable) with the presence of a parent in the room (independent variable).

Defining Variables for the Study

The variables to be studied in quantitative research projects are generally defined in two ways—conceptually and operationally. The conceptual definition is a broad, more abstract definition that is generally drawn from relevant literature, particularly the theoretical literature, the researcher's clinical experience, or, in some cases, a combination of these sources. The conceptual definition is similar to a dictionary definition in that it provides the general meaning associated with the variable, but it is more in-depth and broader in scope. Although considered the starting point, conceptual definitions rarely give direction regarding how the variable will actually be measured for the study. The operational definition, by contrast, stipulates precisely how the variable will be measured, including which tools will be used, if applicable. If a conceptual definition is abstract, an operational definition is concrete. This concreteness is necessary to allow for precise measurement of the variable(s) of interest in the study.

Evidence-Based Practice Considerations

Stommel and Wills (2004) point out that the ability to apply research findings to practice is an expected competency of advanced practice nurses. However, if we accept that it is the desire of all practitioners of nursing to provide "only that care that makes a positive difference in the lives of those whom they serve" (Porter-O'Grady, 2010, p. 1), then it is clear that all professional nurses—from the new graduate to the seasoned veteran—should have the ability to apply research findings to practice. Inherent in this ability is an understanding of how the research process unfolds and what constitutes good research.

Further, Melnyk and Fineout-Overholt (2011) maintain that "the goal of EBP is to use the highest quality of [research] knowledge in providing care to produce the greatest impact on patients' health status" (p. 75). To accomplish this, practitioners—particularly staff nurses who are at the bedside caring for patients on a daily basis—must have the tools to critically analyze research to make appropriate EBP decisions. To critically analyze research, these staff nurses must possess a working knowledge of the language of research; recognize a researchable problem statement; distinguish between and among variables, identifying independent versus dependent variables; determine the population of interest; and, above all, recognize a well-conducted study, one whose findings are worth consideration for applying to practice. In its purest and best form, EBP happens at the bedside. The burden of implementation rests squarely on the shoulders of the staff nurse.

Summary Points

1. Every study begins with a problem the researcher would like to solve.
2. There are many sources for researchable problems, including personal experience, the nursing literature, social issues, and the research priorities of funding bodies.
3. The significance of the problem to nursing and the feasibility of studying the problem are important aspects to consider before embarking on any research project.
4. The problem statement presents the issue or situation to be examined and should identify the population of interest as well as the variables that will be studied.
5. Variables may be classified in a variety of ways: (a) independent versus dependent, (b) continuous versus discrete, (c) extraneous, (d) confounding, (e) categorical, and (f) dichotomous.
6. The problem statement may be written as a question or as a declarative sentence.
7. Placing the problem statement in the PICOT format helps to clarify the population, variables, outcome, and timeframe involved.
8. Hypotheses predict the relationship between or among variables.
9. Hypotheses may take many forms: (a) directional versus nondirectional, (b) simple versus complex, (c) associative versus causal, and (d) null.
10. Variables to be studied are generally defined both conceptually and operationally.
11. For nurses to pursue evidence-based practice, they must understand the research process and all of its components.

RED FLAGS

- Quantitative studies address research problems, research questions, and/or hypotheses.
- Qualitative studies do not use hypotheses, but rather explore research problems and research questions. If a qualitative study discusses a hypothesis, thought should be given to its focus and validity.
- A hypothesis must have at least one independent variable and one dependent variable; it is usually stated in a declarative statement format rather than as a question.
- Key variables within a study should have at least the operational definition provided for consideration.

Multiple-Choice Questions

1. Developing a research study to investigate the availability of health care for minority children whose families are on welfare is an example of a research problem generated primarily from:

    A. Practice.
    B. Social issues.
    C. Healthcare trends in society.
    D. Theory.

2. Problems involving moral or ethical issues are not researchable because:

    A. They are too costly to perform.
    B. Most researchers are not interested in these studies.
    C. They are based on individual values.
    D. Data collection is problematic.

3. Determining if studying the problem will lead to results that are applicable to nursing practice is essential when analyzing the _____ of the problem.

    A. Feasibility
    B. Profitability
    C. Cost
    D. Significance

4. Which of the following topics would be inappropriate for a researchable problem?

    A. The morality of abortion as a form of birth control
    B. The relationship between cigarette smoking and weight loss
    C. The effect of severe dietary restrictions on wellbeing
    D. The relationship between religious beliefs and pain perception

5. Which of the following is the best example of a problem statement containing all parts of the PICOT format?

    A. Children whose parents stay with them experience less pain.
    B. Hospitalized patients who have a relative with them experience less pain than those who do not.
    C. Hospitalized children ages 3–5 years whose parents stay with them during painful procedures experience less pain than those who do not.
    D. Patients who have a relative with them during a transfusion will experience less anxiety than those who do not.

6. Which of the following best represents a well-constructed problem statement?

    A. What affects pain perception?
    B. Obesity negatively impacts self-image in first graders.
    C. This study will compare the effectiveness of antacids.
    D. Does time of day affect appetite?

7. The population and the _____ are the two essential parts of the research problem statement.

    A. Setting
    B. Theory
    C. Concepts
    D. Variables

8. The research question is: "Obesity increases the risk of type 2 diabetes in teenage boys." Which of the following is/are the independent variable(s)?

    A. Teenage boys with type 2 diabetes
    B. Gender and obesity
    C. Obesity
    D. Type 2 diabetes, obesity, and gender

9. The research question is: "Does massage therapy increase satisfaction during cesarean delivery?" Which of the following is/are the dependent variable(s)?

    A. Massage therapy
    B. Satisfaction
    C. Massage therapy and satisfaction
    D. Satisfaction and type of delivery

10. Which statement by a fellow student best describes a confounding variable?

    A. "It can take on a wide range of values."
    B. "A variable that is restricted to whole numbers."
    C. "It describes the characteristics of the study subjects."
    D. "A variable that can't be controlled."

11. Which of the following best represents a dichotomous variable?

    A. Blood pressure
    B. Age at death
    C. Gender
    D. Weight

12. Which of the following represents a simple hypothesis?

    A. Exposure to pet therapy increases appetite in elderly patients.
    B. Family support and positive attitude decrease symptoms of dysreflexia in spinal cord injury patients.
    C. Social support, balanced diet, and regular exercise decrease the incidence of postpartum depression.
    D. Daily exercise and eliminating carbohydrates from the diet will result in a significant weight reduction in obese diabetic patients.

13. What is the difference between a null hypothesis and a directional hypothesis?

    A. One is a declarative sentence; the other is a question.
    B. One assumes a relationship; the other denies that one exists.
    C. One is researchable; the other is statistical.
    D. One includes at least two variables; the other does not.

14. Which statement best represents the relationship between a causal and an associative hypothesis?

A. They are the opposite of each other.

B. One is written as a question, the other as a declarative sentence.

C. One assumes a relationship; the other denies that one exists.

D. They are similar to each other.

15. An operational definition of a variable is one that is:

A. Broad and abstract.

B. Narrow and abstract.

C. Concrete and continuous.

D. Narrow and concrete.

Discussion Questions

1. You work in a cardiology clinic that treats patients who have coronary artery disease and are recovering from a myocardial infarction. Many of these patients have hypertension and are overweight, and you have noticed that some of them have more difficulty following their medical regimens than others. You want to develop a research study to investigate this problem. How would you go about doing so? What would be a possible problem statement?

2. You are a BSN student enrolled in a research course. The instructor has given you the following problem statement: "Does completion of a mandatory health promotion course affect the incidence of smoking cessation among college students who smoke?" Develop four hypotheses that might be drawn from this problem statement: a null hypothesis, a directional hypothesis, a nondirectional hypothesis, and an associative hypothesis. Can all of these hypotheses be developed? If any of them cannot be developed, why not?

3. Read the abstract and then provide the following information:
    a. Identify the population of interest.
    b. Identify the variables.
    c. Construct a research question that could have guided this study.
    d. Construct a null hypothesis.
    e. Construct a directional hypothesis.

Abstract: A major goal in the care of patients with neurological problems is to prevent or minimize episodes of increased intracranial pressure (ICP). Elevations in ICP in response to nursing interventions have been acknowledged since the 1960s when ICP monitoring was first introduced in the clinical setting. Until recently, few studies have specifically examined the effect of oral care on ICP, and oral care and other hygiene measures were combined or not specified, prohibiting a direct interpretation of the influence of oral care alone on ICP. The purpose of this study was to describe the relationship between routine oral care interventions and the changes in ICP, specifically focusing on the effect of intensity and duration of this intervention. Twenty-three patients with a clinical condition requiring ICP monitoring were enrolled over a 12-month period. Oral care provided by neuroscience intensive care nurses was observed and videotaped. Characteristics of the intervention were documented including products used, patient positioning, and duration of the intervention. A subjective scale of 1–5 was used to score intensity of oral care. Wrist actigraphy data were collected from the nurses to provide an objective measure of intensity. Patient physiologic data were collected at 12-second epochs 5 minutes before, during, and 5 minutes after oral care. The mixed-effect repeated measures analysis of variance model indicated that there was a statistically significant increase in ICP in response to oral care ($P = 0.0031$). There was, however, no clinically significant effect on ICP. This study provides evidence that oral care is safe to perform in patients in the absence of preexisting elevated ICP. (Szabo, Grap, Munro, Starkweather, & Merchant, 2014)

Suggested Readings

American Journal of Nursing. (2015). *Evidence-based practice, step by step*. Retrieved from http://journals.lww.com/ajnonline/pages/collectiondetails.aspx?TopicalCollectionId=10

Beitz, J. (2006). Writing the researchable question. *Journal of Wound, Ostomy, & Continence Nursing, 33*(2), 122–124.

Fineout-Overholt, E., Melnyk, B., & Schultz, A. (2005). Transforming health care from the inside out: Advancing evidence-based practice in the 21st century. *Journal of Professional Nursing, 21*(6), 335–344.

Hudson-Barr, D. (2005). From research idea to research question: The who, what, where, when and why. *Journal for Specialists in Pediatric Nursing, 10*(2), 90–92.

Law, R. (2004). From research topic to research question: A challenging process. *Nurse Researcher, 11*(4), 54–66.

University of Washington Libraries. (n.d.). *Research 101* [Archived]. Retrieved from http://guides.lib.washington.edu/content.php?pid=55083&sid=2465031

References

Burns, N., & Grove, S. K. (2001). *The practice of nursing research: Conduct, critique, and utilization* (4th ed.). Philadelphia, PA: W. B. Saunders.

Burns, N., & Grove, S. K. (2007). *Understanding nursing research: Building an evidence-based practice* (4th ed.). St. Louis, MO: Saunders/Elsevier.

Burns, N., & Grove, S. K. (2009). *The practice of nursing research: Appraisal, synthesis, and generation of evidence* (6th ed.). St. Louis, MO: Saunders/Elsevier.

Burns, N., & Grove, S. K. (2011). *Understanding nursing research: Building an evidence-based practice* (5th ed.). St. Louis, MO: Saunders/Elsevier.

Craig, J. V., & Smyth, R. L. (2002). *The evidence-based practice manual for nurses.* London, UK: Churchill Livingstone.

DiCenso, A., Guyatt, G., & Ciliska, D. (2005). *Evidence-based nursing: A guide to clinical practice.* St. Louis, MO: Mosby.

Dichter, M. E., Cerulli, C., & Bossarte, R. M. (2011). Intimate Partner violence victimization women veterans and associated heart health risks. *Women's Health Issues, 21*(4 Suppl.), 190–194. doi:10.1016/j.whi.2011.04.008.

Elliott, A. F., Burgio, L. D., & DeCoster, J. (2010). Enhancing caregiver health: Findings from the resources for enhancing Alzheimer's caregiver health II intervention. *Journal of the American Geriatrics Society, 58*(1), 30–37.

Fain, J. A. (2009). *Reading, understanding, and applying nursing research* (3rd ed.). Philadelphia, PA: F. A. Davis.

Farrell, M. P. (2010). Living evidence: Translating research into practice. In K. Malloch & T. Porter-O'Grady (Eds.), *Introduction to evidence-based practice in nursing and health care* (2nd ed., pp. 99–118). Sudbury, MA: Jones and Bartlett Publishers.

Hanna, K. M., Weaver, M. T., Slaven, J. E., Fortenberry, J. D., & DeMeglio, L. A. (2014). Diabetes-related quality of life and the demands and burdens of diabetes care among emerging adults with type 1 diabetes in the year after high school graduation. *Research in Nursing and Health, 37*(5), 399–408. doi:10.1002/nur.21620

Institute of Medicine Board on Health Care Services. (2003). *Health professions education: A bridge to quality.* Washington, DC: National Academies Press. Retrieved from http://books.nap.edu/openbook.php?record_id=10681

Iverson, K. M., Huang, K., Wells, S. Y., Wright, J. D., Gerber, M. R., & Wiltsey-Stirman, S. (2014). Women veterans' preferences for intimate partner violence screening and response procedures within the Veterans Health Administration. *Research in Nursing and Health, 37*(4), 302–311. doi:10.1002/nur.21602

Karlsson, V., Bergbom, I., & Forsberg, A. (2012). The lived experiences of adult intensive care patients who were conscious during mechanical ventilation: A phenomenological-hermeneutic study. *Intensive and Critical Care Nursing, 28*(1), 6–15.

Ketefian, S., & Redman, R. (2013). Nursing science in the global community. In W. K. Cody (Ed.), *Philosophical and theoretical perspectives for advanced nursing practice* (5th ed., pp. 279–289). Burlington, MA: Jones & Bartlett Learning.

LoBiondo-Wood, G., & Haber, J. (2010). *Nursing research: Methods and critical appraisal for evidence-based practice* (7th ed.). St. Louis, MO: Mosby/Elsevier.

Macnee, C. L., & McCabe, S. (2008). *Understanding nursing research: Reading and using research in evidence-based practice* (2nd ed.). Philadelphia, PA: Lippincott Williams & Wilkins.

Malloch, K., & Porter-O'Grady, T. (2010). *Introduction to evidence-based practice in nursing and health care* (2nd ed.). Sudbury, MA: Jones and Bartlett Publishers.

Melnyk, B. M. (2008). The worldwide epidemic of child and adolescent overweight and obesity: Calling all clinicians and researchers to intensify efforts in prevention and treatment. *Worldviews on Evidence-Based Nursing, 5*(3), 109–112.

Melnyk, B. M., & Fineout-Overholt, E. (2011). *Evidence-based practice in nursing & healthcare: A guide to best practice* (2nd ed.). Philadelphia, PA: Lippincott Williams & Wilkins.

Moorhead, S., Johnson, M., Maas, M., & Swanson, E. (2008). *Nursing outcomes classification (NOC)* (4th ed.). St. Louis, MO: Mosby.

National Institute of Nursing Research (NINR). (n.d.). NINR mission. Retrieved from http://www.ninr.nih.gov/aboutninr/ninr-mission-and-strategic-plan

Norwood, S. L. (2010). *Research essentials: Foundations for evidenced-based practice.* Boston, MA: Pearson.

Polit, D. F., & Beck, C. T. (2008). *Nursing research: Generating and assessing evidence for nursing practice* (8th ed.). Philadelphia, PA: Lippincott Williams & Wilkins.

Polit, D. F., & Beck, C. T. (2014). *Essentials of nursing research: Appraising evidence for nursing practice* (8th ed.). Philadelphia, PA: Wolters Kluwer Health/Lippincott Williams & Wilkins.

Porter-O'Grady, T. (2010). A new age for practice: Creating the framework for evidence. In K. Malloch & T. Porter-O'Grady (Eds.), *Introduction to evidence-based practice in nursing and health care* (2nd ed., pp. 1–29). Sudbury, MA: Jones and Bartlett Publishers.

Reynolds, P. (1971). *A primer in theory construction.* Indianapolis, IN: Bobbs-Merrill.

Schmidt, N. A., & Brown, J. M. (2015). *Evidence-based practice for nurses: Appraisal and application of research* (3rd ed.). Burlington, MA: Jones & Bartlett Learning.

Stommel, M., & Wills, C. (2004). *Clinical research: Concepts and principles for advanced practice nurses.* Philadelphia, PA: Lippincott Williams & Wilkins.

Szabo, C. M., Grap, M. J., Munro, C. L., Starkweather, A., & Merchant, R. E. (2014). The effect of oral care on intracranial pressure in critically ill adults. *Journal of Neuroscience Nursing, 46*(6), 321–329. doi:10.1097/JNN.0000000000000092

West, D. S., Gorin, A. A., Subak, L. L., Foster, G., Bragg, C., Hecht, J., ... Wing, R. R. (2011). A motivation-focused weight loss maintenance program is an effective alternative to a skill-based approach. *International Journal of Obesity, 35,* 259–269.

Wing, R. R., Papandonatos, G., Fava, J. L., Gorin, A. A., Phelan, S., McCaffery, J., & Tate, D. F. (2008). Maintaining large weight losses: The role of behavioral and psychological factors. *Journal of Consulting and Clinical Psychology, 76*(6), 1015–1021.

Chapter 9

Literature Review: Searching and Writing the Evidence

Carol Boswell and Dorothy Greene Jackson

Chapter Objectives

At the conclusion of this chapter, the learner will be able to:

1. Define the concept of literature review.
2. Discuss the purpose of a research/evidence-based practice literature review.
3. Differentiate research articles from nonresearch articles.
4. Recognize the importance of collaboration with a library specialist.
5. Identify steps for conducting a literature review using electronic retrieval methods.
6. Identify guidelines for evaluating research articles.
7. Identify steps for writing a literature review.
8. Relate the literature review to evidence-based nursing practice.

Key Terms

Annotated bibliography	Database
CINAHL	Discursive prose

Literature review

Medical Subject Heading (MeSH)

MEDLINE

Reference librarian

Research articles

Search engine

Introduction

This chapter provides practical guidelines for conducting and writing a **literature review** for an evidence-based proposal and/or research project in nursing. Guidelines and tips are given for selecting appropriate databases for electronic retrieval of research review articles. Steps are given for the process of writing and organizing data based on evidence and issues in nursing practice. Why is this idea of literature review so very important in the current climate of health care? Literature reviews provide the foundation for the advancing of the project and/or proposal toward the inclusion of best practice and evidence confirmation related to the topic being considered. According to Duncan and Holtslander (2012), skills associated with information acquisition are of paramount importance. Klein-Fedyshin (2015) states, "being able to recognize information needs, locate evidence-based knowledge, critically appraise the retrieval, and apply it in practice is vital to nurses" (p. 24). Yet students and practicing nurses declare insecurity and uncertainty in the process of conducting library searches for appropriate materials. When the latest computer-literate generations, the so-called "Generation X" and "Millennials," voice these concerns, more attention must be directed to facilitating the process if evidence-based practice is to be the standard.

Definition and Purpose of the Literature Review

The literature review is a written, analytic summary of research findings on a topic of interest. The Writing Center (n.d.) defines a literature review as anything from a simple summary of the sources to an analysis of the progression of the field, but even the simplest review must have an organizational pattern. It is a comprehensive compilation of what is known about the phenomenon. The work within the literature review is a synthesis of the material, not just a summary. Morgan-Rallis (2014) emphasizes that a literature review should not be an annotated bibliography. The review is guided by the researcher's curiosity about a particular subject and gaps in the knowledge about the subject area. The purpose for developing and presenting a review of the literature emerges from a desire to document the knowledge and ideas currently established concerning the identified topic. The Writing Center (n.d.) states, "while the main focus of any academic research paper is to support your own argument, the focus of a literature review is to summarize and synthesize the arguments and ideas of others" (p. 2). The ensuing document conveys the strengths and weaknesses ascertained from the review of the pertinent literature (Taylor, 2012). Each literature review must be characterized by designated concepts and ideas such as the PICOT (population, intervention, comparison, outcome, time) and/or research objective/purpose.

The literature review is intended to assess the evidence regarding the research topic by identifying and synthesizing studies that examine the subject of interest. Taylor (2012) states that a literature review must not be merely a descriptive inventory of the available information, nor is it to be a collection of synopses. The main purpose of the literature review is to identify what is known and unknown about an area that has not been totally resolved in practice. A second purpose is to determine how an issue can be resolved and managed based on research evidence. The literature review provides the background and the context within which the research is conducted. It lays out the foundation of the study. Specifically, a good review of the literature does the following:

- Identifies a research problem and indicates how it can be studied
- Helps clarify and determine the importance of a research problem
- Identifies what is known about a problem and identifies gaps (what is unknown) in a particular area of knowledge
- Provides examples based on documented studies for resolving a nursing issue
- Provides evidence that a problem is of importance
- Identifies theoretical frameworks and conceptual models for organizing and conducting research studies
- Identifies experts in the field of interest
- Identifies research designs and methodologies for conducting like studies
- Provides a context for interpretation, comparison, and critique of study findings (McGrath & Brandon, 2014; Norwood, 2000; Polit & Beck, 2008)

Taylor (2012) sets out four aspects that need to be identifiable within a literature review. The first is the expectation that the literature review is directed toward an identified topic of interest. The author of a literature review must not ramble in the hope of eventually addressing the needed information concerning a topic of interest. Thought and attention to the flow and appropriateness of each entry into the review are based upon a directed process. Second, the review needs to provide both what is known and what continues to be unknown about the topic. It is critical that a literature review provide both aspects on the topic. The unknown about the topic is as important as the known. By understanding both aspects, the ongoing development of knowledge related to the topic can be effectively developed and structured. The final document should balance these two aspects to provide a complete picture of the current state of the topic under consideration. As a third aspect, controversial perceptions within the literature need to be delineated for consideration. A literature review that does not provide all sides to the question does not effectively consider the entire topic. All subjects have at least two sides to the arguments involved in the process. Finally, the summarization of the complete literature foundation on the topic should facilitate the development of any further needed research or evidence-based practice (EBP) projects. Literature reviews can be provided in either a **discursive prose** format or as an **annotated bibliography**. When provided as discursive prose, the material is provided in sections organized by themes or identified trends, not as a summary of the different research projects identified. The annotated bibliography begins with a succinct discussion of each research report and also includes the themes and concepts embedded within a crucial assessment of the information provided.

The Literature Review Within the Evidence-Based Practice and/or Research Process

Within an evidence-based practice process, the literature review serves to identify the evidence that is currently available related to the challenge identified. For this process, the PICOT question that is determined drives the literature search. The PICOT question from the Hanna, Weaver, Slaven, Fortenberry, and DiMeglio (2014) article would be: What are the:

> (I) demands and burdens of diabetes care in relation to DQOL (Diabetes-Related Quality of Life) in (P) youth during the year (T) after high school graduation to examine the association of DQOL with the (O) predictors of glycemic control, diabetes management, primary diabetes care responsibility, time since graduation, and living independently of parents. (p. 401)

From the evidence that can be located on the topic, a decision concerning the next steps within the process—either research or quality improvement—can be determined. For this PICOT question, a quantitative research study was conducted to obtain the answers to the concerns. From the literature review, which provides the gaps, limitations, or foundation of knowledge on a topic, a person can identify what more is needed within the scientific investigation of the phenomena. Enough evidence may be available to restrict the need for further research. On the other hand, the evidence may be directed into a narrow scope which then demonstrates the need for a broader look at the topic through a directed research process. Using **Figure 9-1**, an article can be ranked to determine the effectiveness of the material. Once the PICOT was developed for the DQOL study (Hanna et al., 2014), the process of ranking it becomes a matter of determining what type of manuscript it represents. The article states that it is a large, longitudinal quantitative study; thus, it would rank as a Level 2, 3, or 4. The sample is not randomized and no intervention was initiated. As a result, this study appears to be a nonexperimental design, which would place it as a Level 4 EBP rank.

The literature review usually happens early during the research process. In qualitative research, however, this step may come at the end of the study. For quantitative studies, the literature review must be started early in the process and continued throughout the process. Initially, the researcher has a hunch or curiosity about something observed in practice. Soon this idea is translated into a research problem or research question. Shortly thereafter, the review of the literature is conducted to see what has happened in other situations where the problem has occurred. In terms of its placement in a research article, the review of the literature usually follows the statement of the research problem or the research

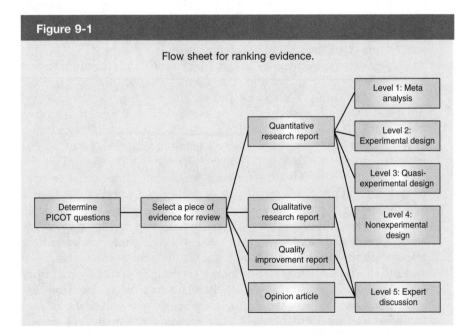

Figure 9-1

Flow sheet for ranking evidence.

question. The reason the review comes early in a quantitative research process is because it sets the stage (lays the foundation) for the rest of the study. As mentioned earlier, the review of the literature provides the theoretical framework for how the current study will be structured, helps to frame the research question into a research hypothesis, and identifies what will be studied and measured in the study.

For example, suppose a unit in a local 340-bed hospital has had no nurse resign or leave the staff in 15 years. This unit exists in a setting where the nursing shortage is rampant. The attrition rate is found to be at an all-time high. A newly hired nursing administrator becomes curious about this unit. She calls the director of the unit to visit and discuss the reason turnover is so low on this unit. From conversations with several other staff members of this unit, the administrator formulates in her mind the theory that a good manager is the most important link to the low attrition rate on the unit. Although a low attrition rate does not seem to be a problem requiring research, this idea can be translated so that some insight is gained to answer the administrator's question, "Is the staff's perception of the nurse manager associated with the attrition or retention rate on a unit?" Searching the literature for studies about managers and retention or attrition can further illuminate this research question. The literature review may then describe what has been found to be true from other similar settings by conducting a survey of nurses who have worked in the same facility or unit for at least 15 years. The new administrator could use this survey or questionnaire to conduct a small research study on her hospital's unit. This hypothetical example illustrates the importance of the literature review and demonstrates how it fits within the rest of the research process. The process used in the study came from the review of the literature.

According to the University Library (n.d.), the formula for commencing a literature review requires that a problem be formulated to drive the selection of materials. Without clearly denoting the problem or challenge, the identifying of materials for inclusion into the review becomes problematic. The second aspect that is needed is the tangible acquisition of the materials relevant for the subject being investigated. Ensuring that each document included in the review addresses a component of the subject is imperative. After the materials are assembled for consideration, each document must be evaluated to ascertain the connection between it and the subject matter under investigation. As the review is being done, four facets are important to consider. Initially within the review, the author's credentials and arguments need to be carefully considered for relevance and provenance. Second, the author's viewpoints should be evaluated for bias. Another area to consider is the inclusion of contradictory data along with the supportive data. Persuasiveness is another facet that should be carefully weighed during a literature review: Are the themes identified and set forth by the author convincing? Finally, the review should ultimately contribute significantly to the understanding of the identified topic. A closing piece of the formula for completing the review entails the documentation of the findings and conclusions as they pertain to the investigated topic. The dissemination of the findings and conclusions is vital for the next steps within either the EBP process or a research endeavor.

Differentiating a Research Article from a Nonresearch Article

Many good sources of very valuable information that may contribute to nursing practice exist. However, for the purposes of illuminating the value of evidence-based knowledge, this text focuses primarily on data from original research. It is often difficult to locate original research, especially when little research has been published in a particular area. If that is the case, the lack of previous studies serves as an opportunity because it can stimulate the development of research data for that particular issue.

The importance of research derives from the fact that it has been conducted using a consistently acceptable scientific method known and respected by the research world. It is not just someone's opinion, but rather has been examined critically. **Research articles** consistently contain components that are required by a scientific decision-making process. **Box 9-1** describes components of a research article.

It is sometimes tempting to choose nonresearch information or evidence when conducting the review of literature. For example, reports from state agencies, various nursing organizations, or websites may present information that is very important to a body of knowledge, yet has not been critically examined in a research study. Some nationally conducted surveys may provide very important information, but may not be considered true research because not all the people in a particular population were included or not enough people returned the surveys. Unless all of the critical components are incorporated in the research process, the information obtained in the investigation should not be considered research. All evidence does have value but each has a different level of value based upon several aspects, which are addressed elsewhere. As these other forms of evidence are considered within a literature review, the level and/or strength of the evidence becomes increasingly important. As indicated earlier, Figure 9-1 is a flow sheet for aiding in the placement of evidence documents toward a level of ranking within the evidence. While this flow sheet uses just one example of ranking methodology, the principles found within the flow chart can be applied to other ranking methods as needed.

Box 9-1

Components of a Research Article

- **Title:** The title describes what the study is about.
- **Abstract:** The abstract is a brief summary of the problem of interest to the researcher. It describes, in approximately 120 words, what took place in the research study and makes a brief statement about the outcome. It helps to determine relevance to the reader who is conducting a search of the literature.
- **Introduction/literature review:** This component gives the background of the research topic and explains why it is important, based on a selective review of relevant literature. It compares and contrasts other research articles and summarizes what is already known and not known about the topic.
- **Purpose of the study/hypothesis/problem statement:** The purpose explains the aim of the study. It is the hypothesis or the research question that the author wants to support or answer.
- **Methodology/procedures/research design:** This component tells what happened. It describes in detail what actions the author took to carry out the study. The method describes the procedure for how the research was conducted and how the information was analyzed or statistical testing was done. It also describes the population, including how it was selected; the setting where the research took place; the number of participants in the study; the type of study, either qualitative or quantitative; and the tools used to collect the data or the method used to attain the information in the study.
- **Major findings/results/analysis/discussion:** This component describes the outcome of the study.
- **Summary/conclusion/ideas for future studies/implications:** This component highlights major findings of the study and identifies the gaps in the study or any areas that need further research. Recommendations for policy or practice are discussed in this section.
- **Works cited/references/acknowledgments:** The reference list should be organized in a recognized literary format (such as APA) or other recognized reference format.

Very often individuals will state that they are "going to research" a topic; searching the literature is not considered research, but rather a mechanism for providing background information for the research project. The use of the word "research" to describe following a line of investigation does not hold the same meaning as the process of conducting a research study. Whether an individual is conducting an EBP review or a research literature review, the person will need to ultimately become very well versed on the evidence available on the topic of interest.

■ Conducting a Literature Review Search

The guidelines presented in this section of the chapter are targeted toward the novice researcher. It is advised that the student researcher seek the help of a professional librarian at the beginning of a research project and throughout the research process when it is necessary to access comprehensive information from appropriate sources. Most literature searches can be done by electronic retrieval. Researchers can find most of the material they need from doing their own personal searches;

❓ THINK OUTSIDE THE BOX

In your current clinical setting, which types of evidence materials are used as the foundation of policies? Discuss the appropriateness and effectiveness of these types of evidence. What levels of evidence are used in the process? How much evidence is needed for a policy to be deemed as "based on evidence" at your facility?

---

however, the most comprehensive searches are done with the help of professional library personnel. Many librarians are credentialed or specially trained in working with particular databases or particular aspects of data management and retrieval.

Some of the special types of librarians include research, law, medical, government documents, and consumer health librarians. Many librarians play an integral role in research. Librarians can provide an effective search within numerous search engines. Nurses need to allow time for these colleagues to provide strength to the dissemination efforts occurring. Nurses must consider their own expertise when starting a research project or conducting research literature reviews. Likewise, they need to embrace the expertise provided by the librarians to ensure that the supportive materials are appropriate, clear, and concise.

■ The Importance of Library Specialists in Conducting a Literature Review

Finding pertinent articles that deal with the topic at hand may be a complex task and may require the expertise of a research librarian. Librarians are able to assist users with finding information in a timely manner. As a result of their education, training, and experience, they are well versed on the databases, including the way in which the information is catalogued and organized. They understand the terminology needed to retrieve the information that is most relevant to the user. Their specialized knowledge may help the user conduct a more comprehensive search from multiple sources. Librarians' search expertise makes them highly skilled at weeding out irrelevant documents that otherwise might inundate the user and cause the researcher to spend unnecessary time chasing down blind alleys. Leedy and Ormrod (2012) strongly encourage all levels of researchers and seekers of evidence to effectively use the **reference librarian**. The world of library resources is exploding with new and innovative means for accessing the evidence available for consideration. The reference librarian must become a key person who is regularly engaged in accessing the evidence to ensure that the materials compiled present the best confirmation and proof available while also providing the other side of the argument. Scholars need to be sure that they are presenting the full picture related to the topic under investigation. All views of the topic need to be supported, thus allowing a strong rationale to be presented for the project being conducted.

Nevertheless, with the advancement of the electronic library, conducting a search is much easier for the beginning researcher than ever before. The beginning researcher must set aside time to learn the process and become comfortable with the search process. With a little help from expert information specialists (librarians) and guidance from a good mentor, the beginning researcher can conduct literature searches and write a literature review that provides evidence supporting a meaningful research proposal or project.

All levels of researchers must understand when and where to ask for help. Anyone can complete an effective literature search, but the key is determining what are effective articles to include, which articles are not needed, and when should an expert such as the resource librarian be used. Developing a collaboration with strategic mentors is paramount within the process.

The Research Idea

The first step in conducting a literature review is brainstorming about an idea or an area of interest with colleagues and mentors. The nurse's practice area is probably one of the most common sources for a research idea in the nursing field. Important issues in nursing provide abundant ideas for research. For example, the nursing shortage, the cost of health care, the quality of care for uninsured persons, and new delivery methods identified in federal legislative bills are all broad areas that may generate a researchable topic. Ideas may also come from reading professional journals or from the news media. As we realize that the majority of research at this time tends to be done within teams of peers who have a common interest, ideas to help provide the foundation for the brainstorming sessions can be determined. During a brainstorming session, every idea should be put on the table for consideration. Once a thorough list of ideas is developed, further development of the selected thinking can be done by the group to clarify and cultivate the research and/or EBP idea.

In addition, articles in professional journals may end with the phrase, "additional research is needed to explore the nature of …" Here is a snapshot of one such article: "Although we did not identify differences in opinions of women with and without IPV [intimate partner violence] history, a more detailed approach to data collection may evoke differences we did not detect" (Iverson et al., 2014, p. 309). In this qualitative example, areas within the current study that would benefit from further investigation are presented to stimulate additional studies. Often, the conclusion of an article marks the starting point for other research ideas.

◼ The Research Question

Most nurses have a hunch or curiosity about some aspect of nursing science or patient care. It is helpful to formulate that idea into a question that, if answered, would contribute to the field of nursing and/or health care. Each research or EBP project should initially answer the question, "So what?" In answering this question, the importance of the project is confirmed before time is wasted on ideas that do not have valid foundations. Formulation of a research question is covered elsewhere. For the purposes of this text, asking a simple question, such as a PICOT, based on the area of interest helps the novice researcher focus on topics and key concepts for conducting the literature search. Utilizing the PICOT format, which is discussed elsewhere, provides crucial components beneficial for conducting a successful literature search. For example, the student researcher may be curious about how long it takes the new baccalaureate-prepared nurse graduate to feel comfortable in a management position. A possible question could be, "What is the role transition time for baccalaureate-prepared nurse graduates in management positions in a small hospital?"

Reading is another very important source of research ideas. In the example provided earlier (Iverson et al., 2014), the author suggested that more research should be conducted to explore other opinions held by women related to IPV screening. Further work on data collection related to this topic, especially for those individuals deployed, was suggested as an area needing additional investigation. This gap resulted from the work completed within this study. Multiple questions could be developed to gain a more thorough understanding of how veteran women consider IPV screening within the provision of health care. Of course, after undertaking further reading, the researcher may have different ideas. Thus, the research question must not be etched in stone. As additional information is acquired from the literature, the evolution of the research project occurs.

Forming an initial question is a good place to start the process of conducting the literature review search. Without the identification of the problem and the development of an initial question, the literature review could become overwhelming and convoluted. This process of stating the initial idea and problem allows for commitment to a specific focus for the preliminary work. To start the literature review, it is important to distinguish between databases and search engines.

Definition of Database

It is appropriate at this juncture to define a **database** and to indicate how it is different from a search engine. Let's start by saying that Google and Yahoo are examples of search engines and MEDLINE is a database. "A **search engine** is a collection of software programs that collect information from the Web, index it, and put it in a database so it can be searched" (Ackerman & Hartman, 2003, p. 47). The job of a search engine is to retrieve the information in a format that is accessible visually on screen at an on-site library or in downloadable, readable (full-text) written format.

Leedy and Ormrod (2012) provide selected broad tactics for conducting useful searches via search engines. To limit the search, utilize at least two key words. One method used to denote crucial words in the search utilizes the addition of the plus sign (+) before the selected word. By using this designation, the search engine concentrates the search on the designated word. A final idea for narrowing the search provided by a search engine is to place quotation marks around any phrase that is principal to the quest. Sources identified by search engines need to be carefully considered concerning the quality and accuracy of the material found within the site. Some websites are closely monitored while others are open to general access and publication of information.

In contrast, a database is an extensive assembly of related information arranged for convenient access and retrieval (Dictionary.com, 2015). A database is a storage location, like a library, where information is stored, catalogued, maintained, and updated systematically. Many of the databases used within literature searches are available online at this time. These sources include indexes, abstracts, encyclopedias, dictionaries, and other universal reference tools. Databases allow an individual to narrow the focus for the search using strategic words, titles, author names, years, languages, and combinations of these elements.

Two main types of databases are available—bibliographic and full text. Bibliographic databases give directions on where to find the information, whereas full-text databases contain the information itself. In other words, the full-text type of database contains the article itself in a downloadable format. In recent years, more major databases have added an increased number of full-text capabilities.

Databases Useful in Nursing

The two most useful databases for nursing literature are Medical Literature Analysis and Retrieval System Online (MEDLINE) and the Cumulative Index to Nursing and Allied Health Literature (CINAHL) (**Box 9-2**). **MEDLINE** provides literature related to medicine, nursing,

Box 9-2

Databases Useful in Nursing

MEDLINE (Medical Literature Analysis and Retrieval System Online)
Cumulative Index to Nursing and Allied Health Literature (CINAHL)
Cochrane Library
Nursing & Health Sciences: A SAGE Full-Text Collection
ProQuest (Health Sciences & Nursing Journals)
Test and measurement databases, theses, and dissertations
PsycINFO

and dentistry. The MEDLINE component of PubMed covers medically related articles for a period from 1946 to the present with some older materials available (National Library of Medicine [NLM], 2012). The focus of information in MEDLINE is biomedicine, but this database also contains the citations that are provided in CINAHL. The **CINAHL** database provides authoritative coverage of the literature related to nursing and allied health.

The MEDLINE database is generally considered the premier bibliographic database for providing access to the North American biomedical literature. It stores and indexes more than 21 million citations and articles from thousands of full-text catalogued titles (ProQuest, 2015). The database is updated more frequently than any other database of its type—daily, Monday through Friday since June 2014 (NLM, 2015b). The NLM website (www.nlm.nih.gov), which contains nursing and medical citations, can be accessed free of charge via the Internet. In other words, library privileges are not required, only access to the Internet. Thus, this website is an excellent place to start a literature search. On the NLM website, individuals can access the Human Genome Project, NIH Roadmap, quality information relevant to toxicology and environmental health, health services research, and public health (NLM, 2012). A wide variety of services are available through the NLM without any changes for the information accessed. It serves as an important reservoir for the healthcare data needed to advance healthcare research and EBP.

The MEDLINE database uses a controlled vocabulary. A controlled vocabulary means that information is catalogued according to specific words or subject headings as in a dictionary or thesaurus. It is arranged in both an alphabetic and a hierarchical format (NLM, 2015b). Although most people start searches using fundamental words, this type of search does not yield the most comprehensive results. The dictionary for finding the words that most appropriately define or match the search term or concept in MEDLINE is the **Medical Subject Heading (MeSH)** database guide. This feature can be accessed from the NLM/PubMed website, adjacent to the left search boxes in most cases. The MeSH home page (www.nlm.nih.gov/mesh) allows individuals to access a "MeSH on Demand" link. Within this link, a person could submit text for which the NLM database can identify a list of MeSH terms relevant to the provided text (NLM, 2015a). To be successful in this process, individuals need to provide well-defined sentences for the site to use. It provides a list of terms usually in less than 1 minute. Once the list of MeSH terms is provided, the site provides a link to a corresponding MeSH browser that can be used to identify articles and documents for consideration (NLM, 2015a). PubMed is a service of the NLM that includes more than 16 million citations from MEDLINE and other life science journals dating back to the 1950s. PubMed includes links to full-text articles and other related resources (NLM, 2015b).

This example illustrates the difference between a key word search and a subject heading search. The key words "patient visitation" might be used to locate journal articles focusing on how nurses perceive open visitation in intensive care units. When the term "patient visitation" was used to search in MEDLINE, 9 citations were retrieved (at the time of this writing). When the subject or controlled vocabulary term found in the MeSH database guide (thesaurus) was used ("visitors to patients"), 1,842 citations were located. In total, 10 MeSH terms were suggested for inclusion in a search along with "patient visitation." When all 11 terms were used, the search identified 5,288,662 potential articles. When only family-related MeSH terms were used out of the 11 (total of 7 terms), the search identified 5,228,018 articles. Knowing how a database stores information is very important in conducting effective and relevant searches. Using dates, types of nursing units, or other strategies can narrow this search.

CINAHL is probably the most popular database used by nurses. It indexes more than 5,300 journals, 1,400 full-text journals and magazines, searchable cited references for more than 1,500 journals, and more than 500,000 records recorded from 1937 to the present (CINAHL Information Systems, n.d.). CINAHL houses nursing publications, including the *American Journal of Nursing* and the publications of the National League for Nursing. It also indexes journals in the allied health fields related to physical therapy, occupational therapy, cardiopulmonary technology, emergency service, physician assistant health education, radiology technology, medical laboratory technology, medical records, surgical technology, and medical assistants. Other selected journals related to biomedicine, consumer health, and librarianship health sciences are also included (CINAHL Information Systems, n.d.).

CINAHL publications can be searched using EBSCO*host* and Ovid and are available for use only through a library. EBSCO*host* provides approximately 700 full-text and secondary databases (EBSCO, n.d.). It accesses databases in business, medical, public, and nursing publications. Many healthcare agencies are finding this resource to be valuable for allowing staff members to access the evidence.

Just as in MEDLINE, records in CINAHL are indexed by a controlled vocabulary or subject headings. Subject headings provide descriptors of the terms listed in the database. Searching by the terms or subjects used in the database yields results that are more relevant to the topic being searched. Subject headings can be viewed by clicking the CINAHL Headings button on the EBSCO*host* toolbar. To begin the search, the subject heading term should be entered in the "Find" field. Searches using this tool can also be done by using key words. The EBSCO*host* system matches articles with appropriate subject terms by a process called mapping.

CINAHL can also be accessed using the Journals@Ovid full-text database. This database contains research articles, book and media reviews, and full-text nursing articles. Information in this database is searched by using key words.

A number of other databases are useful in nursing. These databases include theses and dissertations and free Internet databases (**Box 9-3**), along with the following:

- Cochrane Library: A regularly updated collection of evidence-based medicine databases. These databases include systematic reviews of subjects, including economics, health interventions, controlled trials, and methodologies.
- Nursing & Health Sciences: A Sage Full-Text Collection: Includes full text of 24 journals published by Sage.
- Nursing Journals (ProQuest Nursing Journals): Full-text journals.
- PsycINFO: Includes journals from the social sciences.
- Tests and measurements databases.
- Mental Measurements Yearbook.
- Health and Psychosocial Instruments.

 THINK OUTSIDE THE BOX

Which databases have you used in your literature searches? Discuss the pros and cons of those databases you are familiar with using.

Box 9-3

Full-Text Databases Useful in Nursing

- Academic Search Premier (www.ebscohost.com/academic/academic-search-premier): Designed for academic institutions; contains full-text scholarly publications; source—EBSCO*host* research database.
- AIDSinfo (https://aidsinfo.nih.gov): Federally approved HIV/AIDS research information for patients and healthcare providers.
- CINAHL Plus with Full Text (https://health.ebsco.com/products/cinahl-plus-with-full-text).
- EBSCO*host* (www.ebscohost.com/).
- Cumulative Index to Nursing and Allied Health (CINAHL, https://health.ebsco.com/products/the-cinahl-database).
- The Cochrane Collaboration (www.cochrane.org): Evidence-based medicine systematic reviews.
- Health and Psychosocial Instruments (HaPI, http://bmdshapi.com): Evaluation and measurement instruments in health; available through Ovid Technologies.
- Health and Wellness Resource Center (www.ocls.info/Virtual/OnlineDatabases/db_desc.asp?OnlineDatabasesID=49): Informational sources, magazines, videos, journals, and newspapers on health and disease.
- Journals@OVIDFullText (www.ovid.com/site/about/terms.jsp?top=42): The second generation of Ovid Full Text, which combines all the capabilities of Ovid Full Text Collections with several important features and functions. To access this link, you do need a subscription through a university or library. The link provided allows you to see the terms and conditions for use of this site.
- MEDLINE with Medical Subject Heading (MeSH; www.ncbi.nlm.nih.gov/mesh): Medical Literature Analysis and Retrieval System Online (MEDLINE) is the U.S. National Library of Medicine's (NLM) premier bibliographic database that contains more than 16 million references to journal articles in life sciences, with a concentration on biomedicine.
- Health Sciences: A SAGE Full-Text Collection (http://online.sagepub.com/collection.dtl?coll=HEAL): A searchable database of bibliographic records and full-text journal articles.
- ProQuest Nursing Journals (www.proquest.com/products-services/pq_nursingahs_shtml.html): Designed to meet the needs of students and researchers at academic institutions; includes information on obstetrics, nursing, geriatric care, oncology, and more.

■ Basics of Searching

Any review of published articles about a topic is only as good as what has been searched. In other words, "the first requirement for writing a good literature review ... is to do a good literature search" (Kellsey, 2005, p. 526). An effective place to start is to identify concepts from the research question that can be the focus of the search. For example, the research question, "What is the relationship between nurses' perception of empowerment and retention?", the concepts empowerment and nurse retention could be used as the search terms.

Successful searching takes some planning and thought. According to Duncan and Holtslander (2012), individuals encounter the highest amount of frustration as a result of unsuccessful queries that result in the need for re-querying. Using the incorrect and incomplete terms within the query can result in large, unmanageable search results to work through to get to the key articles. Search engines can locate an enormous number of documents. The results can sometimes be overwhelming.

A clear search strategy is necessary to narrow the results to relevant, usable information. In developing an effective search strategy, it is important to identify the main concepts from the research question, or PICOT question, and/or topic and determine any synonyms for these terms. For the sample research question, "What is the relationship of nurses' perceptions of empowerment and retention?", the concepts are "nurses," "empowerment," and "retention." Other alternate words include "power" and "authority" (for "empowerment") and "retaining" (for "retention"). Duncan and Holtslander (2012) provide several strategies for narrowing the search words, including, "verifying concepts in the course textbook, using thesauri, noting the key words or subject headings identified from located papers, consulting specialized nursing or other pertinent dictionaries, and checking Wikipedia or Google Scholar" (p. 26). These tactics along with the use of selected terms from cited references, retrieved papers, and sources such as Web of Science databases can aid an individual in locating the articles and evidence that are needed to support a change in practice or validate a current practice.

The following steps outline the basics of conducting a search from electronic sources. The researcher should consider the use of MEDLINE while following these steps:

1. Select a topic of interest and identify the concepts or search terms. Think in terms of controlled vocabularies or subject headings for databases when selecting the topic. Subject headings yield more precise results than key words.
2. Access the NLM/PubMed website using an Internet browser.
3. Locate the MeSH database guide to the left of the main PubMed page.
4. Type the search term in the MeSH search box.
5. Select the subject heading from MeSH that matches the search term and place it in the PubMed search box. It will be necessary to switch back from the MeSH database guide to the main PubMed page. This can be done by selecting PubMed from the toolbar drop-down menu.
6. Choose limit options as appropriate by date, author, and title.
7. To combine search strategies, use "and" or "or" in the search box. "And" is more restrictive (reduces the number of citations), and "or" is less restrictive.

■ Other Key Information

When searching for basic information, textbooks can sometimes be helpful and acceptable. A textbook often provides a foundation, a framework, or a gold standard by which other sources are measured. For example, when studying about health disparities, the book that contains the premier report is *Unequal Treatment: Confronting Racial and Ethnic Disparities in Health Care* (Smedley, Stith, & Nelson, 2003). It provides data sources, initial research findings, and suggested models that attempt to explain some of the issues surrounding this problem. From reading this book, it is possible to identify the gaps in the literature and the authors of major articles describing the research in this area. Leedy and Ormrod (2012) recommend a very pertinent idea: Try to access primary sources of material. A primary source is viewed as any "document or physical object which was written or created during the time under study" (Princeton Refdesk, n.d., para. 1). Whenever material is extracted from one source to insert into another source, bias can be introduced. These interpretations and analyses of primary sources are classified as secondary sources (BMCC Library, n.d.). Even when care is given to ensuring accuracy, the interpretation of material reflects a unique view of the material that may be contradictory to the original interpretation. Seeking the primary discussion of the material is imperative for getting the accurate picture that was originally gleaned from the analysis of the information presented. This type of information can also be used as background for the research proposal. If the requirements for the proposal include the use of recent information (e.g., not more than five years old), for example, then research journal articles should be used.

Another point to keep in mind is that the more precise the search, the fewer the number of resources that will be retrieved. The more general the search, the larger the number of articles that will be retrieved. After conducting the initial search, the researcher should review the abstracts of the articles and determine if more or less information is needed. The search should then be modified based on how the materials match the research question.

Evaluating the Literature

Evaluation of what has been published is an important and sometimes complex process. Many sources refer to this process as "critiquing the literature." The term *evaluation* is used here because it is more representative of what takes place and does not seem as overwhelming. Beginning researchers may view this evaluation as an intimidating process because they have far less experience than the authors of the original works. This concern may not always be the case, of course. Many times, the reader has more clinical knowledge than some of the people writing the articles. It is necessary to build on the analytical skills that most nurses have and to draw from the practice experience. The good thing about nursing is that there is enough variety and specialization in practice and academia for every nurse to have something of value to offer. Thus, it is important that beginning researchers believe they have the skills necessary to raise questions about what is published. Accessing and studying the material available on a topic is very important. The other side of that coin is also knowing when to stop accessing and studying to begin the next phases. *Repetition* is the significant term to remember in regard to when to stop. When the material read and analyzed begins to demonstrate a repetitive pattern of material, accessing additional resources can be stopped. At a later time, a further search may need to be done to confirm that no new information has been published since the initial cyclic pattern was found.

A good place to locate information for evaluation of the literature is in the discussion section of an article, where the authors talk about the limitations of the study. Other tools to evaluate articles may be provided in the classroom setting from nursing faculty.

The evaluation process consists of a review of the components of the study and a comparison of the study with other studies related to the same research topic. The driving force behind the evaluation is the need to determine whether the study supports the research question identified and whether it identifies gaps in the literature that support the gap the beginning researcher or student has in mind.

It is generally accepted that the components of the study that should be reviewed include (1) the purpose of the study, (2) the sample size and selection, (3) the design of the study (methods used), (4) the data collection procedures, (5) the analysis of the data, and (6) the author's conclusion. The theoretical framework is also an important section to review, although it is sometimes not included due to space restrictions imposed by the publisher. However, it remains an important part of the study because it provides structure for conducting the study and explaining the results. Conceptual framework is not addressed in this text.

A discussion of the areas selected for evaluation follows. These areas correspond to the headings in the "Gaps in the Literature" table (**Table 9-1**).

Articles

When choosing articles from the literature, the researcher should be aware of the authors' credentials. It is important to identify where they work and how to contact them if you have questions about what they have written. Oftentimes, their email addresses are available. Many authors are helpful and willing to give ideas to beginning researchers on request. The article usually provides some brief background about the authors that informs the reader about their credibility in writing about the research topic. It is important to document the citation of the article and contact information of the author. It may seem painstaking at the time, but it is time well spent to document all the information about how to locate the article, such as the author, date of publication, title of article, title of the work containing the article, volume, and page numbers of the article.

Table 9-1

Gaps in the Literature

Article (Title, author, journal, publication date, contact information for author)	Purpose (Why study was conducted)	Sample (Number of participants, demographics, other characteristics, geographic location)	Methods (Design, instruments or questionnaires, data collection, data analysis)	Major Findings (Results, statistical significance, conclusions)	Limitations (Factors that may complicate the interpretation of the findings)	Gaps (Suggestions for further study that support the research question)

Purpose

The purpose of the study explains why the study is being done. It is distinct from the problem, in that the problem addresses what the study is about (Nieswiadomy, 2012). This section is an appropriate component for the researcher to determine what he or she wants to do with the findings of the study. For example, if the problem of the study is obesity in third-grade students in public schools, the purpose could be to determine if the environment of the school and the age of the children may contribute to food consumption choices. The findings could then be used to make changes in the school or to enhance healthy behaviors in the children while they are at school.

The purpose of the study is usually located in its first few paragraphs. Identifying the purpose may help later in grouping similar types of studies and also in organizing the writing of the literature review.

Sample/Population

The sample is a representation of the entire population of interest. All persons in the world cannot be studied, so a representative sample is selected that may have characteristics similar to the general population being studied. For example, caregivers may be the population of interest. Because it is impossible to study all the caregivers in the world, a sample with similar experiences could be chosen. To choose a manageable sample size, the sample may be narrowed to those caregivers who care for their spouses and live in a particular county of Texas.

The sample/population section of the study describes the study participants. The author describes demographic characteristics (e.g., age, gender, race, ethnicity, educational level, geographic location, income level) of the persons who will be in the study. The description of the sample and how it was selected help the researcher make statements about the generalizability of the study—that is, whether similar findings would be obtained in other locations under the same or similar conditions. How the sample was selected may affect the study findings. If the participants were randomly selected using random tables or computer software, the findings are more likely to be generalizable to other similar subjects. In contrast, if the sample was selected based on who showed up at the

 THINK OUTSIDE THE BOX

Select a topic. Discuss the specific steps you would use to conduct a literature review on that topic. Which words would you use to do the search, and why? Which databases would you use, and why?

announcement of the study (known as a convenience sample), it is less likely that the findings could be generalized to other groups.

This section can be documented by providing just a few statements, such as "persons 65 years of age and older caring for their 65-and-older spouses with Alzheimer's disease in their home in rural west Texas." Other examples of sample statements could be "a convenience sample of registered nurses working in home health agencies" or "a randomly selected sample of diabetics diagnosed within the last 6 months."

Methods

The methods section of the study describes the strategy for how the study is conducted. In quantitative research, the methods section includes (1) the inclusion criteria, explaining how the participants were selected, (2) the exclusion criteria, explaining why subjects were not selected, (3) the sample size and whether it was adequate, (4) the design, (5) the instruments or surveys used, (6) data collection procedures, and (7) data analysis (Portney & Watkins, 2008). Each of these components help the reader to understand the thoughts and rationales used in the planning of the project.

The design describes whether the investigation was a descriptive, correlational, exploratory, or experimental study. (Research study designs are covered elsewhere in this text.) The main points of interest for the reader in the methods section should be whether the methods used to collect the data were controlled for any outside conditions that could confuse the findings of the study and whether the methods affected the accuracy of the findings. For example, if the study focuses on the relationship of weight to blood pressure, the researcher must have ensured that the weight scales and blood pressure machines were calibrated and functioning properly. The procedure for how this was done should also be described in the study. If the condition of the measuring instruments is not standardized, it will be impossible to know whether the findings were accurate. Thus, the methods section of the article should include a description of the conditions under which the weights and blood pressures were measured and the person taking the measurements. If surveys or questionnaires were used, the researcher should discuss how the reliability and validity of these instruments were determined when used with other subjects.

Put simply, the design identifies the number of subjects, the number of groups, the type of intervention, and the conditions under which the intervention was performed (Portney & Watkins, 2008). This section of the study helps the reader interpret the degree of accuracy or validity of the findings.

The analysis of the data describes the statistical tests that were used to test the research hypothesis. For example, if the study sought to determine the relationship between two variables, a correlational test would be done. If the study sought to determine the difference between two variables, the test would be a t-test. The reader should make note of the type of testing and compare it with the testing done in other studies; he or she should also determine if the appropriate test was done to match the research hypothesis. In qualitative studies, the avenues used to control for biases must be listed to provide an understanding of how the researchers attempted to ensure unbiased management of the data collected.

Major Findings

The findings (or results) may overlap with the discussion section of the study, but it is most appropriate for the results to stand alone. The results section should be reported without the researcher's interpretation (Portney & Watkins, 2008). This section is a factual discussion that may be explained with tables and charts. It is important for the reader to determine whether the results match the purpose of the study and the research question. In addition, the reader should make note of any statistically significant results and the tests that were used. When the study discusses qualitative results, the reader should pay attention to how bias and control of the study were managed.

Limitations

The limitations of the study describe the elements that may have complicated the results. For example, suppose a study was done to measure improvement in test scores after an instructive video on electrical safety on small appliances in the workplace was presented to the study participants. A pre-test was given before the video was shown, and a post-test was given 1 week after the video presentation. If the scores were low on the post-test, a limitation could be that too much time had lapsed between the test, the instruction, and the post-test. Discussing this limitation of the study may suggest ways to improve the study if it is later replicated. Limitations may also help to identify gaps in the literature that could be considered in other studies.

Gaps in the Literature

This section is of greatest importance for the review of the literature; however, it cannot be given due diligence unless all the other parts of the research study are examined first. The discussion and conclusion section of the article is generally where most of the suggestions for future research are presented. Suggestions for future research usually represent gaps in knowledge about the research topic. Perhaps a particular group suffers a worse outcome than other populations, relative to a particular disease condition. The gap in the literature might then be that no studies have examined the nature of this problem.

The discussion and conclusion section is where authors most often compare their findings with other studies, offer alternative explanations, or offer support for existing practice (Portney & Watkins, 2008). This section is a reflection of the authors' interpretation and experience, biases, and interests relevant to the findings of the study at hand. The authors discuss unanswered questions and point out gaps in the knowledge on the research topic.

The reader should examine this section very carefully for missing pieces of knowledge and for what is unknown about the research area, looking for information that justifies the research being proposed. This information could be gaps related to unanswered questions regarding gender, age, ethnicity, characteristics of healthcare facilities, geographic locations, differences in disease outcomes, or any combination of variables that have not been examined. These aspects would represent gaps in the literature.

■ Writing the Literature Review

The literature review is not a list of article summaries, but rather a well-written synthesis of information about a topic that includes a discussion on the research that has been done and the evidence gathered, the methodologies, the strengths and weaknesses of findings, and gaps that require more knowledge. The approach to writing the review should be to convince the reader that the information supports the need for the proposed study. Morgan-Rallis (2014) emphasizes the need to "stay on the topic." When directly involved with the writing of the synthesis, it becomes easy to move in directions that are not consistent with the purpose for the document. Staying on track to ensure that the purpose is the outcome for the manuscript is fundamental. The format for writing the review may vary depending on the purpose of the review. If the review is conducted for a class assignment, the student should follow the grading criteria. If the review is part of a grant proposal, it is usually succinct and points out various themes, conceptual models, theories that explain the research question, and gaps in the literature that support the need for the grant.

Unfortunately, it is all too easy to get bogged down while actually writing the review. The researcher usually reads numerous articles before settling on those used in the literature review. Aveyard (n.d.) states the need to be pragmatic when finalizing the review. Each article included in the review must clearly and concisely address the stated purpose for the manuscript and/or review. One manageable tool of organization is an outline. Others have recommended the use of grids or matrices for organizing the review of the articles, or index cards for categorizing the

THINK OUTSIDE THE BOX

Select a research article. Examine which aspects from the article must be documented within the summary provided for a literature review.

materials read (McCabe, 2005; Polit & Beck, 2008). One way of developing headings for an outline is to mark notes on the articles or to use the variables identified for the study. After reading the articles chosen for the review, it is helpful to go back and write in the margins adjacent to pertinent information in the text or to list on the first page of the article the reasons why the article was chosen (e.g., good questionnaire, clearly written design, independent and dependent variables listed and defined, similarities to another study).

Answering Key Questions

A good written review should answer some basic questions. Listed here are questions developed from the information found in most published research studies. These questions are based on experiences of the author from a confluence of reading, conducting, and critiquing research reviews and information learned from graduate courses in nursing and library science:

- What was the main focus of the articles (research question, purpose, objectives)?
- Did the articles represent recent (less than five years old) and classic studies?
- What were the designs of most of the studies (research questions, methodology, sample size, population characteristics, and pertinent conclusion)?
- Which studies did not positively support the research question?
- What were the target populations of most of the studies (e.g., nurses in emergency departments, medical–surgical units, operating rooms)?
- Which models or conceptual frameworks were used to explain the structure of the studies?
- What were the general findings and limitations in most of the studies?
- Which articles were the most similar in findings, design, or other features?
- Which gaps were identified in the articles?
- What was the overall conclusion for the literature review that supports the research question and need for your proposal?

An Outline for Writing the Review

Discussion of the preceding questions should be helpful in providing organization to the review. Organizing the review requires thought and attention. One method for organizing the material is through the use of a table. Tables can be prepared addressing key terms and concepts, research methods, and summary of the research results (Morgan-Rallis, 2014). Another method that can be employed is an outline. An outline provides further guidance for developing headings and completing the written review. The components of the outline include (1) the purpose, (2) a description of the search strategy, (3) the themes or categories of similar types of articles, (4) limitations, (5) gaps in what is known about a research area, and (6) a discussion and conclusion. A more detailed description of an outline for organizing the writing of the review appears in **Box 9-4**.

Other Writing Tips

When writing a literature review for a class, it is important to follow the grading criteria and the objectives of the course. If a review is not for a class assignment, attention should be given to what the audience

---

Box 9-4

Outline for a Literature Review

I. Purpose of the review
II. Description of how search was conducted
  A. Databases used
  B. Key words and subject headings
  C. Rationale or criteria for articles chosen in the review
    1. Articles five years old or less
    2. Classic articles or books
III. Themes of articles
  A. Similarities in articles that support the research question
    1. Purposes, designs, target populations, tools of measurement (e.g., questionnaires, methodologies)
    2. General findings
  B. Conceptual framework, models, or theories that explain the research described in the articles
  C. Inconsistencies in articles
    1. Articles that do not provide positive support for the research question identified
IV. Limitations
  A. Components identified by the authors of the articles that were limitations in the studies
V. Gaps in the articles
  A. Gaps identified by the authors of the articles
VI. Discussion and conclusion
  A. Summary statement of how articles support the proposal
  B. Identification of gaps perceived and how the proposal will meet the needs of some aspect of nursing practice

would find interesting to know about the topic. According to O'Neill (2015), the inclusion of a historical account and/or background materials of the topic help the reader to understand the context for the information provided. The writer needs to ensure that each persuasive argument and articulated point is supported by the findings and clearly verbalized (O'Neill, 2015). The length of the review, in terms of the number of pages, depends on the criteria and purpose of the review. The student should follow the headings and subheadings of the writing style required by the course (e.g., American Psychological Association [APA] or other sources). It becomes critical within the process to be knowledgeable concerning the reference tool to be used. While several reference formats can be used, one that is frequently used within health care is APA format (from the *Publication Manual of the American Psychological Association*, currently in its sixth edition). The referencing framework provides assistance for grammar, font, margin, spacing, and document guidelines, along with how to format the citations and reference list for the different sources used.

Once the required style has been determined, paraphrase the crucial points of the articles and avoid using too many direct quotes. Also, be aware that lengthy writing does not necessarily mean comprehensive writing. Being able to synthesize what is called for in the writing and to give the reader what was promised in the purpose of the writing is what is most important. Staying on point keeps a document meaningful for answering the questions under consideration. For each paragraph and/or section, a summary of how this material supports the purpose for that manuscript/project/study is critical. By using this method of a summary paragraph, it brings the writer back to the idea of how each part connects to the intention of the document.

■ Linking the Literature Review to Evidence-Based Nursing Practice

Evidence-based practice is an important issue in nursing today. Nurses need to know why they do what they do. Although many support the idea of intuition, the profession must provide logical explanations for the actions of nursing based on scientific findings. The literature review provides the foundation for good research. To make sound decisions, today's nurses must be well read. The research presented in the literature review may provide nurses with the background they need to make informed choices in practice. The ability to critically analyze scientific literature is a skill every nurse should develop, and a skill that is central to deciding whether to incorporate new information into practice based on the strength of the evidence.

> **? THINK OUTSIDE THE BOX**
>
> Discuss how you would determine the credibility of information found on the Internet.

Summary Points

1. The literature review is the foundation of the research proposal.
2. A good literature review begins with a good literature search that is assisted by a professional librarian.
3. The assistance of an expert librarian may both enhance the relevance of material found and reduce the amount of time spent conducting the search.
4. A database search using subject headings yields more precise information than a key word search.
5. The literature review identifies what is known and unknown about the research topic.
6. The review should focus on original research studies dealing with the selected topic.
7. The literature review identifies gaps in the literature.
8. The gaps in the literature should support the research question.

RED FLAGS

- Literature summaries should provide enough information about the different sources related to sample size, methodology, and results to allow for a clear understanding of the application of that information to the current project.
- Within the literature review, the sources used should be predominantly primary sources, not secondary sources.
- The current expectation is for references to be within the five-year limit unless the article is a classical/benchmark study.
- When Internet sources are used, the credibility of the information must be reflected in the literature review.
- Gaps in the literature review should be identified.

Multiple-Choice Questions

1. A literature review is:
   A. Everything that is known about a subject.
   B. An analytical summary of research findings.
   C. All approved data on a research topic.
   D. A compilation of all positive results of research.

2. The purpose of the literature review is to:
   A. Identify a problem that has not been resolved.
   B. Clarify the importance of a research problem.
   C. Identify gaps in the literature.
   D. All of the above.

3. The literature review should occur:
   A. Near the end of the research process.
   B. Shortly before the analysis of the problem.
   C. Early in the research process.
   D. None of the above.

4. When conducting a literature review, it is advisable to:
   A. Seek most information from the Internet.
   B. Gather all data from books.
   C. Gather all data from journals.
   D. Seek assistance from a librarian.

5. Evidence-based nursing literature provides the nurse with the ability to:
   A. Choose only those practice activities based on evidence.
   B. Describe and analyze published research results.
   C. Use textbook information.
   D. Solve all nursing issues.

6. A database differs from a search engine in the following manner:
   A. A database stores the information.
   B. A search engine takes you to the information.
   C. Databases are specialized by area of knowledge.
   D. All of the above.

7. Which database is considered the premier bibliographic database for providing access in the North Americas for biomedical literature?
   A. Google
   B. MEDLINE
   C. CINAHL
   D. Yahoo!

8. It is appropriate to use key word searches in which of the following contexts?

   A. Evidence-based medicine
   B. Ovid
   C. MEDLINE
   D. Evidence-based nursing

9. The purpose section of a research study usually:

   A. Tells the geographic location of the study.
   B. Tells why the study was done.
   C. Is the methodology of the study.
   D. Tells what the study is about.

10. The gaps in the literature are:

   A. Missing pieces in the knowledge of the research area.
   B. Questions about the research that have not been explained.
   C. Suggestions for future research made by the author.
   D. All of the above.

11. What is the main difference between a research article and a nonresearch article?

   A. A research article reports statistics on surveys and a nonresearch article does not.
   B. A research article describes research by the original author.
   C. A nonresearch article describes the methods of how the study was conducted.
   D. A nonresearch article conducts analysis and statistical testing on the data presented in the article.

Discussion Questions

1. You are interested in seeing what has been written about using dietary supplements to treat bone loss in postmenopausal women. You have been told that appropriate MeSH headings include "dietary supplements" and "osteoporosis, postmenopausal," but you want to use the MeSH database to verify these terms. You also know that you want only English-language articles, so you limit your search by using the "Limits" function and setting "Language" to English. Execute your search and examine the results. (This exercise was provided by Dr. Jeffrey Huber, personal communication, Texas Woman's University, 2003.)

2. To gain a greater understanding of evidence-based nursing, conduct a search to retrieve references to the published literature about aspirin use for prevention of myocardial infarction. Choose the full-text Nursing Collection produced by Ovid. Develop a search strategy for this topic. Review your results.

Suggested Readings

Ahern, N. R. (2005). Using the Internet to conduct research. *Nurse Researcher*, *13*(2), 55–70.

University of California, Berkeley Library. (n.d.). Finding historical primary sources: Getting started. Retrieved from http://guides.lib.berkeley.edu /subject-guide/163-Finding-Historical-Primary-Sources

University Libraries, University of Maryland. (n.d.). Primary, secondary and tertiary sources. Retrieved from http://www.lib.umd.edu/guides/primary -sources.html

Yale University Library. (2006). Primary sources at Yale. Retrieved from http:// www.library.yale.edu/instruction/primsource.html

References

Ackerman, E., & Hartman, K. (2003). *Searching and researching on the Internet and the World Wide Web* (3rd ed.). Wilsonville, OR: Franklin, Beedle & Associates.

Aveyard, H. (n.d.) Top tips for doing your literature review! Retrieved from http://www.nursingtimes.net/student-nursing-times/top-tips-for-doing -your-literature-review/5018587.article

BMCC Library, (n.d.). Primary vs. secondary sources. Retrieved from http://lib1 .bmcc.cuny.edu/help/sources.html

CINAHL Information Systems. (n.d.). The CINAHL database. Birmingham, AL: EBSCO Industries. Retrieved from http://www.ebscohost.com/nursing /products/cinahl-databases/cinahl-complete

Dictionary.com. (2015). Database. Retrieved from http://dictionary.reference.com /browse/database

Duncan, V., & Holtslander, L. (2012). Utilizing grounded theory to explore the information-seeking behavior of senior nursing students. *Journal of the Medical Library Association, 100*(1), 20–27.

EBSCO. (n.d.). EBSCO Health. Birmingham, AL: EBSCO Industries. Retrieved from http://www.ebscohost.com/biomedical-libraries

Hanna, K. M., Weaver, M. T., Slaven, J. E., Fortenberry, J. D., & DiMeglio, L. A. (2014). Diabetes-related quality of life and the demands and burdens of diabetes care among emerging adults with type 1 diabetes in the year after high school graduation. *Research in Nursing & Health, 37*, 399–408. doi:10.1002 /nur.21620

Iverson, K. M., Huang, K., Wells, S. Y., Wright, J. D., Gerber, M. R., & Wiltsey-Stirman, S. (2014). Women veterans' preferences for intimate partner violence screening and response procedures within the Veterans Health Administration. *Research in Nursing & Health, 37*, 302–311. doi:10.1002 /nur.21602

Kellsey, C. (2005). Writing the literature review: Tips for academic librarians. *College Research Library News, 66*(7), 526–527.

Klein-Fedyshin, M. (2015). Translating evidence into practice at the end of life: Information needs, access, and usage of hospice and palliative nurses. *Journal of Hospice & Palliative Nursing, 17*(1), 24–30. doi:10.1097/NJH.0000000000000117

Leedy, P. D., & Ormrod, J. E. (2012). *Practical research: Planning and design* (10th ed.). Boston, MA: Pearson.

McCabe, T. F. (2005). How to conduct an effective literature search. *Nursing Standard, 20*(11), 41–47.

McGrath, J. M., & Brandon, D. (2014). Searching the literature is NOT for the faint of heart! *Advances in Neonatal Care, 14*(40), 229–231. doi; 10.1097 /ANC.0000000000000111

Morgan-Rallis, H. (2014). Guidelines for writing a literature review. Retrieved from http://www.duluth.umn.edu/~hrallis/guides/researching/litreview.html

National Library of Medicine (NLM). (2012). Fact sheet: The National Library of Medicine. Retrieved from http://www.nlm.nih.gov/pubs/factsheets/nlm.html

National Library of Medicine (NLM). (2015a). Fact sheet: Medical Subject Headings (MeSH®). Retrieved from http://www.nlm.nih.gov/pubs/factsheets/mesh.html

National Library of Medicine (NLM). (2015b). Fact sheet: Medline®. Retrieved from http://www.nlm.nih.gov/pubs/factsheets/medline.html

Nieswiadomy, R. M. (2012). *Foundations of nursing research* (6th ed.). Boston, MA: Pearson.

Norwood, S. L. (2000). *Research strategies for advanced practice nurses.* Upper Saddle River, NJ: Prentice Hall Health.

O'Neill, J. (2015). Literature review guidelines. Retrieved from http://www.apa.org/pubs/journals/men/literature-review-guidelines.aspx

Polit, D. F., & Beck, C. T. (2008). *Creating and assessing evidence for nursing practice* (8th ed.). Philadelphia, PA: Lippincott Williams & Wilkins.

Portney, L. G., & Watkins, M. P. (2008). *Foundations of clinical research: Applications to practice* (3rd ed.). Upper Saddle River, NJ: Prentice Hall Health.

Princeton RefDesk. (n.d.). What is a primary source? Retrieved from http://www.princeton.edu/~refdesk/primary2.html

ProQuest. (2015). Medline/Medline full text: Key facts. Retrieved from http://www.proquest.com/

Smedley, B. D., Stith, A. Y., & Nelson, A. R. (2003). *Unequal treatment: Confronting racial and ethnic disparities in health care.* Washington, DC: National Academies Press.

Taylor, D. (2012). The literature review: A few tips on conducting it. Retrieved from http://www.writing.utoronto.ca/advice/specific-types-of-writing/literature-review

University Library. (n.d.). Write a literature review. Retrieved from http://library.ucsc.edu/help/howto/write-a-literature-review

The Writing Center. (n.d.). Literature reviews. University of North Carolina at Chapel Hill. Retrieved from http://writingcenter.unc.edu/handouts/literature-reviews/

Chapter

10

Population Management

Kathaleen C. Bloom and Lucy B. Trice

Chapter Objectives

At the conclusion of this chapter, the learner will be able to:

1. Compare and contrast a population and a sample.
2. Discuss basic concepts related to sampling.
3. Contrast inclusion and exclusion criteria in the sampling process.
4. Distinguish between probability and nonprobability samples.
5. Identify types of sampling strategies used for qualitative and quantitative research.
6. Discuss approaches to determining sample size.
7. Critically evaluate populations and sampling plans found in research reports for their contribution to the strength of evidence for nursing practice.

Key Terms

Accessible population	Exclusion criteria
Cluster sampling	External validity
Convenience sampling	Inclusion criteria

Internal validity   Sample

Nonprobability sampling   Sampling error

Population   Simple random sampling

Probability sampling   Snowball sampling

Purposive sampling   Stratified random sampling

Quota sampling   Systematic random sampling

Random sampling   Target population

Representative sample   Theoretical sampling

■ Introduction

Keeping in mind that evidence-based practice (EBP) is about integrating the strongest research evidence with clinical expertise and patient needs (Melnyk & Fineout-Overholt, 2014), it is time to examine the research design decisions made in terms of sampling. Regardless of the topic of the research, every investigator must make decisions about which subjects will provide data to answer the research question. This is done through the development of a sampling plan—a process that involves making choices about who or what to include in the sample, how to select the sample, and how many subjects to include in the sample for a particular study. The choices made in developing the sampling plan are critical in designing high-quality clinical studies to build evidence-based nursing practice. Careful appraisal of the sampling plan in a published research study is critical to determining both the quality of the evidence and the applicability of the findings to nursing practice.

A **population** is the entire set of elements that meet specified criteria. An element may be a person, a family, a community, a medical record, an event, a laboratory specimen, or even a laboratory animal. Often called the **target population**, this set encompasses every element in the world that met the sampling criteria, such as all pregnant adolescents, preterm infants, persons with diabetes, or children who are chronically ill. The **accessible population**, by comparison, is that portion of the target population the investigator can reasonably reach. It might include pregnant adolescents enrolled in an alternative high school in the southeastern United States, persons with diabetes who are enrolled in diabetic education at a local hospital, or children with a chronic illness who are enrolled in a summer camp. The **sample**, drawn through a specified sampling strategy from the accessible population, consists of those elements from whom or about whom data are actually collected (**Figure 10-1**).

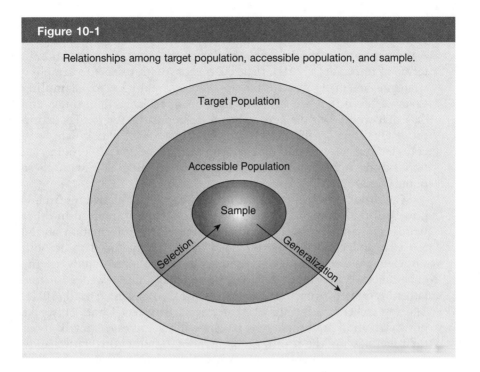

Figure 10-1

Relationships among target population, accessible population, and sample.

Target Population

Accessible Population

Sample

Selection

Generalization

Why Sample?

The purpose of sampling is to accurately draw conclusions about a population based on information from a subgroup of that population, called a sample. It is sometimes possible, even desirable, to obtain data from an entire population. For example, Antwi, Moriya, Simon, and Sommers (2015) performed a population-based study using a nationally representative data base of more than 17 million emergency department (ED) visits to determine the effect of the Patient Protection and Affordable Care Act on ED visits by young adults ages 19 to 25 (the age group targeted by the law). The researchers found that ED visits decreased after the enactment of the law, indicating that young adults seemed to alter their healthcare visit pattern to reflect a more efficient use of medical care.

Researchers, however, usually use samples rather than populations for reasons of efficiency and cost-effectiveness. In most cases, it would be almost impossible, and generally impractical, to conduct a study on the entire population, even though this is the population to which the investigator would like to be able to generalize the conclusions. Sampling strategies, therefore, have been designed to select a subset of the population to represent the entire population.

The overarching concern in evaluating a sample in quantitative research is how well the sample represents the target population. A **representative sample** is one that looks like the target population in terms of important characteristics. Decisions with respect to sampling strategies are made in an effort to reduce sampling error. **Sampling error** is the difference between data obtained from the sample and data that would be obtained if the entire population were included in the study. Thus, to the extent that the sample from which data were collected possesses important characteristics of the accessible and target populations, the findings can be used to develop EBP with these populations.

The major concern in evaluating a sample in qualitative research is how well the sample represents the phenomenon of interest. In other words, the sample must be appropriate to provide information on the research problem. The data provided by the sample need to be both sufficient and relevant. For example, in a qualitative study of the experience of becoming a father, researchers interviewed first-time fathers recruited from prenatal classes (Chin, Daiches, & Hall, 2011). The researchers performed the interviews between 4 and 11 weeks post-birth and found these new fathers willing and eager to talk about their feelings and the realities of fatherhood. Another qualitative study used focus groups consisting of women veterans to determine their attitudes and preferences related to intimate partner violence (IPV) screening within the Veterans Health Administration (Iverson et al., 2014). Researchers found that women believed such screening was important. This screening was true both for women who had experienced IPV and those who had not.

Two key elements in evaluating quantitative research are issues related to the internal and external validity of the findings. **Internal validity** refers to the extent to which the results of the study present an accurate picture of the real world. In other words, did the independent variable make a difference in the outcome, or were there other factors at work? The choice of a sampling strategy is designed to reduce sampling bias, one of the threats to internal validity. Sampling bias is evident when groups of people are either underrepresented or overrepresented in a sample. When assessing the sample in a study, the researcher should ask, "Did any characteristics of the sample influence the outcomes of the study?" Another threat to internal validity is a change in the world or within research participants themselves during the course of the study. Imagine, for example, the effects of the events on and after September 11, 2001, or in the aftermath of the 2015 terror attacks in Paris, on emotional, mental, and physical health and how they might affect study outcomes.

External validity, in contrast, refers to issues with generalizability of the findings from the research beyond the sample and situation that were studied. In other words, to whom and under which circumstances could the findings from this study be applied? When assessing the sample in a study, the researcher should ask, "How well does this group reflect the population as a whole?"

Internal and external validity do not apply in the same way to qualitative research. In qualitative studies, the sample is evaluated as to whether it is representative of the phenomenon of interest, rather than representative of the population as a whole. When assessing the sample in a qualitative study, the researcher should ask, "Did the sample chosen have the ability to talk about a phenomenon or an experience from the perspective of someone who was affected by it?"

■ Whom to Sample?

The responsibility of the investigator is to specify the sampling criteria or the characteristics necessary to be part of the research sample. It is these criteria that determine the target population. Sampling criteria may be very broad or very specific. These criteria are established to minimize bias or to control for irrelevant variability in the sample. Choosing a sample based on carefully selected criteria increases the strength of the evidence, thereby enhancing the ability to generalize the findings.

The researcher must make two different types of decisions—who should be considered for inclusion in the sample and who should be excluded from the sample. **Inclusion criteria** (sometimes called eligibility criteria) are those characteristics that must be met to be considered for participation in the study. Here, the investigator specifies what the sample will look like and which characteristics all study participants will have in common.

Exclusion criteria are not the polar opposite of the inclusion criteria, but rather those characteristics that, if present, would make persons ineligible to be in the sample, even though they might meet all of the inclusion criteria. These exclusions limit the representativeness of the sample and, therefore, the generalizability of the findings. As such, exclusion criteria should be specified after careful consideration. They should represent only those conditions or characteristics that might potentially make a difference in the outcome.

The specification of inclusion and exclusion criteria should not be taken lightly because of potential bias resulting in threats to internal validity and limitation of generalizability. Each criterion should be based on sound reasoning and be grounded in the goal of eliminating a

THINK OUTSIDE THE BOX

What are the potential threats to generalizability in the diabetes-related quality of life example (Hanna et al., 2014) described below?

potentially confounding effect on the outcome of the study. For example, in a study of predictors of diabetes-related quality of life in 17–19 year olds in the last 6 months of high school, the researchers used the following criteria when selecting the sample:

> eligibility criteria: type 1 diabetes for at least 1 year; able to read and speak English; and living with their parent or guardian. Youth were excluded if they had a serious psychiatric disorder or a second chronic illness that could interfere with becoming independent. (Hanna, Weaver, Slaven, Fotenberry, & DiMeglio, 2014, p. 401)

■ How to Sample?

There are two categories of sampling strategies—probability and nonprobability sampling. **Probability sampling** employs specific strategies designed to yield an unbiased (i.e., representative) sample by giving each element the possibility of being selected. The elements, which are each potential members of a sample, are chosen at random (by chance). **Nonprobability sampling** does not include random selection of elements and, therefore, has a higher possibility of yielding a biased (i.e., nonrepresentative) sample. In this case, researchers use elements that are accessible and available, and there is no way of estimating the probability that an element will be included in the sample.

The researcher makes the choice of whether to use a probability or nonprobability strategy based on the problem under investigation and the purpose of the study. Quantitative studies can use either probability or nonprobability sampling strategies. All decisions made about sampling in quantitative studies are based on maximizing the representativeness of the sample. Qualitative studies, because of their very nature, employ nonprobability sampling strategies. All decisions made about sampling in qualitative studies are based on maximizing the representativeness of the phenomenon of interest.

 THINK OUTSIDE THE BOX

Differentiate among the following terms: *target population, accessible population, representative sample, population,* and *sample.*

Probability Sampling Strategies

Probability sampling is the most well-respected type of sampling for quantitative studies, because it is more likely to produce a representative sample. It is not the same thing as random assignment, however. Random assignment is the process of randomly placing subjects in an experimental study in different treatment groups. **Random sampling** involves processes in which each element of the population has an equal chance of being in the sample. Four probability sampling strategies are commonly used: (1) simple random, (2) stratified random, (3) cluster, and (4) systematic random.

Simple random sampling is a process in which the researcher defines the population, lists and consecutively numbers all elements of the population, and then randomly selects a sample from this list.

The most simplistic method of simple random sampling is to put all of the numbers in a "hat" and draw out the desired number of elements. Obviously, this technique would work only for a study with a very small number of elements. For larger lists, the researcher can assign a number to each element and then use a computer program to randomly select the number of elements desired for the sample.

The random selection of the sample may also be accomplished by using a table of random numbers (**Table 10-1**). With this strategy, the researcher begins at any point on the list of numbers and reads consecutive numbers in any direction, choosing those numbers that correspond to the numbered elements in the population until the desired sample size is reached. For example, if you have a list of 50 elements from which to choose a random sample of 15, each element would be numbered from 01 to 50. If you closed your eyes and pointed at the data in Table 10-1 and your finger ended up on the numeral 91254, deciding to go across the rows to the right, the first two-digit number would be 91 (91254), which is not in your range of possibilities. The next two-digit number would be 25 (91254); that element would be selected, as would

Table 10-1				
Excerpt from a Table of Random Numbers				
65321	41047	96423	34988	12015
16523	87651	54210	26792	46234
69874	42036	69723	45631	89063
34702	15423	91254	24090	25752
42831	74369	17961	59467	13265
95032	20348	62349	27478	72159

42 (91254 24090), and 40 (24090). The next two-digit number would be 90 (24090), which is not in your range, followed by 25 (25752), which you have already selected, and 75 (25752), which is not in your range. Thus, the next elements selected would be 24 (25752 42831), 28 (42831), and 31 (42831). This process would continue until 15 elements were selected. Simple random selection is not widely used, because it is rather cumbersome and inefficient. Furthermore, it is rare to have the ability to list every element in the population.

Stratified random sampling is a variation on the simple random sampling technique. When the composition of a population with respect to some characteristic important to the study is known, the population is divided into two or more strata (groups) based on that characteristic. Simple random selection is then used to pick elements from each group. This selection strategy makes each group homogenous as far as the characteristic of interest is concerned. Examples of characteristics upon which stratification may be made include gender, age, ethnicity, occupation, education, and so forth. For example, in a study examining intention to use complementary and alternative medicine before conventional medicine, a two-staged stratified sampling strategy was used to randomly select 1,256 telephone numbers and then one eligible person in the household based on age, gender, and availability (Thomson, Jones, Browne, & Leslie, 2014).

If desired, the researcher may use proportional sampling to ensure that the sample accurately reflects the composition of the population on the characteristic by which the population was stratified. If, for example, 60% of the known population is male, the researcher might want to randomly select 60 males and 40 females for a total sample of 100. Proportional sampling is not generally a wise choice if the strata are of extremely disproportionate sizes. To demonstrate how this technique works, consider a study of variables associated with depression in non-Korean women married to Korean men and living in South Korea (Kim & Kim, 2013). In this study, proportional stratified random sampling was used to select 173 who were receiving services at a government-sponsored service center. Stratification was based on where the participant lived (urban versus rural) and the type of service center (community health service center or multicultural family support center). In this way, the researchers ensured representation of women from all strata without underrepresenting or overrepresenting either urban or rural dwelling women, or those receiving services from either type of service center.

Cluster sampling, also called multistage sampling, is a probability sampling strategy in which not all of the elements of the population need to be known. This strategy employs random selection of first larger sampling units (clusters), then successively smaller clusters, either by simple or stratified random selection techniques. It is a

---

❓ THINK OUTSIDE THE BOX

Why is the use of a randomly selected population a stronger sampling method than the use of a nonrandomized sample? Discuss the value of having the strongest sampling method possible for the research to be conducted.

---

particularly efficient strategy when the population is large and spread out over a large geographic area. For example, in an assessment of radiation emergency preparedness of the citizens of Oakland County, Michigan (population 1.2 million), 30 clusters (census blocks) were identified and 7 households in each cluster were interviewed (Nyaku et al., 2014). Interviewing the entire target population (all households in the county) would have been an impossible task. By identifying and selecting neighborhoods and then households within neighborhoods, however, researchers could conduct an overall assessment in a short period of time (3 days).

Systematic random sampling is a probability sampling technique in which elements are randomly selected from the population at predetermined, fixed intervals. The researcher first determines the desired sample size and then decides on the sampling interval. If the researcher has a list of the elements in the population, the sampling interval is determined by dividing the total population by the desired sample size. Suppose the population includes 750 individuals and the sample size is 50; in this case, the sampling interval would be 15. The researcher selects the first element randomly and then selects every 15th element thereafter to obtain the 50 elements for the sample. If the list is exhausted before the sample size is reached, counting resumes at the top of the list. This technique produces a random sample in a more efficient manner than is possible with simple randomization. For example, in a study of the role of gender in mental health and delinquent behaviors, systematic random sampling was used to select adolescents detained in Connecticut juvenile detention centers (Grigorenko, Sullivan, & Chapman, 2015). Chart reviews were then used to gather data relevant to the research question.

Nonprobability Sampling Strategies

The second broad category of sampling strategies is nonprobability sampling. These techniques are less likely to produce samples that are representative of the population. Nonetheless, they are more widely used in many disciplines, including nursing, because such samples are generally easier to obtain. Commonly used nonprobability sampling strategies include (1) convenience sampling, (2) quota sampling, (3) purposive sampling, (4) snowball sampling, and (5) theoretic sampling.

Convenience sampling is the process of selecting elements to be in the sample simply because they are readily available. Also called accidental sampling, it is the simplest and potentially least representative of all the sampling strategies. It is also currently the most frequently used sampling strategy in nursing research studies. Hanna and colleagues (2014) used convenience sampling in their recruitment of adolescents, and Iverson and colleagues (2014) used convenience sampling in obtaining their sample of women veterans.

Quota sampling begins with the researcher identifying strata of the population and then determining the number of elements in each stratum necessary to proportionately represent the population. Actual selection of elements from each stratum is then accomplished in the same way as in convenience sampling. In a study of the impact of chronic migraine, quota sampling was used to recruit a sample from an Internet research panel that was broadly representative of the U.S. population (Adams et al., 2015).

Purposive sampling, also called judgmental sampling, is a sampling strategy in which participants are handpicked by the researcher, either because they are typical of the phenomenon of interest or because they are knowledgeable about the issues under investigation. This strategy is often used when the researcher desires a sample consisting of experts. McCabe (2011) used this strategy to recruit 100 school nurses and 200 schoolteachers in her evaluation of their perceptions of fatigue among school children.

Snowball sampling, also known as network sampling, is a sampling strategy in which participants already in the study are asked to provide referrals to potential study subjects. Watson Campbell (2015) used purposive snowball sampling to recruit volunteers for her study of individuals who were discharged from a hospice program because of decertification. Tonsing (2015), in describing the recruitment of the 14 women in her study of South Asian women's experience of domestic violence, stated:

> Participants were mainly recruited through social service agencies serving ethnic minorities. The snowball sampling method was utilised [sic] which involved asking the participants to refer other women who had experienced domestic violence. Initially five women were recruited through the social service agencies, which in turn referred nine women. (para. 9)[*]

Snowball sampling is a particularly good strategy to use when potential participants in the study are challenging to find, as might be the case with vegetarians, drug abusers, persons engaged in prostitution, people with a specific disability or rare condition, and homeless individuals, for example.

---

[*]With kind permission from Springer Science+Business Media.

> **? THINK OUTSIDE THE BOX**
>
> Convenience sampling is the most commonly used sampling method. Which steps would you expect to see used within a study to strengthen the study in this type of sampling method?

Theoretical sampling is generally restricted to qualitative research methods, especially in conjunction with grounded theory. It is most analogous to the purposive sampling strategy. As the study unfolds and the interviews conducted with the first few participants are analyzed, conceptual categories and themes are identified. Subsequent decisions as to who will provide data and which data will be gathered are then based on who has already been sampled and which data have already been provided. Sampling and data collection continue until all of the categories and themes are "saturated"—that is, no additional categories or themes are emerging and no new facets of existing categories and themes are uncovered. Busby and Witucki-Brown (2011), for example, used theoretical sampling to select the 15 participants for a grounded theory explanation of how emergency response personnel utilize situational awareness in their management of multiple-casualty incidents.

How Many to Sample?

Once the researcher has decided whom to sample and how the sampling will be done, it is time to make the decision about how many elements need to be in the sample. The question of sample size is a crucial one when the objective is the ability to generalize the findings to a larger population. The generally accepted recommendation is to sample as many elements as possible. It is wise to remember, however, that the validity of a study begins with the design. Even the largest of samples cannot make up for faulty design.

Quantitative Studies

Several factors are taken into consideration when decisions are made about desired sample size in quantitative studies, including factors related to (1) the population, (2) the study design, (3) measurement, and (4) practicability.

Population Factors

Population-related factors that influence required sample size include the homogeneity of the population; the expected rate of the phenomenon, event, or outcome being measured; and the anticipated attrition rate.

In a population that is fairly homogenous (i.e., in which sampling elements are very similar to one another), the required sample size is generally smaller than if the population were more heterogeneous. Similarly, if the phenomenon, event, or outcome occurs frequently, a smaller sample size is needed than if occurrences are infrequent.

In longitudinal studies, attrition may be a problem. When this phenomenon is anticipated to occur, researchers often "over-enroll" participants in the research. If, for example, a study were expected to have an attrition rate of 20% (i.e., if 100 subjects were to begin the study, only 80 would complete it), then the researcher would enroll 125 participants so as to have the desired 100 at completion.

Design Factors

Design factors influencing sample size include the type of study, the number of variables, and the sampling strategy. Quantitative studies, in general, require larger sample sizes than do qualitative studies. Some differences also occur in relation to the quantitative designs themselves. First, a study that is more complex requires a larger sample size. For example, a study employing a longitudinal data collection plan needs to enroll increased numbers of participants at the beginning because of the increased possibility of losing subjects over the course of the study (sample attrition). Second, as the number of variables being measured increases, so does the needed sample size. Third, the sampling strategy itself can affect the required sample size. Stratified random sampling and quota sampling techniques, for example, allow the researcher to use smaller sample sizes than would be needed in studies employing simple random or convenience sampling, because some of the representativeness is already built into the stratification procedure.

Measurement Factors

Measurement factors that influence sample size include the sensitivity of the research instruments and the effect that the process has on the outcome. Data collection instruments in which measurement error is minimal are said to be precise. The less precise the instrument, the larger the sample size might need to be. Because interval-level data are generally more precise, from a sample size perspective it is best to measure at that level if at all possible, because a smaller sample size may be used.

Practical Factors

Practical factors such as cost and convenience also influence sample size. Although population factors, design factors, and measurement factors certainly affect the ideal sample size, it is these practical factors that often prove most influential. When this is the case, adjustments in design and/or sampling strategies need to be made to strengthen the internal validity of the study.

Given these practical factors, how do researchers determine the sample size needed for a particular study? Some use the "rule of 30": There should be 30 subjects for each group or 30 subjects for each variable. This notion is based on the central limit theorem, which asserts that, in a randomly generated sample of 30 or more subjects, the mean of a characteristic will approximate the population mean (Hinkle, Wiersma, & Jurs, 1988). It is essential to remember, however, that representativeness is more important than sample size. The "rule of 30" should, therefore, be considered the minimum acceptable sample size rather than the ideal.

The gold standard in determining sample size is power analysis, a statistical calculation of the number of subjects needed to accurately reject the null hypothesis (Jupiter, 2014). The actual calculation of sample size is beyond the scope of this text. The most commonly used significance level is 0.05 and the standard power is 0.80. The effect size is estimated based on pilot studies undertaken by the researcher or on reports in the literature drawn from previous studies on the same or similar problems. Performing the power analysis prior to conducting a study strengthens the study's credibility concerning the size of the sample utilized. For example, here is the description of the power analysis for a study of the impact of self-management strategies for individuals with long-term indwelling urinary catheters:

> Power calculations were performed ... All calculations employed a significance level of .05 and 80% power.... The analysis indicated that a sample of 220 (160 completers) would provide sufficient power to detect medium effect sizes (15%–30% differences between groups) for the primary health status outcomes. (Wilde et al., 2015, p. 26)

Power analysis formulas are sometimes applied after the fact to determine the power of a test given the sample size and results obtained. Sometimes the formula is used on a post hoc basis to determine the optimal sample size. For example, in a study comparing outcomes of care for an ulcer on a leg in a sample of 104 patients who chose either a nurse-led clinic or home care, the post hoc analysis revealed only a 48% power to find a difference in treatment (Harrison et al., 2011).

Qualitative Studies

Qualitative studies generally employ relatively small, nonrandom samples. Because the aim of qualitative research is to describe and analyze the meanings and experiences of particular individuals or groups, large sample sizes are not generally appropriate or feasible in these scenarios. Instead, the sample size should be sufficient to provide enough information to answer the research question based on the notion of data saturation. Participants continue to be enrolled in a study until no new information is being uncovered; that is, redundancy occurs in all subsequent data collection encounters.

> ### ❓ THINK OUTSIDE THE BOX
>
> What would be the implications of the "rule of 30" applied to qualitative research?

Redundancy may be achieved with a limited number of participants when the sample is homogenous. For this reason, it is not unusual to have very small sample sizes in phenomenologic studies. For example, Fecher-Jones and Taylor (2015) had 11 participants in their study of patients who had laparoscopic colon resection and participated in an enhanced recovery program, and Underhill and Dickerson (2011) interviewed nine participants for their study of the experience of women with a hereditary risk of breast cancer who were participating in a breast surveillance program.

In contrast, for ethnographic or grounded theory studies in which the sample is usually more heterogeneous, larger sample sizes are generally the norm. For example, an ethnography approach was used with 32 women who shared their perspectives on the 1-month postnatal practices in China (Holroyd, Lopez, & Chan, 2011), 30 registered nurses who supplied the data upon which a grounded theory of end-of-life care was developed (McCallin, 2011), and 24 women veterans who provided data with respect to screening for intimate partner violence (Iverson et al., 2014).

◼ Specific Evidence-Based Practice Considerations

Evidence-based clinical decisions are essential for the practice of nursing. Melnyk and Fineout-Overholt (2014) have rightly asserted, "The goal of EBP is to use the highest quality of knowledge in providing care to produce the greatest impact on patients' health status and healthcare" (p. 75). It is imperative, therefore, to have the ability to critically examine the available research and to determine the strength of the evidence. Several guiding questions can help direct reading about and critiquing sampling plans. While these questions are similar in some respects in both quantitative and qualitative research, they differ in many other respects (**Table 10-2**).

Quantitative Evidence Critique

A well-written quantitative research report contains a detailed explanation of the sampling strategy (including sample size determination) and the inclusion and exclusion criteria together with the rationale for their use. Kahre, Fortune, Hurley, and Winsett (2011), for example, provided

Table 10-2	
Guidelines for Critiquing the Sample for Evidence-Based Practice	
Quantitative Research Studies	1. How and when was the desired sample size determined?
	2. Was the sample size adequate to answer the research question?
	3. What were the inclusion and exclusion criteria?
	4. Was the sampling strategy one of probability or nonprobability? Was this strategy appropriate to the research question?
	5. Is the sample for the study clearly described?
	6. Are there potential biases in the sample selection or the sample itself that could have an effect on the outcome of the study?
	7. Is the sample representative of the target population? Is it representative of your own patients?
Qualitative Research Studies	1. Which sampling strategy was used to choose the participants?
	2. Was the sample size adequate to answer the research question?
	3. Is the sample for the study clearly described?
	4. Is the sample representative of the phenomenon of interest?

the following description of the sampling plan in their comparison of measures for pain relief for IV insertion:

> Sample size was calculated using software for power and sample size calculations with estimated standard deviation of change scores at 0.80 power. Nine subjects per group were needed to detect a medium difference. A sample size of 40 healthy adult subjects was estimated to provide an adequate sample size for subgroup analyses. Inclusion criteria for eligibility to participate were licensed registered nurses (RN) aged 21 years or older, palpable veins in hand, forearm or antecubital bilaterally, no allergy to benzyl alcohol or lidocaine, and normal healthy adult as defined in the American Society of Anesthesiologists' (ASA) Physical Status Classification System. (p. 311)[†]

The well-written quantitative research report also thoroughly describes the demographic characteristics of the sample that actually participated in the study:

> The sample included 56 subjects with a mean of 18.6 ± 10.6 years as an RN. Forty-eight (86%) were Caucasian females. Mean years in direct care were 7.5 ± 4.7 years, and the subjects reported a mean of 5.2 ± 4.4 years of IV starts as part of their job description. (Kahre et al., 2011, p. 312)[‡]

[††] Reprinted from Kahre, C., Fortune, V., Hurley, J., & Winsett, R. P. (2011). Randomized controlled trial to compare effects of pain relief during IV insertion using bacteriostatic normal saline and 1% buffered lidocaine. *Journal of PeriAnesthesia Nursing, 26*, 310–314. doi:10.1016/j.jopan.2011.05.009, copyright 2011, with permission from Elsevier.

Descriptions such as these allow the reader to determine the representativeness of the sample for their own population and establish the strength of the evidence for implementing the findings.

Qualitative Evidence Critique

A well-written qualitative research report also contains a detailed explanation of the sampling strategy and a description of the sample obtained. Iverson and colleagues (2011), for example, described the plan they used to recruit participants in their study of women veterans as follows:

> Women VHA [Veterans Health Administration] patients were recruited via fliers in clinics and advertising areas (e.g., bulletin boards) throughout three campuses of the VA Boston Healthcare System. The fliers indicated that the researchers were recruiting women with and without IPV histories and were interested in understanding women patients' attitudes and preferences regarding care for IPV within VHA. Women who did not experience IPV were included because they inevitably would be asked about IPV if VHA providers adopted universal screening. (p. 303)

Evaluating the Evidence for Implementation

Once the sample characteristics and size have been critically analyzed, the next step in determining appropriateness for consideration for EBP is to establish whether this evidence, however good, is applicable in the local situation. For example, in a study of a smoking cessation intervention for pregnant women, Chertok and Archer (2015) employed an intervention using the 5 "A"s program (Ask, Advise, Assess, Assist, Arrange) that was effective in decreasing smoking among pregnant women. Abroms and colleagues (2015) devised a mobile phone smoking cessation program (Quit4baby) in which encouraging and motivational messages were sent to participants via text messaging. The samples in both studies were primarily Caucasian, married or living with a partner, and had at least a high school education.

A nurse who wanted to implement a smoking cessation program with a population that was primarily from ethnic minority groups would need to carefully consider whether the strategy designed by these researchers could be applied in the local setting. An alternative in this situation would be to examine the smoking cessation strategies employed in the studies conducted by Katz and colleagues (2011) and Hennrikus and colleagues (2010), whose samples were predominately from ethnic minorities, unmarried, unemployed, and having a high school education or less. The use of paraprofessional home visits as

THINK OUTSIDE THE BOX

Specific evidence-based practice considerations: Identify the demographic characteristics of a sample that would be representative of the population with whom you are currently working in a clinical course.

described by Katz and colleagues or the mobilization of support within pregnant women's social networks as described in the Hennrikus and colleagues study might be more appropriate for pregnant women in ethnic minorities.

Sampling Decisions for an Evidence-Based Project

After identifying the clinical question or problem on which to build an evidence-based project and deciding, based on the strength of the evidence, on an appropriate intervention or change in practice, a sampling decision must be made. Based on the information contained in this chapter, it should be clear that the best (i.e., the strongest) sampling technique would be a random assignment of patients to either the nursing intervention or the standard of care. If it were not possible to randomize the participants, then a nonrandom sampling plan would be appropriate if efforts to build in representativeness through matching or purposive sampling procedures were used.

■ Conclusion

Although they are only one component in the overall research process, sampling decisions affect the internal validity and the external validity of a study. As such, critical analysis of the sampling strategy, the sample size, and the quality of the sample are essential in determining the relevance of the results of one study, or a group of studies, to EBP for nurses.

Summary Points

1. The population of interest is that group to whom the researcher wants to be able to characterize and generalize.
2. Sampling allows a researcher to draw conclusions about the research problem under investigation based on information from a portion of the population, rather than the whole population.

3. The researcher selects a sample from an accessible population that is representative of the target population to whom the findings may be generalized.

4. Probability sampling strategies employ random selection of elements of the population. Probability strategies include simple random, systematic random, stratified random, and cluster sampling.

5. Nonprobability sampling strategies employ nonrandom selection of elements of the population. Nonprobability strategies include convenience, quota, purposive, snowball, and theoretical sampling.

6. Sampling decisions in quantitative research are made based on the desire to have a representative sample. Sampling strategies include both probability and nonprobability strategies.

7. Sampling decisions in qualitative research are made based on the desire to obtain data that are representative of the phenomenon of interest. Sampling strategies are almost always nonprobability strategies.

8. Critiquing studies to determine their relevance for evidence-based practice (EBP) involves evaluation of the sampling plan, sampling strategies, and sample size for their appropriateness to the research question and the research design.

RED FLAGS

- Randomization of a sample group strengthens a study. Bias within the sampling process is decreased by randomization.

- The appropriate sample size for a quantitative study is best established by performing a power analysis before the study gets underway.

- Convenience and snowball sampling methodologies are weak sampling methods owing to their higher potential for lack of generalizability and potential for bias.

- At the least, inclusion criteria should be documented for review within the research report. Both inclusion and exclusion criteria should be provided.

- Failure to utilize the "rule of 30" can weaken a study.

- Inadequate or unclear description of the sampling strategy results in confusion when others attempt to understand the study's conclusions.

- Failure to use a sampling strategy that would produce a sample size appropriate for the particular research method leads to a limitation for the study.

- Attempts to generalize findings past the representativeness of the sample are inappropriate.

- Failure to acknowledge limitations resulting from sample size or sample selection decisions is problematic.

Multiple-Choice Questions

1. A researcher who wishes to study the impact of having a child with cystic fibrosis on family functioning contacts the local chapter of the Cystic Fibrosis Foundation for assistance in finding parents to interview. Parents of children with cystic fibrosis in the local chapter are the:

    A. Target population.
    B. Accessible population.
    C. Sample.
    D. Participants.

2. A nurse wishes to explore attitudes of critical care nurses toward family presence during resuscitation. She selected for interview 10 nurses who favored family presence and 10 who did not. This is an example of which sampling method?

    A. Snowball sampling
    B. Convenience sampling
    C. Theoretical sampling
    D. Purposive sampling

3. A sample that accurately reflects the characteristics of the population is known as which type of sample?

    A. Random sample
    B. Purposive sample
    C. Representative sample
    D. Probability sample

4. Which of the following types of studies would require the largest sample size?

    A. A study in which the population is homogeneous
    B. A study involving multiple variables
    C. A study measuring interval-level variables
    D. A study using cluster sampling

5. A researcher has decided to conduct a satisfaction survey among all of the patients who presented to the emergency department over a 2-month period of time. This is an example of which sampling method?

    A. Stratified random sampling
    B. Cluster sampling
    C. Convenience sampling
    D. Purposive sampling

6. In a study of nursing students' attitudes toward caring for patients with hypertension who are noncompliant with their medications, the researcher randomly selected a sample of nursing students from a list of all students enrolled in each of five nursing programs that had been randomly selected from one state. Because the sample was randomly selected, to which population can the findings be generalized?

   A. Nursing students in the programs that were randomly selected
   B. Nursing students in the state from which the programs were randomly selected
   C. Nursing students in the United States
   D. All nursing students

7. A power analysis determined that a sample size of 196 would provide a power of 0.80 with an alpha less than 0.05. The study enrolled 202 subjects. Is the sample size adequate, and why?

   A. No; the power achieved with a sample size of 196 is only 0.80.
   B. No; the sample size is inadequate to prevent a Type I error.
   C. Yes; the sample size was supported by a power analysis.
   D. Yes; 202 subjects were included, way more than the minimum of 30.

8. When is determination of an adequate sample size in qualitative research determined?

   A. A power analysis indicates the power is 0.70.
   B. The sample size is large enough to identify differences in groups.
   C. Saturation and redundancy of data are achieved.
   D. A sample size of 30 is obtained.

9. Which of the following would be the strongest method for assigning 50 subjects to treatment and control groups in an experimental study?

   A. Group subjects according to attending physician.
   B. List subjects alphabetically, divide the list in half, place the first 25 names in the treatment group and the last 25 in the control group.
   C. Assign each participant a number, place even-numbered participants in the treatment group and the odd-numbered in the control group.
   D. Assign each participant a number, place the numbers in a box, and draw numbers from the box, alternating placement in either the treatment group or the control group.

10. In interpreting quantitative research results, the representativeness of the sample is most closely tied to which of the following?

   A. Internal validity
   B. External validity
   C. Sample validity
   D. Research validity

Discussion Questions

1. You are a nurse working in the labor and delivery suite in an academic medical center. You are interested in nonpharmacologic pain management for your patients and would like to implement an evidence-based change project on your unit. Which particular sampling concerns will you examine in the research studies about nonpharmacologic pain management for laboring patients?

2. You are a BSN student enrolled in a research course. The instructor has given you the following problem statement: "Does music affect the perception of pain in patients who have undergone hip replacement?" Describe one probability sampling plan and one nonprobability sampling plan for answering this question.

3. Read the excerpt that follows from an article describing a study testing a self-management intervention for long-term indwelling catheters and answer the following questions:
    a. What is the sampling strategy used?
    b. What were the inclusion and exclusion criteria?
    c. What are the sample characteristics?
    d. Is this sample representative?
    e. How could the sampling strategy be improved?

    > Participants consisted of community-dwelling individuals recruited in two distinct regions by two study sites: (a) a university in a large northeastern U.S. state and (b) a home care agency that conducts research in a large metropolitan area in the same state. For the university site, participants were recruited through nurses or physicians ... In the home care agency, their database was used to identify potential participants ... Screening for eligibility and interest in participation was conducted by phone ... Eligible participants were adults aged 18 and above. Inclusion criteria were as follows: (a) expect to use an indwelling urethral or suprapubic catheter for at least 1 year and will be in the study region for at least 4 months; (b) can complete study measurements alone or with the help of a caregiver; (c) speak English; and (d) have access to a telephone... Individuals were excluded for terminal illness or cognitive impairments. Children under 18 were not included ... Ages ranged from 19 to 96 years (Mdn = 61). The range in duration of catheter use was 1–470 months (39 years). Self-reported diagnoses involved spinal cord injury (40%), multiple sclerosis (23%), diabetes (12%), stroke (2%), prostate (10%), spina bifida (1%), neurogenic bladder not otherwise reported (8%), Parkinson's disease (2%), and others (3%). (Wilde et al., 2015, pp. 25, 28)

Suggested Readings

Cleary, M., Horsfall, J., & Hayter, M. (2104). Data collection and sampling in qualitative research: Does size matter? *Journal of Advanced Nursing*, *70*(3), 473–475. doi:10.1111/jan.12163

Kandola, D., Banner, D., O'Keefe-McCarthy, S., & Jassal, D. (2014). Sampling methods in cardiovascular nursing research: An overview. *Canadian Journal of Cardiovascular Nursing*, *24*(3), 15–18.

References

Abroms, L. C., Johnson, P. R., Heminger, C. L., Van Alstyne, J. M., Leavitt, L. E., Schindler-Ruwisch, J. M., & Bushar, J. A. (2015). Quit4baby: Results from a pilot test of a mobile smoking cessation program for pregnant women. *Journal of Medical Internet Research, 3*(1). doi:10.2196/mhealth.3846

Adams, A. M., Serrano, D., Buse, D. C., Reed, M. L., Marske, V., Fanning, K. M., & Lipton, R. B. (2015). The impact of chronic migraine: The Chronic Migraine Epidemiology and Outcomes (CaMEO) Study methods and baseline results. *Cephalalgia: An International Journal of Headache, 35*(7), 563–578. doi:10.1177/0333102414552532

Antwi, Y. A., Moriya, A. S., Simon, K., & Sommers, B. D. (2015). Changes in emergency department use among young adults after the Patient Protection and Affordable Care Act's dependent coverage provision. *Annals of Emergency Medicine, 65*(6), 664–672.

Busby, S., & Wituki-Brown, J. (2011). Theory development for situational awareness in multi-casualty incidents. *Journal of Emergency Nursing, 37,* 444–452. http://dx.doi.org/10.1016/j.jen.2010.07.023

Chertok, I. R., & Archer, S. H. (2015). Evaluation of a midwife- and nurse-delivered 5 A's prenatal smoking cessation program. *Journal of Midwifery & Women's Health, 60,* 175–181. doi:10.1111/jmwh.12220

Chin, R., Daiches, A., & Hall, P. (2011). A qualitative exploration of first time fathers' experiences of becoming a father. *Community Practitioner, 84*(7), 19–23.

Fecher-Jones, I., & Taylor, C. (2015). Lived experience, enhanced recovery and laparoscopic colonic resection. *British Journal of Nursing, 24*(4), 223–228. http://dx.doi.org/10.12968/bjon.2015.24.4.223

Grigorenko, E. L., Sullivan, T., & Chapman, J. (2015). An investigation of gender differences in a representative sample of juveniles detained in Connecticut. *International Journal of Law and Psychiatry, 38,* 84–91. doi:10.1016/j.ijlp.2015.01.011

Hanna, K. M., Weaver, J. E., Slaven, J., Fortenberry, D., & DiMeglio, L. A. (2014). Diabetes-related quality of life and the demands and burdens of diabetes care among emerging adults with type 1 diabetes in the year after high school graduation. *Research in Nursing & Health, 37,* 399–408. doi:10.1002/nur.21620

Harrison, M. B., VanDenKerkhof, E., Hopman, W. M., Graham, I. D., Lorimer, K., & Carley, M. (2011). Evidence-informed leg ulcer care: A cohort study comparing outcomes of individuals choosing nurse-led clinic or home care. *Ostomy Wound Management, 57*(8), 38–45.

Hennrikus, D., Pirie, P., Hellerstedt, W., Lando, H. A., Steele, J., & Dunn, C. (2010). Increasing support for smoking cessation during pregnancy and postpartum: Results of a randomized controlled pilot study. *Preventive Medicine, 50,* 134–137. doi:10.1016/j.ypmed.2010.01.003

Hinkle, D., Wiersma, W., & Jurs, S. (1988). *Applied statistics for the behavioral sciences* (2nd ed.). Boston, MA: Houghton-Mifflin.

Holroyd, E., Lopez, V., & Chan, S. W. (2011). Negotiating "doing the month": An ethnographic study examining the postnatal practices of two generations of Chinese women. *Nursing & Health Sciences, 13,* 47–52. doi:10.1111/j.1442-2018.2011.00575.x

Iverson, K. M., Huang, K., Wells, S. Y., Wright, J. D., Gerber, M. R., & Wiltsey-Stirman, S. (2014). Women veterans' preferences for intimate partner violence screening and response procedures within the Veterans Health Administration. *Research in Nursing & Health, 37,* 302–311. doi:10.1002/nur.21602

Jupiter, D. C. (2014). Counting your chickens before they're hatched: Power analysis. *Journal of Foot and Ankle Surgery, 53,* 519–520. doi:10.1053/j.jfas.2014.05.001

Kahre, C., Fortune, V., Hurley, J., & Winsett, R. P. (2011). Randomized controlled trial to compare effects of pain relief during IV insertion using bacteriostatic normal saline and 1% buffered lidocaine. *Journal of PeriAnesthesia Nursing, 26,* 310–314. doi:10.1016/j.jopan.2011.05.009

Katz, K. S., Jarrett, M. H., El-Mohandes, A. A., Schneider, S., McNeely-Johnson, D., & Kiely, M. (2011). Effectiveness of a combined home visiting and group intervention for low income African American mothers: The pride in parenting program. *Maternal and Child Health Journal, 15*(Suppl.1), S75–S84. doi:10.1007/s10995-011-0858-x

Kim, H. S., & Kim, H. S. (2013). Depression in non-Korean women residing in South Korea following marriage to Korean men. *Archives of Psychiatric Nursing, 27,* 148–155. doi:10.1016/j.apnu.2013.02.005

McCabe, M. A. (2011). Perceptions of school nurses and teachers of fatigue in children. *Pediatric Nursing, 37,* 244–250, 255.

McCallin, A. M. (2011). Moderated guiding: A grounded theory of nursing practice in end-of-life care. *Journal of Clinical Nursing, 20*(15–16), 2325–2333. doi:10.1111/j.1365-2702.2010.03543.x

Melnyk, B. M., & Fineout-Overholt, E. (2014). *Evidence-based practice in nursing and healthcare: A guide to best practice* (3rd ed.). Philadelphia, PA: Lippincott Williams & Wilkins.

Nyaku, M. K., Wolkin, A. F., McFadden, J., Collins, J., Murti, M., Schnall, A.,... Bayleyegn, T. M. (2014). Assessing radiation emergency preparedness planning by using community assessment for public health emergency response (CASPER) methodology. *Prehospital and Disaster Medicine, 29,* 262–269. doi:10.1017/S1049023X14000491

Thomson, P., Jones, J., Browne, M., & Leslie, S. J. (2014). Why people seek complementary and alternative medicine before conventional medicine: A population based study. *Complementary Therapies in Clinical Practice, 20,* 339–346. doi:10.1016/j.ctcp.2014.07.008

Tonsing, J. C. (2015). Domestic violence: Intersection of culture, gender and context. *Journal of Immigrant and Minority Public Health.* Advance online publication. doi:10.1007/s10903-015-0193-1

Underhill, M. L., & Dickerson, S. S. (2011). Engaging in medical vigilance: Understanding the personal meaning of breast surveillance. *Oncology Nursing Forum, 38,* 686–694. doi:10.1188/11.ONF.686-694

Watson Campbell, R. (2015). Being discharged from hospice alive: The lived experience of patients and families. *Journal of Palliative Medicine, 18*(6), 495–499. doi:10.1089/jpm.2014.0228.

Wilde, M. H., McMahon, J. M., McDonald, M. V., Tang, W., Wang, W., Brasch, J., ... Chen D. G. (2015). Self-management intervention for long-term indwelling urinary catheter users: Randomized clinical trial. *Nursing Research, 64*(1), 24–34. doi:10.1097/NNR.0000000000000071

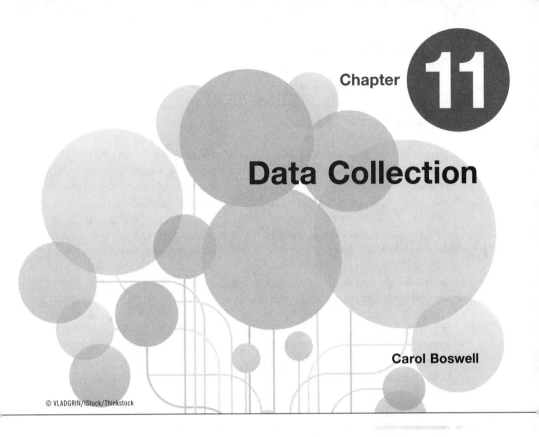

Chapter **11**

Data Collection

Carol Boswell

Chapter Objectives

At the conclusion of this chapter, the learner will be able to:

1. Contrast a researcher's decision to use accessible data versus new data.
2. Distinguish various forms of data collection processes.

Key Terms

Accessible data	Novel data
Biophysiological data	Observation
Closed-ended questions	Open-ended questions
Data collection	Primary data
Focus group	Questionnaire
Interview	Secondary data
In vitro	Systematic review
In vivo	Tests
Meta-analysis	

■ Overview of Data Collection Methods and Sources

Data come in many forms and are obtained through multiple methodologies. **Data collection** is a foundational piece of all aspects of the research process. The data collection process should drive the tool selection, aid in the determination of the research methodology, speak to the questions about sampling, and drive the selection of the statistical/evaluation process for the study. As a result, the process of collecting data essentially establishes boundaries for a project. As a researcher begins to conceptualize the implementation of a research project, the question of the appropriate facts required for addressing the PICOT (population, intervention, comparison, outcome, time) question(s), research question(s), research purpose(s), and/or hypothesis(es) becomes critical. According to LoBiondo-Wood and Haber (1998), "The major difference between the data collected when performing patient care and the data collected for the purpose of research is that the data collection method employed by researchers needs to be objective and systematic" (p. 308). The independence and organization of the data collection practice provide for generalizability of a research project's resulting outcomes to a broader population. By carefully building the research project around the data that will best address the question raised within the study, each aspect of the research process becomes increasingly appropriate to gather the information needed to answer the burning question.

The specification of the outcome for each phase of the data collection plan is mandatory. When all aspects and/or variables of the data required for the study are established prior to the initiation of the study, the selection of the appropriate data collection method can be effectively addressed as part of this specification. This process decreases the potential for unintentionally omitting a key component of the data. Data collection is fundamental to the entire process, resulting in the need to carefully consider the use of different types of data and/or processes when making the decisions about data collection methods. The nature of the data needed within the study must be reflected in the final section of the methods to be used to collect the needed data successfully.

Before delving into a discussion of the functions of data collection sources and data collection tools/instruments, it is helpful to have an understanding of the definitions of selected concepts. The term *source* within the data collection process of research focuses on the processes used to collect the data. These sources can be any tool or instrument or any process, such as interviewing, observation, or focus groups, by which information can be accessed. The sources for data collection can be varied but require a connection with the participants. Data collection "tools/instruments" comprise the actual physical devices employed to collect the information that is under investigation. The use of a tool/ instrument does not mandate a direct connection with the participants, as these tools could be delivered by mail or through the Internet. Tools and instruments can be hard copy collection forms such as tests and questionnaires, but can also be tools that provide physiological data such as laboratory equipment, weight scales, and x-ray reports.

There are several major methods of data collection:

- Tests
- Questionnaires
- Interviews
- Focus groups
- Observations
- Biophysiological data
- Systematic reviews
- Existing or secondary data

The data set identified by the researcher for any selected study can usually be accessed by one or more of these methods.

According to Polit and Beck (2008), the researcher must try to determine which data will effectively address the question under investigation, describe the sample characteristics, establish methods for controlling extraneous variables, analyze impending biases, recognize subgroup effects, and check for manipulation of the data. Creswell (2003) reinforces this notion by identifying the data collection steps, including (1) establishing the boundaries for the study, (2) accumulating the data through the appropriate methodologies, and (3) clarifying the process for recording and managing the data collected. As a result, the researcher has the responsibility to understand the different formats of data collection, the strengths and weaknesses of the different methods, and the specific needs recognized for the topic under evaluation.

Accessible Data Versus Novel Data

As the researcher begins the process of clarifying the data collection process, a key question arises concerning the type of information that will be used to satisfy the question being investigated. Two types of data can be identified—accessible (existing) or new (novel). The aspects of each of these data types need to be conscientiously considered as the researcher determines the data collection process.

Accessible data may also be called existing data; they provide an essential source for use in research endeavors. This information may be located in preexisting reports (e.g., hospital records, databases, narrative journaling documents, historic documents). It can be used as the basis for a secondary analysis of the data gathered in a previous study or as records developed for some other reason, such as hospital patient records and national databases. The use of preexisting records, often called a retrospective chart/record review, is common in nursing research because these documents are an economical and convenient source of information. Questions do arise with this form of data. The records' biases and incompleteness raise concerns because the data must be used "as is." Accessible data cannot be expanded or further clarified. Secondary analysis of data allows for the use of data collected for a prior project to test one or more different hypotheses and illuminate fresh relationships located within the data. When preexisting data can be used, this practice does eliminate the time-consuming and costly process of collecting the data before beginning the analysis process. The use of accessible (existing) data serves as the foundation for evidence-based practice. Meta-analyses, synthesis analyses, and meta-syntheses, which use obtainable research reports as their underlying data base, integrate the material to provide the foundation for evidence-based protocol guidelines.

New or **novel data** comprise original information collected for a specific study. This type of data is unique to the question or questions under investigation. The researcher needs to judiciously determine each component of data needed for the particular question(s). Within the time sequence allocated for the research project, all of the various pieces of data must be collected. The data collection plan should address each aspect of the needed information so that at some point during the process, it is all collected for use during the analysis process. It is helpful during the process to consult a statistician to ensure that the data will address the key questions being investigated.

Another way to classify data is either as primary data or secondary data. Primary (novel) data are data generated through the actual conducting of an original study. **Primary data** provide direct access into the actual process being reported. The information comes from the source without any additional interpretations or modifications. In contrast, secondary (accessible) data are pulled from existing data and documents (Management Study Guide, 2013). **Secondary data** are information interpreted by the alternative reviewer or investigator. Each reviewer tends to include their individualized analysis of the information as it applies to a given situation. Thus, additional biases from the further interpretation of the materials may be introduced. This process of using accessible or secondary data is termed "data mining."

■ Key Categories of Data for Nursing Studies

Within any research design, the data collection process must be matched to the stated study aims and/or purpose and reflect the particular strategies implemented during the study. Many data sources are available for use.

> **❓ THINK OUTSIDE THE BOX**
>
> Using the following examples of research questions, select a data collection method and justify your selection:
> 1. What information has been used to determine the use of 6-hour NPO (nil per os, or "not by mouth") status prior to an outpatient surgical procedure versus a 12-hour NPO status level?
> 2. What information serves as the basis for the range of blood sugars used within newly diagnosed adolescent diabetics?
> 3. What information could be used to determine the cause of patient falls?

They include secondary data from national surveys and other secondary data sources such as Medicaid, demographic indicators, nonclinical program data, clinical program data, public comments, informant groups, questionnaire/interview surveys, screenings, and epidemiology surveys. Researchers must carefully and thoroughly contemplate the various methods of data collection and the various sources of data, thereby ensuring they select the most appropriate options.

Orcher (2005) identified two feasible incentives for using established instruments. Established tools are identified as validated tools based on the number of times that the tool has been successfully used while fostering a reliable body of research. By using a validated tool for a study, the results can be compared and contrasted to the prior studies that used the tool. As tools are used in subsequent studies, the validity and reliability of the tool are further established for different populations. Each of the two incentives can have a profound impact on the quality of the research study outcomes:

- Initially, time and energy should be expended to ensure that the data collected are appropriate for the study question(s) and the methodology is effective in capturing the total picture needed to address the research problem.
- Care should be given to identifying any confounding variables that could adversely affect the research outcomes.

◼ Significant Facets of Data Collection Schemes

As the investigator establishes the data collection methodology for a study, questions concerning the consistency of the data collected from each participant become of paramount importance. The basic idea is that the data should be collected in the same manner for each of the participants so that unique environmental, societal, and physical effects are diminished. One aspect impacting research projects is what has been labeled the Hawthorne effect. The original study was conducted at the Hawthorne Works to determine the effect lighting had on worker's productivity (New World Encyclopedia, 2014). The Hawthorne effect refers to the susceptibility of some individuals to labor harder and/or function better when being observed such as in a research study. As Cherry (2015) states, "individuals may change their behavior due to the attention they are receiving from researchers rather than because of any manipulation of independent variables" (para. 1). Concerns related to the Hawthorne effect, for example, must be carefully thought about to minimize the potential of participants modifying their behaviors because they are affected—either positively or negatively—by being included in a study. As studies of the Hawthorne effect have shown, the simple act of being selected to participate in a project can result in the modification of the behavior being evaluated. This effect is real. Researchers must carefully consider all aspects of the data collection process to diminish the likelihood that the resulting modifications will be so pronounced that the data collected are of little value.

Another important aspect within the data collection process is interrater reliability. In studies that employ more than one data collector, the goal is to ensure accuracy, such that each of the data collectors accumulates the information in the exact same way. According to Melnyk and Fineout-Overholt (2005), it is critical to prepare data collectors to use the instrument planned for use in a study. This planning allows for interrater reliability, or consistency, in the paradigm that is being observed at least 90% of the time (Melnyk & Fineout-Overholt, 2005). If the 90% rate cannot be accomplished, the researcher and data collectors must establish a level of agreement for the specific project that considers the element of chance. Items that have to be carefully considered within this process are the need to use the same questions by each data collector, the ordering of the question delivery, and the acceptability of providing interpretations to the participants. If one data collector does these items but another does not, the results could be affected.

Now let's turn our attention to the types of data collection methods. In the remainder of this chapter, for each method, an overview of the method expectations, strengths of the method, and limitations resulting from its use are discussed.

■ Test Methods

Overview

The use of **tests** within the research process is a fairly common methodology for ascertaining the explicit intelligence, talents, behaviors, or cognitive endeavor that is under investigation. Frequently, the terms tool, instrument, and *standardized test* are used interchangeably to describe this research method. These devices are used within research to appraise characteristics, aptitude, accomplishments, and performance. The use of self-reporting strategies when the goal is collection of vast amounts of research information appears to be an effective process. Directness and versatility are two key benefits associated with the use of tests (especially standardized tests) to discover the information that is sought within a research project.

The Educational Testing Service (ETS) Testlink Test Collection Database (2015) contains descriptions of more than 25,000 instruments, including research and unpublished instruments. By searching the ETS database for available tools, a researcher can determine the related material prior to downloading any test. Should a tool not have all of the material needed for inclusion in a study, the author or publisher information is provided to allow for direct engagement with the individual to determine the appropriateness of the tool. Another resource for locating possible tools is a review of literature on a topic. As research articles are reviewed with the literature review process, tools used in prior studies can be identified and evaluated. Other research reports may also provide insight concerning tools that have been used in other research projects about an identified topic. A final place to look when attempting to locate a tool is the Internet. Due to the constant expansion of the Internet, entering key words related to evaluation tools into a search engine can provide potential instruments to consider.

When a tool cannot be located to address a particular topic, the following eight steps identified by Orcher (2005, p. 121) for building an appropriate instrument can be used:

1. Develop a plan.
2. Have the plan reviewed.
3. Revise the plan in light of the review.
4. Write items based on the plan.
5. Have the items reviewed.
6. Revise the items in light of the review.
7. Pilot test the instrument.
8. Revise the instrument in light of the pilot test.

Because an instrument is essential in addressing a topic, the development of a unique instrument can be a suitable alternative when the researcher cannot locate an appropriate one for data collection.

Strengths

Because tests are structured, a comparable motivation encouraging completion of the tool is presented for each participant, thus allowing for consistency during the data collection process. Each potential participant is offered the same benefits for agreeing to participate in the study. The equivalency of the measurement across research populations is another benefit from using this form of data collection. According to Bouffard and Little (2004), tests and assessments provide additional valid and reliable data because they tend to reduce the identification of perceptions and opinions. Because the functionality of a test is established through its validity and reliability, the usability of the tool within multiple population samples certifies the effectiveness of that tool. As tools are used repeatedly, the availability of reference group data grows, providing additional support for the tool and the data collected via use of that tool.

Another advantage to using tests relates to the administration process for the tool. Frequently, tests can be dispensed within a group setting, which saves time, expense, and energy. When the data can be collected in a group setting, the response rate is higher, due to the greater control exerted with this type of administration. Interrater reliability is improved since the instructions for the tool completion are given to the group rather than repeated for each individual.

An additional reward for using tests within the data collection process is the accessibility of an extensive assortment of tests. The wide variety of tests available for use in research projects reflects the many content areas that might be investigated. For this reason, the identification of a functional tool that is appropriate for use within a research project requires a persistent quest for the most applicable instrument. The same instrument/tool can be used both prior to and after an intervention has been delivered to allow for comparison of the changes in the results from both phases.

The final advantage of tests within the research process derives from the practicality of undertaking data analysis. The quantitative features of the data accumulated through use of this methodology allow for the structured, organized process. Because quantitative data are numerical in nature, those data can be easily used within the calculations used for statistical analysis.

Limitations

Although tests have multiple strengths related to their use in research, several limitations must also be considered with this methodology. If a test requires that a fee be paid for each individual taking the test, the

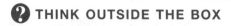

? THINK OUTSIDE THE BOX

Discuss the ethical aspects of using covert data collection methods.

expense can be excessive should a large sample be required. In addition, standardized tests must be evaluated for the presence of biases within the construction of the tool. These biases may be directed toward a certain group of individuals or a unique population. Because tests are structured, this data collection method does not lend itself to open-ended and probing types of questions as easily as other methods do.

Another area the researcher must consider is the management of incomplete test documents. Will these incomplete forms be omitted from the data analyzed, or will the answered questions still be included? Does the inclusion of incomplete forms skew the results? When no responses are provided for selected aspects within any research instrument/tool, the appropriate management of the potential distortion of the results should be considered.

A final area of potential weakness or limitation with the use of tests relates to the problems encountered when an instrument/tool lacks psychometric data. Psychometric data are the validity and reliability measurements for the tool/instrument. It is the process of validating the tool for the anticipated use. If the tool does not measure what is being evaluated, then the use of the tool would be a limitation since the results could not be authenticated. In such cases, the project does not guarantee the validity or reliability for the device. When a tool lacks the foundational psychometric data, the use of the tool in other projects can provide validity and reliability of the tool, but it cannot certify the appropriateness of the tool for all uses.

◼ Questionnaire Methods

Overview

When a questionnaire is the tool used for data collection, the data collection method is a survey process. A survey necessitates the querying of individuals through the use of some device that contains questions to be answered. A **questionnaire** is a data collection tool completed by a participant, where the researcher has the intent to discover what the individual thinks about a specific item. Questionnaires can be employed to gather information concerning knowledge, attitudes, beliefs, and feelings. A questionnaire, which is a self-reporting device, can be provided as a paper-and-pencil device, a telephone survey, or a structured document uploaded to or created on the Internet, such as those generated through companies such as SurveyMonkey. As a result, the device can be administered in person, by mail, by telephone, or via the Internet.

According to Brink and Wood (2001), questionnaires limit the replies possible because they involve directed answers to prearranged questions. Several types of questions can be incorporated into the questionnaire format, including dichotomous (yes/no), multiple choice, cafeteria, rank order, forced-choice ratings, checklists, calendar, and visual analogue (Polit & Beck, 2008). The researcher should consider the question format while assessing the applicability of different tools. In one example, Hanna, Weaver, Slaven, Fortenberry, and DiMeglio (2014) utilized a questionnaire to assess diabetes-related quality of life (DQOL) within their study. In their article, they provide information related to the number of questions along with the scoring process for the DQOL questionnaire. Another tool that they used was entitled the Emerging Adult Diabetes Management Self-Report, which they adapted (as described in the article), because the population was emerging adults within 1 year of high school graduation. As can be seen within the discussion of the tools in this article, the thought process concerning the use of tools along with the management of the administration of the tools was provided.

Should a researcher elect to develop a tool specific for the topic under investigation, several facets of the instrument should be vigilantly contemplated in designing the questionnaire (**Box 11-1**). Of course, the entire tool must address the research focus and be appropriate for the target population. These two items are fundamental to the process of developing the questions and the format for the tool. The language

---

Box 11-1

Design Tenets for Questionnaires

- Ensure that the tool addresses the research purpose, objectives, goals, and questions.
- Carefully consider the target population who will use the questionnaire so that the tool is easy to use.
- Use simple, familiar language without jargon and with correct grammar.
- Compose each question to be understandable, concise, and reasonably brief.
- Consider sequencing the questions from impersonal to personal, less sensitive to more sensitive, and broad to specific.
- Avoid using questions that hint at or direct responses, use double negatives, or embarrass the participant.
- Verify that each question addresses only a single topic.
- Structure the tool by beginning with questions that stimulate interest and group questions by topics.
- Cautiously word questions dealing with painful situations.
- Incorporate into the question all information necessary to address the issue under investigation.
- Construct the tool with the questions in the same order for each testing session to provide consistency in delivery and data collection.
- Ascertain the necessary format to accumulate the appropriate information: open-ended questions, closed-ended questions, mutually exclusive and exhaustive response categories, or response categories for closed-ended questions (rating scales, ranking, semantic differential, checklists).
- Use various items and approaches to appraise conceptual ideas.
- Carefully consider the use of reverse wording on some of the questions to eliminate the possibility of a "response set."
- Determine the coding and/or weighting of the responses prior to the administration of the tool.
- Conduct a pilot test of the tool with a select group of the target population to confirm the applicability of the tool.

employed within the instrument must be free of jargon, use familiar words, and be easily understood by the potential participants. Each statement should be short and specific, while addressing only one concept. Care must be given to the wording to prevent any leading of the participants toward a specific response.

According to Boswell (2010), "Good questions endeavor to scrutinize, evaluate, translate, illuminate, and reflect relationships about the multiple fragments of data assembled on any given topic" (para. 1). While neutral wording for each statement should be the goal, the use of active verbs in the statement is conducive to analysis, synthesis, and evaluation of the situation, thus resulting in an optimal response (Boswell, 2010). Careful thought must be given to each step in the development of questions to be used in any type of query. The questions must connect back to the PICOT question, research question/hypothesis, or research purpose. While some demographic questions are frequently included, the primary questions are to be developed to address the problem/challenge being answered by the project.

The type of questions (open-ended versus closed-ended) is one of the initial concerns to be addressed in terms of the format of the instrument. **Open-ended questions** leave the direction of the answer up to the individual participant. This type of questioning is more frequently used to assess qualitative types of issues and exploratory research. In contrast, **closed-ended questions** force a response because the researcher provides the answers. Closed-ended questions lend themselves to the collection of quantitative data and quantitative (confirmatory) research.

When developing closed-ended questions, the tool developer must ensure that the categories used for the answers are mutually exclusive and exhaustive. An example of a mutually exclusive category is the classification of years of service to an organization. The potential choices must not overlap because overlapping of categories would cause confusion. Therefore, the ranges would need to be stated as follows: "Years of service: Less than 3, 4–6, 7–9, 10–12."

For categories to be exhaustive, every possible option must be presented as a potential selection piece. In the ranges provided in the preceding example, individuals who had worked 13 or more years would not be provided with an option that they could select. However, keep in mind that the researcher may not want a certain range. In such a case, the researcher will need to provide a rationale for the exclusion. An example of when a lack of a specific range might be appropriate is when the researcher opens the year range to include every year possible.

The tool developer needs to carefully consider the information that is being sought through the use of the questionnaire. As that decision is confirmed, the tool should then address each and every potential aspect of the information being collected. For example, the types of response categories are an important consideration with closed-ended questionnaires. The instrument developer should consider several types of responses, including rating scales, ranking, semantic differential, and checklists (**Table 11-1**). Ultimately, the type of information that is being collected should drive the choice of response categories used for the tool.

Strengths

The use of questionnaires for data collection has several advantages. A primary reason for using this methodology is the ability to access a larger sample in a group setting at a minimum expense. Participants also seem to favor the use of questionnaires because this method of data collection provides a greater sense of anonymity. The use of questionnaires can also be time-sensitive to the participant. As the process is begun, the researcher can state that the completion of the questionnaire should take a designated amount of time. Thus, the participant can then

Table 11-1	
	Types of Questionnaire Responses
Type of Response	**Example of Response**
Rating scales	On a scale from 0 to 10, with 10 being the most severe pain you can imagine and 0 being no pain at all, where does your current pain level fall? 0 1 2 3 4 5 6 7 8 9 10 No pain Most severe pain
Ranking	Nurses rank different things at different levels. The following is a list of items that many nurses value in the workplace. Please designate their order of significance to you by placing "1" beside the most significant, "2" beside the next most significant, and so on. _____ Salary _____ Competent peers _____ Effective workplace _____ Management workload _____ Opportunities to advance
Semantic differential	On each of the combinations provided, place an "X" to reflect how you see yourself function related to the two associated terms. Competent |_|_|_|_|_|_|_| Incompetent Pleasant |_|_|_|_|_|_|_| Unpleasant Responsible |_|_|_|_|_|_|_| Irresponsible Successful |_|_|_|_|_|_|_| Unsuccessful
Checklists	Please check all of the applicable characteristics you think a nurse should have in order to participate in evidence-based practice (EBP). _____ Critical thinking abilities _____ Energy _____ Knowledge about searching _____ Years of nursing experience _____ Desire for EBP

determine if they have that amount of time to use for the process. Another advantage identified by Brink and Wood (2001) is the potential to collect an enhanced quantity of data with an extensive variety of topics using a standard format. A final advantage to the use of this data collection method is the opportunity to determine the validity and reliability of the tool, thereby strengthening the overall design of the research project.

Limitations

The use of questionnaires as a data collection method does present some notable problems, however. To ensure adequate sampling, the tool must be short and to the point. Long, cumbersome questionnaires result in individuals electing not to complete the tool, which in turn requires enrollment of additional sample participants to complete the research project and can delay the project.

Another limitation resulting from the use of questionnaires in data collection is the potential for participants to be nonresponsive to selected items within the tool. This nonresponsiveness to items results in a dilemma for the researcher because the inclusion of an incomplete questionnaire becomes an important question to address prior to the actual use of the tool within a study.

A final limitation resulting from the use of this method is the time-consuming nature of the data collection process. For open-ended questions, the differences within the verbal responses must be carefully considered and correlated. This process is time consuming because the verbal responses are not preselected responses. Determinations concerning the comparability between terms must be made carefully and supported by documentation to reflect the thought processes used. For closed-ended questions, the establishment of the data set, the process of data input, and the actual inputting of the quantitative data must be considered and planned because it requires focused time to manually enter each piece of data.

■ Interview Methods

Overview

Brink and Wood (2001) identified the key variation between a questionnaire and an **interview** as the presence of an individual to conduct the interview; this "personal touch" is the basic difference between the two data collection methods. Otherwise, the expectations and concerns about interview questions are the same as arise in the development of a questionnaire or survey.

Within this compilation design, the use of an interviewer to direct the questioning process requires that trust and rapport be developed between interviewer and interviewee. The interviewer has to present a positive, supportive manner to engage the individual being queried. If the individual does not perceive the environment to be appropriate, the data collected may be skewed. Thus, the environment selected for the session is of paramount importance. Because the questions are presented by the interviewer, the ordering of the questions and the environment wherein the questions are presented should allow for openness from the interviewee and the increased depth of the resulting responses. If a room is too hot, too cold, too noisy, or too open, the participant may elect not to continue the interview or may be less open to engaging in dialogue. According to Bouffard and Little (2004), "Questions [in an interview] are generally open-ended and responses are documented in thorough, detailed notes or transcription" (p. 3).

Interview data collection can pull together information from both the quantitative and qualitative realms. When quantitative information is sought from the interview process, the questions are completed through the use of a structured format. Frequently, closed-ended questions are administered by means of a standardized test. Each question is asked in the same pattern or flow. The environment of the interview is controlled in an attempt to reduce the effect of confounding environmental variables.

If the purpose of the planned data collection is to seek qualitative information, the entire process can be managed in a less structured manner. Often, the questions used for this type of interview are geared more toward the open-ended type. When an informal conversational interview format is used, the process is impulsive and freely structured. An interviewer serves as a mediator who guides participants as they move between topics. To better facilitate the process, the interviewer should initiate the discussion with a subject matter that is significant but not problematic.

The flexibility of the interview process is perceived as both an advantage and a disadvantage for this data collection method. With the openness of the data collection process, the interviewer collects not only verbal data, but also nonverbal data. By juxtaposing the nonverbal communication with the verbal statements, clarification related to the meanings of the comments and data is improved and facilitated. The disadvantage is related to the wealth of data that can be collected and then must be utilized or analyzed to determine the appropriateness of the material. The volume of data collected can make the data analysis process overwhelming and cumbersome.

Strengths

One of the initial strengths noted with the interview data collection design is the resulting powerful and abundant information accumulated, which paints an extensive portrait of the issue at hand and may have far-reaching implications. Another benefit gained from using this design is the ability, through the use of communication, to highlight issues that may present themselves only during the course of discussion as the interview progresses. The ability to measure attitudes, probe feelings, pose follow-up questions, gather internal meanings and ways of thinking, and control the depth of information amassed are other advantages associated with the use of the interview data collection method. An extra advantage is that interviews allow for the collection of data without the requirement that the participant be able to read or write.

Limitations

The interview data collection process does present some limitations that must be considered as a researcher decides which method to use. This methodology for gathering information can be both expensive and time consuming. Conducting individual interviews requires time-intensive interactions and close observation of the nonverbal communication that helps to clarify the verbal responses. The interviewer must be able to elicit the information expected for the research project. Related to this limitation of the interviewer is interrater reliability. When more than one interviewer is used to collect the data, the interviewer could alter and/or transform the data collected by the use of various processes. When the data are not collected in the same manner by each interviewer or data collector, bias may be introduced. Another weakness to consider is the potential for the participants to say what they perceive is appropriate or socially desirable, instead of what they actually believe. In addition, the sample size is often small when the interview methodology is used, making generalizations to a larger population more difficult. Finally, analysis of the open-ended, subjective data collected via interviews requires time and thought to ensure that the results are valid and supported by the information.

◼ Focus Group Methods

Overview

Although focus groups share many of the characteristics discussed in relation to interviews, a **focus group** entails a type of "coordinated interview," in which approximately 6 to 12 homogeneous individuals are led in the discussion of a selected topic at the same time. According to Shaha, Wenzel, and Hill (2011), "focus groups—moderated group discussions designed to allow research participants to exchange, discuss, agree, or disagree about opinions, attitudes, and experiences—are an increasingly popular way of eliciting the attitudes or opinions of populations regarding sensitive, under-investigated topics" (p. 78).

Each focus session tends to last approximately 1 to 3 hours. To facilitate the data collection process, the sessions typically are audio- or video-recorded for analysis at a later time.

The focus group leader should understand where the session should come together in regard to the data to be collected. This leader must ensure that the research topic is adequately covered during the discussion. The focus group leader's challenges are to persuade everyone to share in the dialogue, motivate conversation, channel the progression between the different topics, stay impartial, and endeavor not to interject any biases into the discussion while maintaining control of the discussion.

Many different features within the process need to be controlled and manipulated. The participants must understand that their opinions and experiences are important, such that no answers are inappropriate within the context of the subject under investigation. Care concerning the setting for the focus group should address comfort, privacy, and convenience. Although the session is recorded in some manner, the focus group leader and researcher must ensure that the participants feel secure in the knowledge that the recording will be used only to pull out the information provided.

The researcher should also give thought and consideration to the membership of the group. Shaha and colleagues (2011) suggest that the researcher should consider group members' educational background, job positions, and/or work environments. For example, Iverson and colleagues (2014) used focus groups within their research project. The inclusion criteria for the focus group were presented to provide a clear understanding of who was included within the project. When these items are not taken into consideration, problems with feasibility, power, confidentiality, and integrity can develop. A homogeneous grouping with regard to gender, age, and socioeconomic status enhances the generalizability of the resulting data. Putting thought into the size and composition of each focus group is essential to maximize the effectiveness of the data collection process.

Iverson and colleagues (2014) used the recommendations for effective focus groups within their project. They used informed consent to address the ethical aspects. Five focus groups were conducted, which led the research team to determine that data saturation had been reached. The questions posed addressed the research purpose and were provided as open-ended queries. Each of these aspects reflects thought and attention to the overall needs of data collection within a focus group process.

As the focus group is pulled together, the focus group leader should begin the session with a personal introduction concerning the research team members, purpose for the session, discussion about why the session is important, and what type of administrative support is in place. It is also important that the members of the focus group understand that any participation is completely voluntary on their part. For the session to be successful, members must feel comfortable in discussing their attitudes and opinions on the topic without fearing any type of repercussions. During the session, the focus group leader and/or research team member must make sure that distractions such as background noises are removed. Time must be allowed for the initial development of trust between the members of the focus group and the group leader. Without this trust, the information obtained can be biased and compromised.

Strengths

Many of the same advantages listed previously for interviews also hold true for the focus group data collection method. The collection of data is done in an open and revealing manner that allows for the growth and exploration of ideas and concepts. As members of the focus group discuss the different aspects presented through the process, the moderator can probe the in-depth information for additional understanding of the phenomenon. Each individual is allowed to react to other participants without having to carry the entire data collection process by himself or herself.

Limitations

Limitations of this design process relate to the sizing and management of the focus groups. The moderator must be adept at conducting the process. Getting the right moderator, organizing the appropriate focus group members, conducting the session, and completing the management of the data can also be quite expensive. Within each group, extrovert personalities must be controlled, while involvement of introvert personalities is encouraged.

Observation Methods

Overview

According to Wood and Ross-Kerr (2006), "**Observation** is a method of collecting descriptive, behavioral data and is extremely useful in nursing studies because one can observe behavior as it occurs" (p. 171). The entire process of observing individuals results in an interactive engagement. Frequently, what a person says and what a person does can be two different pieces of information. Observation allows for the confirmation of what is said by the viewing of specific behaviors and activities. It is an articulation of individualism, character preconceptions, and beliefs. Each individual assesses a situation based on his or her unique background and philosophy of life. As a result, the selectivity of this type of data collection must be highly patterned by the expectations of the study. Clarity related to the behavioral information under investigation is imperative.

LoBiondo-Wood and Haber (1998) specified four conditions needed for the use of observation as a data collection method:

- "Observations undertaken are consistent with the study's specific objectives,
- Standardized and systematic plan for the observation and the recording of data,
- All of the observations are checked and controlled, and
- Observations are related to scientific concepts and theories" (p. 312).

The complexity of the process requires attention to be given to the operationalization of the variables. The variables are frequently the behaviors being observed. Consequently, the individual characteristics and conditions (traits, symptoms, verbal communications, nonverbal conditions, activities, skills, or environmental aspects) should be clearly and distinctly documented for the integrity of the data collection process. Another issue that arises with this type of data collection process is whether the observer will be directed to try to provoke some behavior/action by the individuals being observed.

Both quantitative and qualitative observations can be used within this research effort. Because generalizability of the results is desired, a checklist of the behaviors/observations is frequently used to provide a structure for the analysis phase of the process. Put simply, quantitative observations require the standardization of those items to be counted or not counted. Likewise, clear directions related to the operational definitions of the selected behaviors must be given. When these behaviors are unmistakably defined, the observational sessions produce the quantitative data expected from the research process. The definition should include the "who, what, when, where, why, and how" for the behavior on which data are to be collected within the study. As an example, if one piece of data that a researcher wants to collect is the number of times a person made eye contact during a lecture presentation, clarification is needed as to what duration of eye contact would be

---

❓ THINK OUTSIDE THE BOX

After selecting an evidence-based topic, develop open-ended and closed-ended questions that could be used to address the topic. Debate the benefits of using open-ended versus closed-ended question formats.

counted. In this case, the researcher might establish that each time the lecturer made eye contact with a student for at least 45 seconds, the contact would be counted. In contrast to quantitative observation, qualitative observation is investigative and open ended. The resulting information provides massive amounts of field notes to analyze.

Four diverse observer roles create a continuum of data collection with the observation methodology:

- *Complete participant.* The observer takes the role of member within the sample; the data are collected via a covert (hidden) process; the members of the group are not informed about the data collection process.
- *Participant-as-observer.* The observer continues to work from within the group but collects the data through an overt (informed) process; the members of the group are aware that the observer is taking on the dual roles of member of the group and spectator.
- *Observer-as-participant.* The observer does work from within the group but spends more time in the role of spectator, instead of member of the group; data are collected in an overt manner.
- *Complete observer.* The observer is totally in the role of watcher; covert observations are used to collect the data.

For each data collection session, the researcher takes time to conscientiously consider which of these depths of observation is appropriate for the study population. Because some of the methods require covert (undercover) data collection, the researcher must also justify why this clandestine method is needed. In these situations, the question is raised as to the necessity of collecting information without the individual's knowledge and the ethics of that undisclosed process. The researcher must diligently document the manner in which the individuals would be protected from harm.

On the other side of the picture, when the participants know they are being watched, the researcher has to work to ensure that behaviors are not modified due to this knowledge (the Hawthorne effect). Frequently, the course of action used to ensure that individuals are behaving naturally is related to the length of time the observations are occurring. The researcher/observer may have to be immersed in this

❓ THINK OUTSIDE THE BOX

Using a PICOT question format, describe how you would collect data for the topic you addressed in the PICOT question.

situation of being observed for a long period of time so that the participants become comfortable with him or her being there. As their comfort with the researcher's presence increases, the individuals return to their normal behaviors, allowing the observer to then see the normalcy of the situation.

Strengths

According to Bouffard and Little (2004), the observation method provides "highly detailed information from an external perspective on what actually occurs in programs" (p. 3). The depth of the information obtained is the primary benefit from collecting data in this manner. Having someone watch the activity under investigation allows events that might otherwise be undetected in everyday life to be identified and discussed. Observation as a data collection process is seen as an effective method for understanding important related items of a designated setting. Another advantage of this method is that it can be used with any individual regardless of educational preparation. Thus, the behaviors, attitudes, and involvement of individuals who may have weaker verbal skills can be evaluated and researched.

Limitations

The limitations of this data collection practice flow from the time-consuming, labor-intensive, and expensive nature of completing the observation process. Interrater reliability of the observers and the training of these individuals have equally important implications for the quality of the resulting data. Without the assurance that the observers are knowledgeable about the entire process, the excellence of the data may be questioned.

Bias is a major problem that must be addressed throughout the observation period. Researchers and observers should be up front about the presence of any biases that might potentially compromise the integrity of the study results. It becomes imperative that all biases are identified and reported. Biases cannot be completely removed; therefore, the acknowledgment of the existence of the predispositions provides validation of the results. Consumers of the research results can then be aware that these preconceptions were recognized.

■ Secondary (Existing) Data Methods

Overview

The data collection process using secondary (existing) data builds on the information collected from another study. The use of secondary data takes the data compiled for another reason and applies it in a different manner; as a result, this method of reevaluating should be carefully considered and contemplated. The researcher must explain which pieces of the primary data will be used in reassessment of the information. Within this process, the researcher reconsiders a part of the information accumulated through some other manner in an attempt to address a follow-up type of question.

The data used for these secondary assessment projects might include documents, physical data, and/or archived research data, for example. When documents are used, they could include personal documents, such as letters, diaries, or family pictures, and official documents, such as attendance records, budgets, annual reports, newspapers, yearbooks, minutes, or client records.

Strengths

The advantages of using this method to assess existing records result from the availability of the records. A data collection process that relies on secondary data can be completed without any intrusion into the lives of people. The extra time gained by using the sources already assembled can be devoted to collecting key pieces of information that previously were overlooked or not valued.

In addition, the reevaluation of documents allows for exploration of alternative conclusions. The environmental aspects and historic perceptions can augment the interpretation of the data. A fuller evaluation of the information can be completed, thereby providing a more comprehensive understanding of the phenomena under investigation. By using previously collected records, researchers can identify trends because the entirety of the incident can be manipulated. For the most part, the use of secondary (existing) data is also less expensive than collection of primary data.

Limitations

Some of the weaknesses of this data collection method revolve around the restrictiveness of the data sources. The only data that can be collected and analyzed are the data that were initially amassed. The researcher cannot add questions and can access only the information that has been compiled. Among the other barriers presented by the use of secondary data is the potential for the data to be out of date.

Another obstacle a researcher may encounter related to this type of data collection results from the restriction on accessing certain documents. If the documents are controlled to protect individual privacy, access to the information could be problematic.

An additional hindrance ensuing from this method is the limitation resulting from the sample used for the initial data collection. Specifically, the original sampling inclusion and exclusion criteria could negatively affect the secondary assessment of archived research data.

A final problem with the use of secondary (existing) data is the lack of open-ended or qualitative data related to the question. The researcher would need to acknowledge the unavailability of this type of data, which might or might not affect the quality of the project. If the project did not require the inclusion of qualitative data, then a secondary assessment of data would be appropriate. If qualitative data were desired to paint the total picture of the occurrence under investigation, the likelihood of accessing the original sample to gain further data would be highly problematic, if not impossible. Thus, the reevaluation of secondary sources for additional results can pose difficulties because of the lack of initially collected information relating to the topic under current discussion.

■ Biophysiological Methods

Overview

The final type of data collection method is the use of biological indicators to organize the data being sought for the research activity. The research community views biophysiological measures as objective data. Researchers may use the **biophysiological data** collection process either alone or in combination with other methods.

This method of data collection necessitates the use of specialized equipment to establish the physical and/or biological condition of the subjects. Two types of biophysiological methods are possible:

- **In vivo**: Requires the use of some apparatus to evaluate one or more elements of a participant. Examples of the types of items evaluated include blood pressure measurements, electrocardiograms, temperatures, muscular activity, and respiratory rates and rhythms.
- **In vitro**: Requires the extraction of physiological materials from the participants, frequently via a laboratory analysis. Examples of the types of items within this realm include bacterial counts and identifications, tissue biopsies, glucose levels, and cholesterol levels.

As an example of the use of in vitro data, Hanna and colleagues (2014) document the use of glycemic control (HbA1C), which requires the extraction of a small amount of blood to determine glycemic levels. Within the article, they speak to the levels that they used to control for bias.

This type of data collection process is frequently used with experimental and quasi-experimental research designs. Typically, the data are used to advance the implementation of specific nursing actions. Because

THINK OUTSIDE THE BOX

Discuss the challenges involved in using in vitro and in vivo data collection methods.

of the type of information collected through this method, the research projects gathering biophysiological data tend to be more structured and controlled.

Strengths

The advantages of using this kind of data collection are the objectivity, precision, and sensitivity of the information compiled. The facts acquired from the use of specialized equipment have the tendency to be viewed as having increased independence from bias and subjectivity. As a result, the research community views this level of data with enhanced respect.

Limitations

The disadvantages related to the use of the specialized apparatus include the cost of obtaining the measurements and calibrating the instruments, which can be enormous with some data collection processes. Also, the acquisition of data by instrumentation requires specialized knowledge and training to be able to accurately gather the data. Additional research assistants may be required to perform the testing processes, leading to escalating costs, greater time commitments, and concerns related to interrater reliability.

A final problem resulting from this type of data collection is the potential reluctance of the accessible population to participate in such a study. Some members of the accessible population may decline to allow the physiological and biological measurements. The researcher must obtain informed consent from each individual prior to the collection of data and/or samples for analysis.

◼ Systematic Analysis

With the increasing focus on evidence-based practice, systematic reviews and meta-analysis reviews are becoming commonplace in the literature. These different forms of pulling the evidence together provide a clean synthesis of current knowledge about a topic. The Institute of Medicine (2011) defines a **systematic review** as a process of identifying, selecting, assessing, and synthesizing the findings from similar but individualized studies. This process of data collection allows for the clarification of what is known and not known about an identified topic. Robertson-Malt (2014) notes the international standard for systematic reviews is the Preferred Reporting Items for Systematic Reviews and Meta-Analyses (PRISMA). This document holds as a vital and fundamental tenet for PRISMA to be the recording of the material in plain and transparent language. The PRISMA statement holds six items as essential within the flow diagram:

> unique records identified by the searches, records excluded after preliminary screening, records retrieved in full text, records or studies excluded after assessment of the full text, studies meeting the eligibility criteria for the review, and studies contributing to the main outcome. (Robertson-Malt, 2014, p. 49)

Within the data collection process, another method utilized within evidence-based practice is **meta-analysis**. According to materials developed by Northern Arizona University (2001), a meta-analysis is a process of merging the outcomes from multiple studies related to one primary topic. The strength of each set of conclusions is determined to provide an overall view of the evidence available on the identified topic. The methods used within the various studies, along with the quantification of the findings from the studies, are condensed into a summary document related to the topic under investigation. The effect size within a meta-analysis seeks to establish the relevance of the tests, treatments, and methods used in the research studies under consideration. These documents are then used to provide the context for the next steps in the research process and the determination of the reliability of the evidence related to that topic.

The Institute of Medicine (2011) developed Standards for Systematic Reviews to provide direction to individuals for completing a systematic review using an effective and manageable approach. Hemingway and Brereton (2009) identified five aspects that demonstrate a high-quality systematic review. To generate an effective review, all relevant published and unpublished evidence should be included within the document. Porritt, Gomersall, and Lockwood (2014) strongly endorse the idea that the study selection process is the vital stage within the review process. Determining which types of studies will be included is critical to the overall success of the review. After all the evidence is compiled, inclusion criteria as to which pieces of evidence are to be included in the review must be determined. It is not possible to include everything, so care must be given to the determination of the inclusion criteria to allow for effective evidence to be included. After the selection of the evidence to be included in the review, each piece and report must be assessed for the quality of that evidence toward the goal of the review. As the appraisals are completed on each of the studies, incorporation of the results into an unbiased report of those findings is imperative. Porritt and colleagues (2014) identified the different types of bias to consider, including selection biases, performance biases, detection biases, and attrition biases. Following the synthesizing of the results, an interpretation of the findings in a balanced and impartial summary is the culmination of the review. Effective consideration of any flaws in the evidence must be noted within a high-quality systematic review.

Systematic reviews must be completed with a peer-reviewed protocol to allow for replication of the review as needed. Hemingway and Brereton (2009) stated that, looked "at individually, each article may offer little insight into the problem at hand; the hope is that, when taken together within a systematic review, a clearer (and more consistent) picture will emerge" (p. 2). The process for completing a review requires that each member of the review team carefully and appropriately assess each of the selected articles/documents utilizing the agreed upon criterion. To effectively conduct a systematic review, five steps should be followed. The first step within the process is the formation of a suitable and fitting review question. Within the healthcare question, attention to the principal objective, along with the phenomena of interest, is critical. Once the question is clearly worded, a search of the literature and other sources of evidence is initiated. Because systematic reviews need to be unbiased, the search for evidence must be accomplished in any venue where the evidence for that topic could be located. Furthermore, it is essential that each and every view of the topic is included in the search. The third component within the review process is an assessment of the studies. Using the inclusion criteria, specific documents are selected to be included in the review. From this point, the researcher performs a critical appraisal of each document to determine the strength of the evidence based on the methodological quality of that study. Some questions that can be used to drive the appraisal of each document are:

- Is the subject defined adequately to allow the development of the review?
- How thorough was the search for studies and evidence?
- Did the inclusion criteria provide a clear and concise description to be used that allowed for the fair application of the criteria?
- Is the review conducted as a blinded or independent review to decrease biases?
- How was missing information managed within the review?
- Do the included studies and documents reflect similar effects? If not, why?
- Did the review speak to the idea of robustness of the process?
- Were the recommendations supported by the strength of the quality of the evidence? (Hemingway & Brereton, 2009).

Once the overview of the documents is determined, the combining of the findings is carefully and thoughtfully integrated into the review. Care and attention to the depth and quality of the review must be established. Two types of systematic reviews used in the research field are meta-synthesis and meta-analysis. A meta-synthesis is a review that primarily focuses on qualitative data. A meta-analysis utilizes quantitative data to address a clinical effectiveness problem. The process for either type of analysis includes the same steps listed earlier. The difference between these two is the types of studies and evidence considered within the review. The analysis would be directed by the research method used in the different documents included in the review.

■ Achievement of the Data Collection Strategy

Each of the data collection strategies profiled in this chapter has both benefits and limitations. The researcher must carefully consider the PICOT question, research purpose, research question/hypothesis, research design, sampling method, cost considerations, and time restrictions as he or she identifies the appropriate data collection plan. According to Bouffard and Little (2004), "Using multiple methods to assess the same outcomes [e.g., using surveys and document review to assess program management] provides a richer, more detailed picture" (p. 5). Although it certainly adds to the richness of the results, the use of multiple methods of data collection also increases the resources (cost, personnel, and tools) required to carry out the project.

Each researcher must carefully consider the many different strategies available for accessing the information needed to address the identified research problem. In singling out the appropriate data collection process, justification for those choices needs to be documented. Because each method has its own set of strengths and limitations, the primary objective for the researcher is to substantiate the rationale for the choices made to dispatch the research challenge.

In determining the strategy, the objectives of the project, along with the type of data required, should be taken into account during the decision-making process. If the strategy for a research or evidence-based project has been determined to be the use of a tool, several aspects must be considered. The selection of a tool, the questions that need to be developed, and the method for implementing the tool/questions must all be contemplated. In addition, the environment of the data collection process is just as important as the individual questions to be addressed. Within the environment, the participants must be made to feel secure with the process, or the resulting data could be compromised.

■ Evidence-Based Practice Considerations

Within the realm of evidence-based practice (EBP), the focus is more on the idea of outcome measures. According to Melnyk and Fineout-Overholt (2005):

> The effectiveness and usefulness of outcomes measurement is affected by: the quality of the data, the consistency and accuracy of the data collection process, the commitment and ability of those collecting the data and making decisions based on findings, and the timing of data collection. (p. 306)

The principal issues for data collection, as viewed from the EBP perspective, are the quality of the process and the content of the data collected. Each choice made by a researcher concerning the data to be collected, the method or methods to be used, and the environment used to collect the data must be founded on reliable, sensible judgments. The rationales for these decisions can make or break the study by determining the validity and reliability of the results produced by the study. If the decisions are not supported by appropriate thought processes and planning, then the entire inquiry is in jeopardy.

A researcher need not select the strongest data collection methods possible, but researchers must select the optimal strategies for getting the data needed to answer the questions asked and provide an appropriate justification for each of those decisions. The key is to make a decision and justify the selection with sound reasoning and a sound decision-making process. The entire research or evidence-based process rests on the quality of the data. The data form the foundation on which the results, recommendations, and outcomes of a study are based; the merit of the data becomes the underpinning for the research or evidence-based conclusions. The researcher must provide a sound rationale and strong support for the decisions made concerning the data collection process.

Summary Points

1. Data come in many varieties, and data collection is achieved through numerous methodologies.
2. Data collection sources are items or strategies for accumulating the information desired.
3. Data collection tools are the tangible devices used to complete the collection of the data.
4. The major methods of data collection are tests, questionnaires, interviews, focus groups, observations, secondary (existing) data, and biophysiological data.

5. Attention must be given to the information that actually exists and the information that is accessible. These two types of data may not be the same.

6. The basic objective in research is to collect the data in the same manner for each of the participants so that unique environmental, societal, and physical dimensions are diminished.

7. Another key aspect of the data collection process is the establishment of interrater reliability when more than one data collector is used to gather evidence.

8. Tests are used to ascertain the specific knowledge, talents, behaviors, and/or cognitive capabilities under investigation.

9. A questionnaire/survey is a data collection tool that is completed by a participant and allows the researcher to discover what the individual thinks about a specific item.

10. When interviews are used as the data collection process, establishing trust and rapport between interviewer and interviewee is essential.

11. Environmental aspects of the study setting must be taken into account when planning to conduct interviews and/or focus groups.

12. Observation allows for the confirmation of what is said by viewing the participant's specific behaviors and activities.

13. Several ethical issues need to be carefully considered as the method of observation is determined.

14. A data collection process that uses secondary (existing) data builds on the information collected from another study or document.

15. Systematic reviews are key components within the documentation of evidence.

16. A systematic review is a process of identifying, selecting, assessing, and synthesizing the findings from similar but individualized studies.

RED FLAGS

- Tools used for quantitative data collection should have documentation of their validity and reliability indices.
- If desired, effective discussion of the entire data collection process should be provided in the report of the study results to allow for replication of the study.
- The use of appropriate tools to collect the information being sought must be addressed.
- The type of information needed to satisfy the research question must be reflected in the study design.
- The potential for a Hawthorne effect must be evaluated.
- If two or more data collectors are used within a study, interrater reliability must be established.
- Systematic reviews should document the different steps taken to ensure the quality of the review process.

Multiple-Choice Questions

1. Which of the following processes is not a major method of data collection?
   A. Observations
   B. Open-ended questions
   C. Secondary (existing) data
   D. Tests

2. When considering the different data collection schemes, researchers must be careful to contemplate the presence of the Hawthorne effect. The Hawthorne effect is defined as a process in which the:
   A. Participant does not modify his or her behavior to meet the expectations of the study.
   B. Researcher modifies his or her behavior because of conducting the study.
   C. Researcher modifies the participants' behavior based on the data collected.
   D. Participant modifies his or her behavior as a result of engagement in the study.

3. Which of the following are tenets for use when designing a questionnaire?
   A. Use a variety of items and approaches to appraise conceptual ideas.
   B. Ensure that each question addresses the entire scope of the topic.
   C. Use simple but appropriate jargon for the designated topics.
   D. Both A and B.

4. Which of the following is a method of data collection?
   A. Experimental
   B. Grounded theory
   C. Observation
   D. Cross-sectional

5. When developing questions for an instrument, a researcher should be careful in the wording to:
   A. Provide hints toward the response.
   B. Use jargon as needed.
   C. Use single-topic questions.
   D. Use cultural aspects to provide context.

6. Open-ended questions provide primarily _____ data.
   A. Confirmatory
   B. Exhaustive
   C. Qualitative
   D. Quantitative

7. Which of the following statements is true concerning observation?

   A. Clear directions related to the operational definitions of the selected behavior must be determined.

   B. Ethical considerations are a minor concern within this method of data collection.

   C. Observation data collection strategies result in manageable amounts of field notes to analyze.

   D. Within observational sessions, the observer is always known to the participant.

8. When creating a questionnaire, it is essential to do each of the following except:

   A. Be concise and reasonably brief.

   B. Code and weight the responses prior to the administration of the tool.

   C. Conduct a pilot testing of the tool with a select group of the target population.

   D. Use double-negative questions regularly within the tool.

9. A researcher decides to use observation as the data collection method for a study. To effectively collect the needed data from college-age students, the researcher enrolls in a selected college course to be able to observe and collect data about the behaviors of the students. The researcher is using which observation role?

   A. Complete participant

   B. Participant-as-observer

   C. Observer-as-participant

   D. Complete observer

10. Which of the following terms best describes data compiled for another reason and applied in a different manner?

   A. Primary data

   B. Secondary data

   C. Novice data

   D. Experimental data

11. Which of the following biophysiological tests is an example of in vivo data?

   A. Complete blood count

   B. Urinalysis

   C. Respiratory rate

   D. Bacterial count

12. A systematic review considers:

   A. Reports about clinical standards

   B. Research and other documents that address the topic being reviewed

   C. Only opinion documents that address a topic of interest

   D. Only quantitative research reports

Discussion Questions

1. A researcher begins to develop the demographic section for use within a project. The three questions developed are the following:

    a. How many years have you been practicing professional nursing?
    - 0–5 years
    - 5–10 years
    - 10–15 years
    - More than 15 years

    b. What is your highest nursing degree?
    - ADN
    - BSN
    - MSN
    - Doctorate

    c. I have never been identified in a legal case.
    - Yes
    - No

    Which problems are present within these three questions that need to be corrected?

2. A researcher initially planned to use covert data collection techniques (observing a class of teenagers via a one-way mirror) for a research project designed to determine the aggressive behaviors of boys and girls. Neither the parents nor the students were to be informed about the research project because no intervention was planned. Which other observational role might the researcher use to make the data collection process an overt one?

3. A researcher has decided to conduct a structured interview with nursing students concerning their perceptions of what tasks constitute the provision of spiritual care within an acute care setting. Write three open-ended questions and three closed-ended questions related to this idea.

Suggested Readings

Ahern, N. R. (2005). Using the Internet to conduct research. *Nurse Researcher, 13*(2), 55–70.

Colling, J. (2004, June). Coding, analysis, and dissemination of study results. *Urology Nursing, 24*(3), 215–216.

Duffy, M. E. (2005). Systematic reviews: Their role and contribution to evidence-based practice. *Clinical Nurse Specialist, 19*(1), 15–17.

Halcomb, E., & Andrew, S. (2005). Triangulation as a method for contemporary nursing research. *Nurse Researcher, 13*(2), 71–82.

Happ, M. B., Dabbs, A. D., Tate, J., Hricik, A., & Erlen, J. (2006). Exemplars of mixed methods data combination and analysis. *Nursing Research, 55*(2), S43–S49.

Holopainen, A., Hakulinen-Viitanen, T., & Tossavainen, K. (2008). Systematic review—A method for nursing research. *Nurse Researcher, 16*(1), 72–83.

Institute of Medicine. (2011). *Standards for systematic reviews: Report at a glance.* Retrieved from http://iom.edu/Reports/2011/Finding-What -Works-in-Health-Care-Standards-for-Systematic-Reviews/Standards .aspx

Kuipers, P., & Hartley, S. (2006). A process for the systematic review of community-based rehabilitation evaluation reports: Formulating evidence for policy and practice. *International Journal of Rehabilitation Research, 29*(1), 27–30.

Priest, H., Roberts, P., & Woods, L. (2002). An overview of three different approaches to the interpretation of qualitative data. Part 1: Theoretical issues. *Nurse Researcher, 10*(1), 30–42.

Vishnevsky, T., & Beanlands, H. (2004). Qualitative research. *Nephrology Nursing Journal, 31*(2), 234–238.

Examples of Data Collection

Questionnaires
Palese, A., Tomietto, M., Suhonen, R., Efstathiou, G., Tsangari, H., Merkouris, A., ... Papastavrou, E. (2011). Surgical patient satisfaction as an outcome of nurses' caring behaviors: A descriptive and correlational study in six European countries. *Journal of Nursing Scholarship*, *43*(4), 341–350.

Interviews
Adhiambo Onyango, M., & Mott, S. (2011). The nexus between bride-wealth, family curse, and spontaneous abortion among southern Sudanese women. *Journal of Nursing Scholarship*, *43*(4), 376–384.

Focus Groups/Interviews
Wood, E. B., Hutchinson, M. K., Kahwa, E., Hewitt, H., & Waldron, D. (2011). Jamaican adolescent girls with other male sexual partners. *Journal of Nursing Scholarship*, *43*(4), 396–404.

Secondary Data Analysis
Nantsupawat, A., Srisuphan, W., Kunaviktikul, W., Wichaikhum, O. A., Aungsuroch, Y., & Aiken, L. H. (2011). Impact of nurse work environment and staffing on hospital nurse and quality of care in Thailand. *Journal of Nursing Scholarship*, *43*(4), 426–432.

References

Boswell, C. (2010). Questioning students to develop critical thinking. In L. Caputi (Ed.), *Teaching nursing: The art and science* (2nd ed., Vol. 2, pp. 423–453). Glen Ellyn, IL: College of DuPage Press.

Bouffard, S., & Little, P. M. D. (2004). Detangling data collection: Methods for gathering data. *Harvard Family Research Project, 5*, 1–6. Retrieved from http://www.hfrp.org/publications-resources/browse-our-publications/detangling-data-collection-methods-for-gathering-data

Brink, P. J., & Wood, M. J. (2001). *Basic steps in planning nursing research: From question to proposal* (5th ed.). Sudbury, MA: Jones and Bartlett Publishers.

Cherry, K. (2015). What is the Hawthorne effect? Retrieved from http://psychology.about.com/od/hindex/g/def_hawthorn.htm

Creswell, J. W. (2003). *Research design: Qualitative, quantitative, and mixed method approaches* (2nd ed.). Thousand Oaks, CA: Sage Publications.

Educational Testing Services. (2015). *Testlink test collection database.* Retrieved from http://www.ets.org/test_link/find_tests/

Hanna, K. M, Weaver, M. T., Slaven, J. E., Fortenberry, J. D., & DiMeglio, L. A. (2014). Diabetes-related quality of life and the demands and burdens of diabetes care among emerging adults with type 1 diabetes in the year after high school graduation. *Research in Nursing & Health, 37*, 399–408. doi:10.1002/nur.21620

Hemingway, P., & Brereton, N. (2009). What is a systematic review? *Hayward Medical Communications.* Retrieved from http://www.whatisseries.co.uk

Institute of Medicine. (2011). *Finding what works in health care: Standards for systematic reviews.* Retrieved from http://iom.edu/Reports/2011/Finding-What-Works-in-Health-Care-Standards-for-Systematic-Reviews.aspx

Iverson, K. M., Huang, K., Wells, S. Y., Wright, J. D., Gerber, M. R., & Wiltsey-Stirman, S. (2014). Women veterans' preferences for intimate partner violence screening and response procedures within the Veterans Health Administration. *Research in Nursing & Health, 37*, 302–311. doi:10.1002/nur.21602

LoBiondo-Wood, G., & Haber, J. (1998). *Nursing research: Methods, critical appraisal, and utilization* (4th ed.). St. Louis, MO: Mosby.

Management Study Guide. (2013). Secondary data. Retrieved from http://managementstudyguide.com/secondary_data.htm

Melnyk, B. M., & Fineout-Overholt, E. (2005). *Evidence-based practice in nursing and healthcare: A guide to best practice.* Philadelphia, PA: Lippincott Williams & Wilkins.

New World Encyclopedia. (2014). Hawthorne effect. Retrieved from http://www.newworldencyclopedia.org/entry/Hawthorne_effect

Northern Arizona University. (2001). Module 2: Methods of data collection: Chapter 2 [Online lesson]. Retrieved from http://www.prm.nau.edu/prm447/methods_of_data_collection_lesson.htm

Orcher, L. T. (2005). *Conducting research: Social and behavioral science methods.* Glendale, CA: Pyrczak Publishing.

Polit, D. F., & Beck, C. T. (2008). *Nursing research: Generating and assessing evidence for nursing practice* (8th ed.). Philadelphia, PA: Lippincott Williams & Wilkins.

Porritt, K., Gomersall, J., & Lockwood, C. (2014). Study selection and critical appraisal: The steps following the literature search in a systematic review. *American Journal of Nursing, 114*(6), 47–52.

Robertson-Malt, S. (2014). Presenting and interpreting findings: The steps following data synthesis in a systematic review. *American Journal of Nursing, 114*(8), 49–54.

Shaha, M., Wenzel, J., & Hill, E. E. (2011). Planning and conducting focus group research with nurses. *Nurse Researcher, 18*(2), 77–87.

Wood, M. J., & Ross-Kerr, J. C. (2006). *Basic steps in planning nursing research: From question to proposal* (6th ed.). Sudbury, MA: Jones and Bartlett Publishers.

Chapter **12**

Reliability, Validity, and Trustworthiness

James Eldridge

Chapter Objectives

At the conclusion of this chapter, the learner will be able to:

1. Identify the need for reliability and validity of instruments used in evidence-based practice.
2. Define reliability and validity.
3. Discuss how reliability and validity affect outcome measures and conclusions of evidence-based research.
4. Develop reliability and validity coefficients for appropriate data.
5. Interpret reliability and validity coefficients of instruments used in evidence-based practice.
6. Describe sensitivity and specificity as related to data analysis.
7. Interpret receiver operand characteristics (ROC) to describe validity.

Key Terms

Accuracy

Concurrent validity

Consistency

Construct validity

Content-related validity

Correlation coefficient

Criterion-related validity

Cross-validation

Equivalency reliability

Interclass reliability

Intraclass reliability

Objectivity

Observed score

Predictive validity

Receiver operand
   characteristics (ROC)

Reliability

Sensitivity

Specificity

Stability

Standard error of
   measurement (SEM)

Trustworthiness

Validity

■ Introduction

The foundation of good research and of good decision making in evidence-based practice (EBP) is the **trustworthiness** of the data used to make decisions. When data cannot be trusted, an informed decision cannot be made. Trustworthiness of the data can only be as good as the instruments or tests used to collect the data. Regardless of the specialization of the healthcare provider, nurses make daily decisions on the diagnosis and treatment of a patient based on the results from different tests to which the patient is subjected. To ensure that the individual makes the proper diagnosis and gives the proper treatment, the nurse must first be sure that the test results used to make the decisions are trustworthy and correct.

Working in an EBP setting requires the nurse to have the best data available to aid in the decision-making process. How can an individual make a decision if the results being used as the foundation of that process cannot be trusted? Put simply, a person cannot make a decision unless the results are trustworthy and correct.

This chapter presents five concepts to help the nurse determine whether the data upon which decisions are based are trustworthy: reliability, validity, accuracy, sensitivity, and specificity. Each defines a portion of the trustworthiness of the data collection instruments, which in turn defines the trustworthiness of the data, ensuring a proper diagnosis or treatment.

Reliability and validity are the most important qualities in the decision-making process.

- Reliability = the instrument consistently measures the same thing.
- Validity = the instrument measures what it is intended to measure.

If either of these qualities is lacking in the data, the nurse cannot make an informed decision and, therefore, is more likely to make an incorrect decision. An incorrect decision in the medical field can have catastrophic consequences for the patient. Thus, one can see why reliability and validity are so important. What do these concepts mean? What would happen if the same test was run on a person several times but the results were different each time? In the case of varying results, a decision becomes ambiguous because the results are unclear.

Reliability is defined as the consistency or repeatability of test results. Other descriptors used to indicate reliability include "consistency," "repeatability," "objectivity," "dependability," and "precision." Accuracy is a function of reliability: The better the reliability, the more accurate the results. Conversely, the poorer the reliability, the more inaccurate are the results, which increases the chance of making an incorrect decision. Furthermore, accuracy is affected by the sensitivity and specificity of the test. **Sensitivity** can be defined as how often a test measures a "true" positive result, while **specificity** determines the capability of the test for determining "true" negative results. The greater the sensitivity and specificity is for a test, the more accurate the test results. The concepts of sensitivity and specificity are discussed in more detail later in this chapter.

Validity is defined as the degree to which the results are truthful. It depends on the reliability and relevance of the test in question (**Figure 12-1**). Relevance is simply the degree of the relationship between the test and its objective, meaning that the test reflects what was reported to be tested.

An example of relevance is the measurement of the height of a patient. A nurse uses a stadiometer (a ruler used to measure vertical distance) to establish a patient's height. Is the stadiometer a relevant height measurement device? Height is the vertical distance from the floor to the top of the head, and a stadiometer measures vertical distance from the floor to any point above the floor; thus, the stadiometer is a relevant measure of height.

Validity cannot exist without reliability and relevance, but reliability and relevance can exist independently of validity. **Figure 12-2a** depicts the case in which there is a high degree of reliability and a low degree

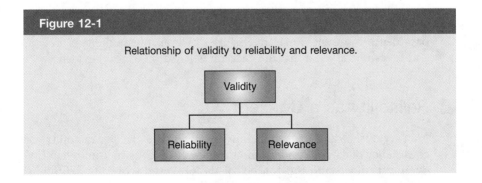

Figure 12-1

Relationship of validity to reliability and relevance.

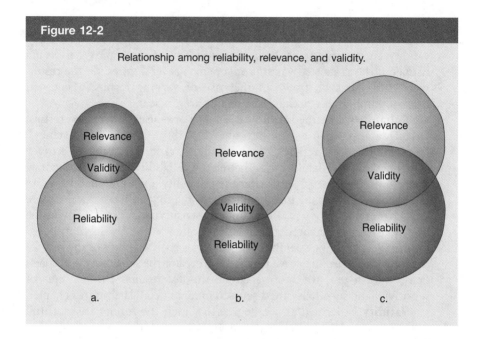

Figure 12-2

Relationship among reliability, relevance, and validity.

of relevance. In this representation, even when reliability is high, validity is low due to the lack of relevance. This figure shows that under the most reliable test, a low degree of relevance decreases the validity of the test.

Figure 12-2b depicts the situation in which there is a high degree of relevance and a low degree of reliability. In this representation, even when relevance is high, validity is low due to the lack of reliability. Even when a nurse uses what might be considered the most relevant test for the situation, if the instrument has a low degree of reliability, it will also have a low degree of validity.

Figure 12-2c shows the desired capacity for an instrument—to have both a high degree of reliability and a high degree of relevance, thereby creating a high degree of validity. Whereas the other examples show that a test can be reliable but not relevant, or relevant but not reliable, a valid test will always have some degree of reliability and relevance. When validity is absent, the results of the testing are not truthful and making an informed or evidence-based decision is impossible. However, when validity is present, a nurse can be assured that the decision is based on truthful evidence.

■ Reliability as a Concept

As previously described, reliability focuses on the repeatability or consistency of data. To understand the theoretical constructs of reliability, one must understand the concept of the **observed score**. By definition, the observed score is the score that is seen; stated in other terms, the observed score is the actual score printed on the readout of an instrument.

An example of an observed score is the measurement of a patient's blood pressure. The systolic and diastolic pressures are determined based on the aneroid dial or digital liquid crystal display (LCD) readings associated with the first sound (systolic) and the last sound (diastolic) heard in the brachial artery. If the first sound occurs at a reading of 130 mmHg, this is the systolic observed score. If the last sound occurs at 85 mmHg, this is the diastolic observed score. These observed scores for blood pressure are not the true blood pressure scores for the patient, as those scores ultimately depend on factors such as the amount of error incorporated in the type of sphygmomanometer, the quality of the stethoscope, the quality of hearing of the person taking the blood pressure, the experience of the person taking the measurements, and placement of the cuff over the artery.

A second example that may help in understanding the reliability of an observed score is the measure of quality improvement of a specific program. For instance, consider a hospital that wants to determine whether a specific pain management protocol helped reduce hospital days for patients. It used a pain scale that patients completed every 6 hours, and patient release was determined by the patient achieving an observed score of 3 on a 10-point pain scale. In this case, the scale would need very little error, because a change of 1 point on the scale might determine the release or premature release of a patient. If the scale had a high error rate—for example, 2 points of error—and the patient scored a 3 on the scale, then it would not be possible to know if the score was a 3, as high as 5, or as low as 1. The scale number may be affected by time of day the question was asked, the way the question was asked, the type of pharmaceuticals the patient is receiving, the patient's language skills, the patient's tolerance, and the severity of the initial injury causing the pain.

Each of these nuances can add or subtract error from the true score, which increases the variability between the observed score and the true score. This variability can be described as the error score, thereby defining the observed score as the sum of the true score and the error score. As shown in **Figure 12-3**, any error within the measurement decreases the degree to which the observed score reflects the true score. Note that the net effect of an error score can be positive or negative, depending on the nature of the error.

The true score exists only in theory, because all data collected are observed score data. A nurse can think of the true score as the perfect score of a test—that is, a score without any error and void of any misinterpretation. Of course, the world is not perfect and, therefore, neither are any data that might be collected. Thus, a true score exists and never changes for a given period of time; changes occur only in the error score, which then determines the observed score.

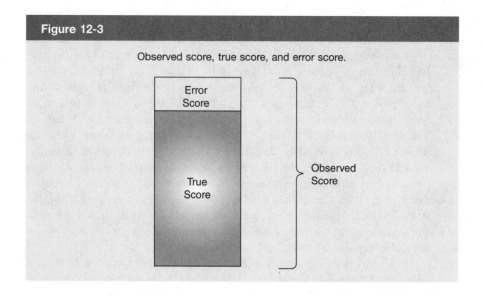

Figure 12-3

Observed score, true score, and error score.

Error
Score

True
Score

Observed
Score

❓ THINK OUTSIDE THE BOX

Discuss the elements of trustworthiness as related to making decisions about the data found in the study by Iverson and colleagues (2014). Where might error occur within the screening process and questionnaire used in this study?

Reliability is the degree to which the observed score of a measure reflects the true score of that measure. Therefore, reliability could theoretically be calculated as the proportion of observed score variance that consists of true score variance (**Figure 12-4**). In this equation, if no error exists, then the observed score variance and the true score variance are equal, and the reliability coefficient is 1.0. Conversely, when the observed score variance and the error score variance are equal, the reliability coefficient is 0. Thus, reliability always falls within the range of 0–1.0, with perfect reliability equaling 1.0 and no reliability equaling 0. For research

Figure 12-4

Theoretical calculation of reliability.

$$\text{Reliability} = \frac{S^2\,\text{true}}{S^2\,\text{observed}} = \frac{S^2\,\text{observed} - S^2\,\text{error}}{S^2\,\text{observed}}$$

purposes, high reliability measures are desired if at all possible. The general rule is that reliability coefficients greater than 0.80 are considered to be high. Note that if the reliability coefficient is calculated to be greater than 1 (e.g., 1.15), a calculation error has been made, because the range of reliability is always between 0 and 1.0.

Forms of Reliability

Although the purpose of the theoretic concept of reliability is to determine the relationship between the true and observed scores of a measurement, practical use of this concept allows a nurse to determine the relationship only between two or more observed scores. The relationship between these observed scores allows an individual to estimate reliability and to determine a range for the true score. The outcome of the calculation of the relationship between two or more observed scores is known as the correlation coefficient. The **correlation coefficient** is the practical calculation of the theoretic expression of the proportion of observed score variance that consists of true score variance, as described previously.

Given this basic understanding of reliability as a concept, it is now time to learn about the forms of reliability. Globally, reliability can be described as either **interclass reliability** or **intraclass reliability**. The most basic description of interclass reliability is the reliability between two and only two variables or trials, whereas intraclass reliability is the reliability between more than two variables or trials. The limiting factor that separates the two forms of reliability is the number of variables or trials that can be used in the calculation of the correlation coefficient. The number of variables also determines which statistical equation is used to develop the correlation coefficient. Each of these considerations has its place in EBP depending on the number of variables a nurse uses to calculate the reliability coefficient.

Interclass Reliability

Interclass reliability is the reliability between two measures that are presented in the data as either variables or trials. Four types of interclass reliability are distinguished:

- Consistency
- Stability
- Equivalency
- Internal consistency

Each of these reliability coefficients is developed using a Pearson Product Moment (PPM) correlation. Most statistical packages or spreadsheet software can calculate PPM correlations; therefore, the actual equation is not included in this text. Although each interclass reliability coefficient uses the same formula, the calculated reliability coefficient is defined by the type of variables to be compared and the methods used for interpretation of the results. This concept becomes more evident as the types of interclass reliability are further defined.

Consistency

One type of interclass reliability to report is the consistency of a measure. **Consistency** simply describes the degree to which you can expect to get the same results when measuring a variable more than once on a single day. Consistency reliability is sometimes described as test–retest reliability, because it compares two trials of a single measure. An example of testing for consistency would be running two tests on a single blood sample from each subject to measure hemoglobin using a single hemoglobin analyzer. The question is whether the results from the hemoglobin analyzer are consistent within a single day. In **Table 12-1**, the subjects' hemoglobin from a single sample of blood was measured twice, and the reliability coefficient was calculated to be 0.996.

This coefficient simply means that 99.6% of the observed score variance is true score variance. Because the reliability coefficient is close to 1.0, the reliability of the instrument is high. The initial question with this data was whether or not the machine was consistent. The results demonstrate that it was consistent, with a consistency reliability coefficient of $r_{xx}' = 0.996$.

Table 12-1

Consistency and Stability of the Ac•T diff Analyzer

Subject Number	Test 1 (g/dL)	Test 2 (g/dL)
1	14.10	14.00
2	12.20	12.10
3	11.90	11.90
4	14.50	14.40
5	13.80	13.90
6	13.20	13.10
7	13.50	13.60
8	14.00	14.10
9	11.10	11.00
10	9.60	9.90
		$r = 0.996$

Stability

When results of trials or tests are collected over 2 or more days, consistency becomes **stability**. Suppose we take the same data from Table 12-1, this time imagining that the samples were tested over a 2-day period. The question now becomes whether a blood sample is stable over a 2-day period. Notice that the results remain constant, because nothing has changed except the theoretical timing of the tests. The reliability coefficient is still 0.996, but this time a nurse would interpret the results as the samples being stable over a 2-day period, with a stability reliability coefficient of $r_{xx}' = 0.996$.

Both consistency and stability have their place in EBP. In the current example of hemoglobin testing, the consistency of the measures is described by determining that, for any time during a single day, the data would be repeatable. A nurse can expect the same results as long as no other factors have occurred in the interim, such as acute onset of anemia. In other words, the nurse is sure that the hemoglobin analyzer will give the same measure of hemoglobin for the same sample within the same day. Notice that nowhere in this example of consistency do we assume that the measurement gives the correct amount of hemoglobin, only that it indicates the presence of the same amount of hemoglobin. To determine if this is the correct amount of hemoglobin, the relevance and the validity of the instrument would have to be known.

When discussing this example in terms of stability, the key determination relates to the length of time that the blood samples remain stable. Hemoglobin analyzers usually have instructions that indicate the timeframe for running samples before differing results would be seen. In most instances, the timeframe is usually 24 hours. A question might arise concerning how the manufacturer determined this timeframe. The answer simply is that the manufacturer developed a stability coefficient using the same techniques described previously.

Again, notice that nowhere in the example of stability is there any mention of the correctness of the amount of hemoglobin over a 24-hour period; the only consideration is that it is the same amount of hemoglobin measured for a 24-hour period. To determine whether this is the correct amount of hemoglobin over the 24-hour period, the relevance and the validity of the instrument and the measures would need to be determined.

Equivalency

Another type of interclass reliability to report is equivalency. This kind of reliability allows a person to report whether one type of test is equivalent to another. **Equivalency reliability** is calculated in the same manner as the consistency and stability coefficients described previously, except that a PPM correlation between two forms of a single test is calculated, rather than a single variable over two trials.

An example of testing for equivalency reliability would be comparing two methods of blood pressure measurement to determine if they are equivalent. In this case, the question is whether the systolic blood pressure results determined by an automatic blood pressure cuff are equivalent to those recorded from manual blood pressure measures using a stethoscope and sphygmomanometer. As shown in **Table 12-2**, subjects' systolic pressure was measured once with an automatic cuff and once using manual methods. The reliability coefficient was calculated to be 0.959.

This coefficient simply means that 95.9% of the observed score variance consists of true score variance. The reliability coefficient is close to 1.0 reflecting the reliability between the instruments is high. The initial question with these data was whether automatic cuff readings are equivalent to manual readings of systolic blood pressure. A person can now report that the two methods are equivalent, with an equivalency reliability coefficient of $r_{xx}' = 0.959$. These results indicate that either an automatic cuff or manual methods are acceptable for measuring systolic blood pressure, because they are equivalent. No matter which method is used, a nurse can expect to get similar measures from a single individual. Notice again that there is no mention of the correctness of the data, only the similarity of the data. To determine if the blood pressure measures are correct, the relevance and the validity of the measures would need to be determined.

Table 12-2

Equivalency of Automatic Versus Manual Systolic Pressure Readings

Subject	Automatic Cuff Systolic (mmHg)	Manual Method Number Systolic (mmHg)
1	150.00	155.00
2	130.00	128.00
3	125.00	129.00
4	124.00	120.00
5	122.00	125.00
6	148.00	144.00
7	133.00	135.00
8	146.00	143.00
9	117.00	120.00
10	121.00	120.00
		$r = 0.959$

Internal Consistency

The final type of interclass reliability discussed here is the internal consistency of written tests. Internal consistency reliability is sometimes described as split-halves reliability, because it entails comparing two halves of a written test. To calculate the internal consistency of a written instrument, the instrument responses are divided into two equal halves. The sum of each half is calculated to make the comparison.

The simplest means for dividing a test in half is to compare the sum of the odd-numbered question responses with the sum of the even-numbered question responses. If possible, the questions should be matched between each half, based on their content and difficulty. Another possible method is to make the *a priori* assumption that both halves are equal because the questions were randomly placed in order during the development of the written test. As with the other types of interclass reliability, the PPM correlation is used to develop the reliability coefficient.

Data for a 10-item pain questionnaire are presented in **Table 12-3** to demonstrate the principle of internal consistency. Each item of the pain questionnaire is scored from 0 (strongly disagree) to 5 (strongly agree). The questionnaire is then divided into odd and even scores, with the sum of the scores for the odd-numbered items and the sum of the scores for the even-numbered items presented in the table. The question under

Table 12-3		
Internal Consistency of a 10-Item Pain Questionnaire		
Subject	Odd-Numbered Item Scores	Even-Numbered Item Scores
1	25.00	21.00
2	18.00	14.00
3	16.00	18.00
4	12.00	14.00
5	10.00	10.00
6	18.00	19.00
7	15.00	18.00
8	12.00	9.00
9	14.00	15.00
10	17.00	13.00
		$r = 0.761$

> ### ❓ THINK OUTSIDE THE BOX
>
> Look around your clinical setting. Which tools or instruments are present, and how are they typically used for data collection? Do they include surveys of employees, patients, or consumers? Are the tools or instruments used appropriately?

consideration is whether this questionnaire has internal consistency. As with the previous types of reliability, the reliability coefficient is reported; here, it is 0.761. This coefficient simply means that 76.1% of the observed score variance consists of true score variance. Notice that the internal consistency is lower than in previous examples. The fact that the reliability coefficient is lower does not mean that the questionnaire is not reliable—just that it is less reliable than it could be.

The initial question for these data was whether the pain questionnaire was internally consistent. We can now report that it has some internal consistency, with a reliability coefficient of $r_{xx}' = 0.761$, but there is at least some error present in the questionnaire. In other words, the questionnaire is not perfectly consistent internally, so the results from using the questionnaire will not be an accurate reflection of the true score. This does not mean that this questionnaire should not be used, but rather that a person needs to be careful in the interpretation and use of the results of the questionnaire. When using written item tests, individuals can actually estimate how reliability will change as a result of adding items to the questionnaire. To estimate a new reliability for a written questionnaire with added items, the Spearman–Brown prophecy formula (**Figure 12-5**) could be used.

Where r_{kk}' is the new reliability coefficient, r_{xx}' is the original reliability coefficient, and k is the total items on the new questionnaire divided by the number of items on the original questionnaire, the Spearman–Brown prophecy can be determined. In the example given in Table 12-3, the reliability coefficient was 0.761. To calculate the reliability of the questionnaire if 10 questions were added, a person would solve for r_{kk}' using the information shown in **Figure 12-6**.

The original reliability coefficient is 0.760 and the number of total items on the new questionnaire divided by the total items on the original

Figure 12-5

Spearman-Brown prophecy.

$$r_{xx'} = \frac{k \times r_{xx'}}{1 + r_{xx'}(k - 1)}$$

Figure 12-6

Spearman-Brown prophecy example.

$$r_{xx'} = \frac{2 \times 0.761}{1 + 0.0761(2 - 1)}$$

---

test is 2. Notice that by increasing the number of items on the questionnaire to 20, the new reliability coefficient for the questionnaire becomes 0.864. This coefficient is higher than the original value. Thus, adding items to the questionnaire improves this tool's internal consistency and strengthens the interpretation of its results. As discussed earlier, as reliability and relevance increase, so does validity. If the questionnaire being used has a high degree of relevance, the addition of more questions to the questionnaire (assuming they are relevant) would increase the reliability of the questionnaire, thereby improving the validity of its results.

In the article by Hanna, Weaver, Slaven, Fortenberry, and DiMeglio (2014), Cronbach's alpha coefficients were provided for both of the instruments used within the study. The diabetes-related quality of life (DQOL) tool demonstrated Cronbach's alpha coefficient scores of the subscales of 0.84, 0.83, and 0.90 during T1 and 0.85, 0.84, and 0.90 during T2. For the second tool, the Emerging Adult Diabetes Management Self-Report, the Cronbach's alpha coefficient was 0.81 at T1 and 0.85 at T2. As can be seen, each of these scores are close to the 1.0 level which implies a high internal consistency. As was stated earlier, a common interpretation of the reliability coefficient scores reflects that any level greater than 0.80 is considered to be high. All eight of these Cronbach's alpha coefficient scores exceed this level. The article does discuss the covariates for the depressive symptoms as measure by the Beck Depression Inventory (BDI-II). In-depth discussion related to the internal consistency was not provided within the article. The discussion centered on providing the statistical levels, which were found for the different tools.

Intraclass Reliability

Now that we have an understanding of interclass reliability, it is time to move on to intraclass reliability. As discussed earlier, the basic difference between interclass reliability and intraclass reliability is the number of variables that can be analyzed. Interclass reliability testing allows for the reliability analysis of only two variables, whereas intraclass reliability testing allows a researcher to develop a reliability coefficient for more than two variables.

Suppose we wanted to measure the reliability of three different pain scales. One of the scales requires only 2 minutes for completion, the second scale requires 10 minutes for completion, and the third scale requires 30 minutes for completion. The nurse would prefer to use either the 2-minute or 10-minute scale for efficiency, but the 30-minute scale is currently being used. Although the data could be analyzed using three PPM correlations to determine the equivalency reliability coefficients for these tools, this kind of analysis would miss a very important portion of the error: In the PPM interclass analysis, the statistic estimates only the error between the items, but it ignores the error within the item that reflects the differences in individuals taking the test.

In contrast, the intraclass reliability coefficient uses analysis of variance (ANOVA) to determine not only the error between the tests, but also the error within the tests. Using ANOVA allows for construction of a better estimate of the overall reliability of the scales and the errors that reduce the observed score variance, which is the true score variance. Thus, whereas PPM analysis allows for only a two-dimensional view of reliability, ANOVA supports a three-dimensional view of reliability. Notice that the basic terms of reliability remain the same. In the current example, a nurse is still estimating the equivalency of the scales, but now an error that might exist within each individual scale is included.

Figure 12-7 shows the equation used in determining a reliability coefficient using ANOVA. In this equation, a reliability coefficient is developed using the mean square between scales and the mean square within scale data from the ANOVA table.

Table 12-4 presents data for the example of the three pain scales. These ANOVA data include the between-cells mean square of 2908.233 and the within-cells mean square of 35.100. As shown in **Figure 12-8**, the reliability coefficient is determined by substituting the numbers represented in the table into the ANOVA equation for reliability (Figure 12-7).

In this example, the equivalency reliability is 0.988 for the three scales. We can now state that the 2-minute pain scale is equivalent to the 10-minute pain scale and the 30-minute pain scale. The evidence for replacing the longer 30-minute test with the more efficient 2-minute test is now documented, because the tests are equivalent. The same ANOVA reliability equation can be used to determine consistency, stability, and equivalency, depending on the intended use of the data.

Figure 12-7

Intraclass reliability coefficient using ANOVA.

$$r_{xx'} = \frac{MS_{between} - MS_{within}}{MS_{between}}$$

Table 12-4

Intraclass Reliability Using ANOVA

Subject Number	2-Minute Scale	10-Minute Scale	30-Minute Scale
1	15.00	35.00	60.00
2	12.00	30.00	51.00
3	9.00	22.00	40.00
4	10.00	25.00	42.00
5	11.00	19.00	43.00
6	14.00	31.00	45.00
7	6.00	20.00	38.00
8	3.00	15.00	33.00
9	12.00	22.00	45.00
10	11.00	21.00	45.00

Source of Variation	SSq	DF	MSq	F
Between cells	5816.467	2	2908.233	82.86
Within cells	947.700	27	35.100	
Total	6764.167	29		

Note: DF = degrees of freedom; F = F-distribution; MSq = mean square; SSq = sum of squares.

Objectivity

An area of intraclass reliability that is often overlooked is the measure of **objectivity**. Objectivity is the reliability of scores assigned by judges, multiple observers, or reviewers. In theory, if three individuals see the same performance, they should score the performance based on the merits of the performance, such that their scores are not affected by internal biases that each may possess. When no bias is evident, the scores should be similar among the judges.

A good example of objectivity (or lack of objectivity) comes from the 2002 Winter Olympics figure skating competition, in which three

Figure 12-8

Intraclass reliability coefficient using ANOVA.

$$r_{xx'} = \frac{2908.233 - 35.10}{2908.233} = 0.988$$

judges rated the performance of the Canadian skating pair. Two of the judges assigned scores of 9.9 and 9.8 for the pair's performance, but a third judge scored the pair at 7.8. If no biases were associated with the scoring method, then the third judge should have been expected to score the performance in the 9.7–9.9 range.

Objectivity also has relevance for EBP. The Apgar score—a tool for assessing the health of newborn infants—offers an example of objectivity in healthcare practice. If three medical professionals are in the delivery room, the Apgar scores each assigns to the newborn should be equivalent. This factor can be tested using the same ANOVA techniques described in the previously given pain scale example, albeit with scores for each observer, rather than each scale, being used. A researcher could determine if the Apgar scores are objective. If they are not, the researcher could meet with the observers to determine where differences occurred.

By now, it should be clear that the same formula (either PPM or ANOVA, depending on the number of trials) is used to determine the reliability of any measure. The only difference in the results relates to the interpretation based on the intended use of the data.

Accuracy

Another item that is important when determining the intraclass reliability of a test is the test's **accuracy**. The measure of the accuracy of a test is known as the **standard error of measurement (SEM)**. The SEM reflects the fluctuation of the observed score attributable to the error score. Computing the SEM allows a researcher to determine confidence intervals for the observed score based on the standard deviation of the test and its reliability. The relationship between the true score and the observed score was discussed earlier in this chapter. The SEM allows a researcher to provide a range for which the true score is present.

The equation shown in **Figure 12-9** is used to calculate the SEM. Notice that in this equation, the reliability coefficient of the test and the standard deviation of the sample are used.

The SEM can be determined for any of the prior examples. For Table 12-1, the standard deviation of the sample is 1.496, and the reliability coefficient is 0.996. Using the equation in Figure 12-9, we can compute the SEM as $\pm$ 0.0946 mg/dL (**Figure 12-10**).

 THINK OUTSIDE THE BOX

On most clinical units, many different tools are regularly used, such as thermometers, glucometers, sphygmomanometers, and weight scales. Are these tools accurate? How can you be sure that they are reliable and valid for what they are being used to evaluate? Are they valid and reliable tools?

Figure 12-9

Standard error of measurement.

$$SEM = s \sqrt{1 - r_{xx'}}$$

In a normal distribution, 68% of the sample scores fall between ± 1 standard deviation of the mean. Thus, for this example, we have 68% confidence that the hemoglobin scores will fall between ± 0.0946 mg/dL of the measured score. If a ± 2 standard deviation from the mean is used, a 95% confidence interval for the scores is expected. To find the SEM for ± 2 standard deviations from the mean, we multiply the SEM by 2 (the number of standard deviation units). In our example, we have 95% confidence that the true hemoglobin score will fall between ± 0.1892 mg/dL of the measured score. If a blood sample is run in the analyzer and the hemoglobin level is found to be 14.0 mg/dL, we would therefore have 95% confidence that the true score is between 13.1080 mg/dL and 14.1892 mg/dL. Notice that as the standard deviation increases for a set of scores, the SEM increases. Also, as the reliability of a set of scores decreases, the SEM increases. To proclaim a tool as giving an accurate measure, test scores need a relatively low standard deviation and a high reliability coefficient.

Up to this point, we have examined accuracy as it relates to continuous data. But what happens when a test uses nominal data—how do we determine its accuracy? In the case of nominal data, we use the χ^2 (chi-square) statistic and its corresponding phi coefficient as a measure of accuracy. Think of the phi coefficient as a correlation or reliability coefficient for nominal data. A χ^2 statistic and its corresponding phi coefficient would most likely be used when you are trying to determine whether a new test is equivalent to a "gold standard" test. All of the same rules apply just as they have in the previous discussion of reliability for continuous data; however, now you are simply determining the accuracy of the new test based on its "pass or fail" performance compared to the "gold standard" test.

Be aware that reliability and accuracy can be sensitive to situational changes; although a test is reliable in one situation or within one group,

Figure 12-10

SEM for consistency of a hemoglobin analyzer.

$$SEM = 1.496 \sqrt{1 - 0.996}$$
$$= \pm 0.0946 \text{ mg/dL}$$

it may not always be reliable when the situation or group changes. This consideration is especially important concerning written items. Factors that can affect reliability and accuracy include the following issues:

- *Fatigue.* Fatigue of the person taking the test or collecting the data can decrease reliability.
- *Practice.* The more practiced a person becomes at taking a test or in collecting data, the more reliability is improved.
- *Timing.* The more time that passes between test administrations, the more the reliability of the test is decreased.
- *Homogeneity of the testing conditions.* The more homogeneous the testing conditions (e.g., same room, same time taken to collect data, same time of day), the better the reliability.
- *Level of difficulty.* The more difficult a test or data collection procedure, the lower the reliability.
- *Precision.* The more precise the measurement (e.g., 1/100 vs. 1/1000 decimal), the better the accuracy.
- *Environment.* Environmental changes such as ambient pressure or temperature variations can decrease reliability.

The more control maintained over these factors, the better the reliability and accuracy of the resulting data. Accuracy and reliability improve the decision-making process in EBP.

Receiver Operand Characteristics (ROC) and Accuracy

When discussing nominal data, historically the use of the χ^2 statistic determines accuracy; however, newer statistical methods such as **receiver operand characteristics (ROC)** curves are being implemented in the field of nursing to determine accuracy of test results (Zou, O'Malley, & Mauri, 2007). ROC analyses were first developed for the armed services during World War II as a method for determining the accuracy of radar signals. More recently, this statistical method is being adapted to the medical field for defining the accuracy of diagnostic tests. ROC analysis determines the sensitivity and specificity (accuracy) of a diagnostic test to predict a specific outcome of disease the test is reported to measure. Most of the time, ROC analysis uses dichotomous variables much like a 2×2 χ^2 statistic; however, the analysis can also be used when an ordinal grading system is available for determining disease severity. The most basic form of ROC analysis uses a 2×2 method for determining accuracy of positive and negative results from a specific diagnostic test compared to whether or not the patient actually possesses the disease. **Table 12-5** represents the conceptual nature of a dichotomous diagnostic test comparing the positive and negative test results to actual disease state of a patient (nondiseased or diseased).

In Table 12-5, a perfectly accurate test would indicate only true negative results and true positive results; however, as discussed previously, there is always some inherent measurement error in diagnostic tests.

Table 12-5

Conceptual Nature of a Dichotomous Test

	Disease State	
Test Result	**No Disease**	**Disease**
Negative test result	True negative	False negative
Positive test result	False positive	True positive

The ROC analysis allows the medical provider a means to quantify this error and determine in which area of the figure the error is greatest. Unlike the SEM, which gives the researcher a global characterization of the measurement error, ROC analysis allows the researcher to determine the sensitivity (rate of true positive results) and the specificity (rate of true negative results) for any diagnostic test.

Calculations for sensitivity and specificity are fairly simple to develop. The researcher needs to know the rates or number of individuals within each of the four groups (true negative, false negative, true positive, and false positive). **Table 12-6** simplifies the variables necessary to calculate sensitivity and specificity.

In Table 12-6, TN represents the number of individuals who do not have the disease and have negative test results on the diagnostic test (true negatives). FP represents the number of individuals who do not have the disease but have positive results on the diagnostic test (false positives). FN represents the number of individuals who have the disease but have negative test results on the diagnostic test (false negative). TP represents the number of individuals who have the disease and have positive results on the diagnostic test (true positives). To calculate sensitivity (the probability of the test to correctly predict true positive

Table 12-6

Variables for Calculating Sensitivity and Specificity

	Disease State		
Test	**No Disease**	**Disease**	**Total**
Negative	TN	FN	TN + FN
Positive	FP	TP	FP + TP
Total	TN + FP	FN + TP	n

Note: FN = false negative; FP = false positive; TN = true negative; TP = true positive.

scores), the formula used is TP/(TP + FN). To calculate specificity (the probability of the test to correctly predict true negative scores), the formula used is TN/(TN + FP). Many reasons might be discussed for why ROC analyses might be used, but one of the most common reasons is to determine if a less invasive and less expensive diagnostic test will provide as good or better results when compared to the "gold standard" diagnostic test for a given disease.

For an example of calculating sensitivity and specificity of a diagnostic test, let's assume a new diagnostic test was developed for assessing the presence of carpal tunnel syndrome. The test uses a tactile response of the index fingers by touching the fingers with a thin monofilament line while conducting a modified Phalen's test (MPT) for carpal tunnel syndrome. The response from the patient is simply YES, they feel the thread (positive MPT) or NO, they do not feel the thread (negative MPT). Previously each patient was diagnosed for the presence (positive electrodiagnostic neural conduction study [EDS]) or absence (negative EDS) of carpal tunnel syndrome via an EDS. The data for the test are provided in **Table 12-7**.

To determine the sensitivity of the modified Phalen's test, the equation would be 39/46, where 39 represents the number of individuals who reported a positive MPT and a positive EDS score, and 46 represents the total positive EDS scores. The sensitivity of the modified Phalen's test is 0.848, or 84.8% probability of predicting true positive tests. To determine the specificity of the modified Phalen's test, the equation would be 20/21, where 20 represents the number of individuals who reported a positive MPT and a negative EDS score, and 21 represents the total negative EDS scores. The specificity of the modified Phalen's test is 0.952, or 95.2% probability of predicting true negative tests. The conclusion from these data is that the modified Phalen's test can accurately predict both true positive and true negative tests.

The philosophical discussion that occurs when using ROC analysis in the healthcare field is what should be considered acceptable values for sensitivity, specificity, and overall accuracy. Acceptable values are often

Table 12-7

Sensitivity and Specificity of the Modified Phalen's Test

Neg	Negative EDS	Positive EDS	Total
Negative MPT	20	7	27
Positive MPT	1	39	39
Total	21	46	66

Note: EDS = electrodiagnostic neural conduction study; MPT = modified Phalen's test.

dependent on the severity of the disease state. If the disease is life threatening, then sensitivity values should be above 85%, while specificity values may be somewhat lower. If the disease or diagnosis is mundane, then sensitivity values may be lower, but specificity values should be higher. The overall accuracy of a test should still follow the general rules of reliability and exceed 80%.

▮ Validity

To this point in the chapter, the knowledge necessary to understand the reliability and accuracy of the data collected has been provided. The fact that a test has accuracy and reliability does not mean that the test is valid, however. A valid test is defined as a test that truthfully measures what it purports to measure. Validity can be classified as either logical or statistical in nature. Logical validity requires inference and understanding of the subject being measured. Statistical validity uses statistical formulas to compare the test in question with a specific criterion or known valid measure. In EBP, validity is further delineated into three types: content-related validity, criterion-related validity, and construct-related validity. Depending on the measure, either one type or several types of validity can be used to determine if a measure is valid.

Content-Related Validity

Content-related validity is based on the logical thought process and interpretation of the measure. Many people refer to this quality as face or logical validity. The American Psychological Association (APA, 1985) defines content-related validity as "demonstrating the degree to which the sample of items, tasks, or questions on a test is representative of some defined content" (p. 10). A humorous restating of this concept is the cliché, "If it looks like a duck and quacks like a duck, then it must be a duck." A valid test using content-related validity should logically measure the content being reported.

Consider the pain scale example introduced earlier in this chapter. Content-related validity would assume that if it logically asks questions concerning the specific nature and degree of pain for a patient, then it must be measuring the pain of the individual. Another example arises with the stadiometer: If the stadiometer is a ruler, and a ruler measures distance, then it must logically be able to measure height. Both of these examples show the use of a logical thought process to validate the measure as a truthful representation of what the instrument purports to measure.

The fact that a test has content validity does not always mean that the test is valid. Other nuances may add error to the test and negate the test's content validity. Consider the practice of measuring blood pressure at the arm, which is an accepted, valid method for measuring blood pressure. But what happens when the person obtaining the measurement is inexperienced or does not place the cuff in the proper position? The result will be an invalid measurement owing to the use of an improper measurement procedure. Any deviations in measurement procedures decrease the reliability of the test, thereby invalidating the data collected with the instrument.

The criteria for content-related validity can be traced back to the process used in developing the test, the interpretation of the results, and a well-defined protocol for collection of the data. In developing content-related validity, the researcher needs to be aware of extraneous factors that can affect the outcome of the test and render the test invalid. Whenever content-related validity for an instrument is relied upon, a set of strict guidelines concerning the use and collection methods of the instrument need to be in place to ensure that the validity of the instrument is not rendered useless by these factors.

Criterion-Related Validity

Criterion-related validity is based on a comparison between the test being used and some known criterion. According to the APA (1985), criterion-related validity involves "demonstrating test scores are systematically related to one or more known criteria" (p. 11). Criterion-related validity is the statistical validity identified earlier in this chapter. (Terms such as *statistical validity* and *correlational validity* are sometimes used as synonyms for *criterion-related validity*.) The same statistical technique used to determine reliability (i.e., PPM) is used to develop a validity coefficient.

Consider the following example: measurement of oxygen saturation of arterial blood in patients. The criterion for arterial saturation would be blood gas analysis from an arterial line; however, this type of measurement brings the risk of complications and should not be used during a routine office visit. An alternative method for measuring oxygen saturation is via an infrared monitoring device that attaches to the fingertip. The infrared monitor is minimally invasive, can be used with the general population without risk, and is supposedly valid for estimating arterial oxygen saturation. To verify that the alternative method of infrared monitoring is valid, a researcher would identify a small sample of patients, subject those patients to both tests, and compare their actual blood gas results with the infrared monitoring scores. The PPM would be calculated to quantify the comparison, which would be between the alternative test to be used and the known criterion. The results would have a validity coefficient associated with the infrared monitoring model instead of a reliability coefficient. Interpretation would be done in the same manner used to interpret the reliability coefficient.

Criterion-related validity can be subdivided into **concurrent validity** and **predictive validity**, based on the time between the collection of data using the alternative method test to be validated and the criterion measurement. Concurrent validity can use the PPM statistic for validity coefficient development. With predictive validity, however, the researcher is not limited to using the PPM correlation; a linear or logistic regression can be used to develop a validity coefficient. Concurrent validity coefficients are developed simultaneously for the criterion and the alternative method test, whereas predictive validity is not limited by time.

The arterial blood oxygen saturation testing described previously is an example of concurrent validity. In this example, both criterion and alternative method measures are collected at the same time to develop the validity coefficient.

The criterion in predictive validity can be measured years after the collection of alternative method test data. Testing for the occurrence of heart disease is an example of predictive validity. A patient's total cholesterol, high-density lipoprotein (HDL) cholesterol, and low-density lipoprotein (LDL) cholesterol levels, along with other measures, are used to predict the future occurrence of atherosclerosis. Atherosclerosis—the criterion in this example—does not occur until later in life, whereas the lipid profiles, which are the alternative method test, are collected years earlier. In the predictive validity example, if a PPM correlation is used, the validity coefficient might be low because the criterion measure is a nominal value. In this case, a researcher might use logistic regression techniques to predict the probability of occurrence and develop the validity coefficient from the probability of occurrence, rather than simply from the dichotomous variable (i.e., either a person does or does not have heart disease). A good point to remember is that whenever the criterion is a continuous variable, there is a better chance of having a high validity coefficient due to the possibility of improved true score variance and lower error score variance.

When a dichotomous or nominal variable is used as the criterion, a researcher should expect to have a lower validity coefficient due to a decline in true score variance and an increase in error score variance. An example of this mystery is presented in **Table 12-8**.

❓ THINK OUTSIDE THE BOX

Discuss how you could make sure that each person who collects data as part of a research project does the collection in the same manner to ensure reliability of the study results.

Table 12-8

Effects of Variable Scale on Validity Coefficient

Subject Number	Heart Disease (Yes or No)	Probability of Heart Disease	Total Cholesterol Level
1	0	40%	145
2	1	75%	200
3	1	89%	225
4	0	45%	170
5	0	30%	160
6	1	65%	195
7	0	40%	165
8	1	85%	250
9	1	88%	300
10	0	50%	180

Heart disease and total cholesterol $r = 0.777$

Probability of heart disease and total cholesterol $r = 0.879$

In this example, the criterion measure of atherosclerosis is presented both as a dichotomous variable and as a probability of occurrence based on a logistic regression formula. The alternative test for the validity coefficient is the total cholesterol levels of the subjects collected when they were 40 years of age. Notice that when a continuous variable is used as the criterion in this example, the validity coefficient is 10% higher compared with use of a dichotomous criterion. When using dichotomous variables as measures of validity, a researcher can expect to have lower validity coefficients than when using continuous variables. This decline in the validity coefficient reflects the lack of variability within the dichotomous measure—the lack of variability decreases the effectiveness of determining the true score of the measure. If the true score measure is decreased, then the error score measure is increased, which also affects reliability.

Many times, **cross-validation** techniques are used to develop a validity coefficient from a predictive validity criterion. Cross-validation simply implies that the researcher uses one group of subjects to develop the regression equation to predict the criterion and then gathers data from a second separate, but similar, group to develop the actual validity coefficient. Cross-validation techniques are generally used in developing new prediction models for a criterion.

ROC Analysis for Determining the Criterion-Related Validity of Diagnostic Exams

Because predictive analysis as a subsidiary of criterion-related validity compares an alternative method test to a criterion measurement for developing a validity coefficient, one can logically infer that ROC analysis may be used not only to describe the accuracy of a diagnostic test, but also as a measure of the validity of a diagnostic test. When using ROC analysis for validation of testing, the evidence-based practitioner can develop an inherent validity coefficient that quantifies the predictive quality of the alternative test to predict the presence or absence of the disease. An inherent validity coefficient quantifies the ability of the alternative diagnostic test to identify true positive and true negative results. The inherent validity coefficient is calculated using the following equation:

$$(\text{True positive tests} + \text{True negative tests}) / n$$

In the case of the modified Phalen's test from Table 12-7, the inherent validity is $(20 + 39)/66 = 0.893$, or 89.3% probability of correctly identifying true positive and true negative disease states (Bilkis et al., 2012).

Construct Validity

The most abstract of validity procedures is construct validity. **Construct validity** refers to the concept of "focusing on test scores that are associated with a psychological characteristic" (APA, 1985, p. 9). In practice, construct validity attempts to develop validity for measures that exist in theory but are unobservable.

The best example of this type of validity in EBP is the measure of pain perceived by a patient. Although we know pain exists, direct measurement of pain is somewhat convoluted and is affected by the psychological traits, tolerance levels, and perceptions of the patient. The tool most commonly used to measure pain today is the analog pain scale, which measures pain on a one-dimensional scale of 1 to 10. To develop a more precise pain scale that measures several dimensions of pain and has a high validity coefficient, constructs must be developed that can measure these traits associated with pain. Thus, we can think of construct validity as the combination of content validity and statistical validity to develop a validity coefficient for an abstract variable such as pain.

To develop construct validity of a variable, the variable must first be defined as specifically as possible. The researcher would then need to identify all of the constructs associated with the variable and to define them as specifically as possible. These definitions would prove helpful in developing the measurement scales and tools to quantify the variable. In the case of the pain example, pain might be defined as the degree to which a physical symptom causes discomfort at greater than normal levels for a patient. In using this definition, the constructs associated with this variable need to be identified and defined. Notice in the definition of pain that the term *degree* is used, which assumes that some type of quantifiable scale with specific unit differences is available to quantify the intensity and severity of the variable. Also, the term *discomfort* is used in the definition, which assumes that some type of non-wellbeing exists. In this case, intensity is one construct, severity is another construct, and discomfort is the final construct that needs to be defined and measured.

To start the process of developing a pain scale, think about the physical pain that you have experienced previously in relation to the constructs of intensity, severity, and discomfort. If your experience with pain is limited, you might seek the help of others who have more experience with pain or investigate current publications in pain research to help you with the definition and development of these constructs. For the current example, assume the definitions for your constructs are as follows:

- Intensity is the degree of pain.
- Severity is the degree of debilitation associated with pain.
- Discomfort is the degree of the measure associated with the patient's pain tolerance.

In this example, it is assumed that these three constructs are measurable and part of the content that defines the overall construct of pain.

Once you have defined the constructs, you need to determine the type of scale that can be used to measure each one. For intensity, you might decide to use a scale of 0 to 10, where 0 is defined as the absence of pain and 10 is defined as the most excruciating pain imaginable. For severity, you might have to develop a scale using terms that reflect a decline in functional capacity associated with debilitation. For discomfort, you might use a scale that reflects the type of pain, such as sharp, dull, or throbbing.

After developing the scales for the constructs that are included in the measurement of pain, you must determine how each scale should be weighted to reflect the absolute construct of pain. Again, you might want to rely on personal experience when developing your construct weights; alternatively, you might wish to seek expert opinions or explore previous research to help in developing your weighting system.

When you have accomplished this last step, you have a measure that logically measures pain (content validity). You are ready to test the merits of the measure by applying it to comparable groups to determine the statistical validity of the measure. In using statistical validation measures, you are attempting to prove the following hypothesis: Those individuals with diseases that are not associated with pain should score low on the new pain scale, and those individuals with diseases or disorders associated with a high level of pain should score high on the new pain scale.

By combining the logical validation of the pain scale with the statistical interpretation of the pain scale, you have developed construct validity for a measure of pain. As you become more comfortable with the process of developing construct validity for abstract or unobservable measures, you will find that the greater the number of definable constructs, the greater the validity gained by the measure.

■ Conclusion

This chapter focused on two key principles that determine trustworthiness of research data: reliability and validity. Whereas reliability and relevance can exist independently of each other, validity cannot exist without the presence of both reliability and relevance.

The two basic statistical techniques used to determine reliability and validity are the PPM correlation and the ANOVA test. As with most techniques, the selection of which to use is based on the number of variables being compared. When there are only two variables, a researcher would use PPM; when more than two variables are being compared, the ANOVA technique would be used. Both techniques generate a coefficient between an absolute value of 0 and 1.0, and the presence of a coefficient greater than 1.0 signifies an error in the calculations.

The interpretation of the coefficient is the only change that should occur regardless of the technique used. In the case of reliability, the coefficient can be used to interpret the consistency, stability, equivalency, or objectivity of the measure depending on which aspects were used to determine the estimate. A researcher can also use the reliability coefficient in conjunction with the standard deviation of the sample to determine the accuracy of the measure using the SEM equation. With reliability and accuracy determined, a nurse can be sure that comparable measures are similar and can be interpreted as consistent, stable, equivalent, or objective within a defined range of error. In the case of validity, these techniques can be used to develop a validity coefficient for concurrent validity or predictive validity based on the time between the collection using the alternative method test, or a validity coefficient for construct validity to improve the interpretation of the measure beyond simple content validation.

Summary Points

1. Trustworthiness of study data is only as good as the instruments or tests used to collect the data.
2. Reliability and validity are the most important concepts in the decision-making process when designing research studies.

3. Reliability is the determination that an instrument consistently measures the same thing.

4. Validity is the determination that an instrument measures what it is supposed to measure.

5. Validity cannot exist without reliability and relevance.

6. Reliability and relevance can exist independently of validity.

7. The correlation coefficient is the degree (positive or negative) of the relationship between the variables.

8. Interclass reliability is the consistency between two measures that are presented in the data as either variables or trials.

9. The three types of interclass reliability are consistency, equivalency, and internal consistency.

10. Intraclass reliability allows for the development of a reliability coefficient for more than two variables.

11. Within intraclass reliability, objectivity and accuracy need to be considered.

12. The three types of validity are content-related validity, criterion-related validity, and construct-related validity.

13. Content-related validity is the level at which a sample of items, tasks, or questions represent the defined content.

14. Criterion-related validity reflects the demonstration that test scores are systematically related to one or more identified measures.

15. Criterion-related validity is subdivided into concurrent validity and predictive validity.

16. Construct-related validity concentrates on the test scores that are associated with a psychological characteristic.

17. A receiver operand characteristics (ROC) analysis can be used for determining the criterion-related validity of diagnostic exams.

RED FLAGS

- If reliability and validity are missing from the data, an informed decision concerning the trustworthiness of the results of a research study cannot be made.

- If validity is documented in a study without any indication of reliability and relevance, concerns about the trustworthiness of the results should be raised.

- If a tool is documented as being used within a study, the report should provide information concerning the validity and reliability indices for the tool.

Multiple-Choice Questions

1. When making good decisions in evidence-based practice, the _____ of the data is necessary.
   A. Confirmability
   B. Trustworthiness
   C. Independence
   D. Timing

2. Reliability is defined as the case in which an instrument:
   A. Consistently measures the same thing.
   B. Measures what it is supposed to measure.
   C. Measures demographic data.
   D. Consistently measures the same sample.

3. Reliability and relevance may exist:
   A. With dependence on validity.
   B. With only independence of validity.
   C. Independently of validity.
   D. None of the above.

4. A valid test will _____ have some degree of reliability and relevance.
   A. Never
   B. Sometimes
   C. Frequently
   D. Always

5. When measuring blood pressure, the actual score is the:
   A. Observed score on the instrument.
   B. Estimated score determined by the nurse.
   C. Perfect score without error.
   D. First sound heard by the nurse.

6. Reliability coefficients greater than _____ are considered to be high.
   A. 0.50
   B. 0.60
   C. 0.70
   D. 0.80

7. As an example of consistency and stability in EBP, when a urinalysis is done four times in a 24-hour period, the urine sample needs to be the _____ amount.

   A. Correct
   B. Same
   C. Smallest
   D. Largest

8. Dividing scores on a pain questionnaire (with 0–5 items) into odd-numbered and even-numbered scores is a mechanism that can be used to determine:

   A. External consistency.
   B. Relevance.
   C. Internal consistency.
   D. Validity.

9. A research study was developed to consider the assessment of skin color. Nurses on a medical–surgical unit were asked to record their judgments of the skin color from four pictures of individuals with differing skin tones. This process is an example of which area of reliability measurement?

   A. Accuracy
   B. Objectivity
   C. Feasibility
   D. Equivalency

10. Which test is used to establish the measurement of the accuracy related to reliability?

   A. ANOVA
   B. Standard error of measure (SEM)
   C. Pearson Product Moment (PPM) correlation
   D. Reliability coefficient

11. To establish a test as an accurate measurement of reliability, the test scores need a relatively _____ standard deviation and a _____ reliability coefficient.

   A. High; high
   B. Low; low
   C. Low; high
   D. High; low

12. Factors that can affect the reliability, objectivity, and accuracy of a tool or test include:

   A. Practice, timing, and environment.
   B. Fatigue, subjects, and environment.
   C. Precision, homogeneity of the test conditions, and the researcher.
   D. Sequencing, practice, and level of ease.

13. Validity can be classified as:

    A. Universal.

    B. Concise.

    C. General.

    D. Logical.

14. A criterion for content-related validity determination is:

    A. The inclusion of extraneous variables.

    B. Establishment of brief guidelines for using the tool.

    C. A well-defined protocol for data collection.

    D. The clarification of nuances that might add errors.

15. A researcher was comparing alternative methods for establishing a child's core body temperature for a study. The testing included the measurement of anal, oral, and aural temperatures. This example reflects which type of validity determination?

    A. Construct-related validity

    B. Criterion-related validity

    C. Content-related validity

    D. Predictive validity

16. A study presented the results from the development of a new tool. This tool was established to measure the level of anxiety perceived by children. Which type of validity would this study need to document for the tool?

    A. Content-related validity

    B. Criterion-related validity

    C. Construct-related validity

    D. Concurrent validity

Discussion Questions

Use the following data to answer questions 1–4.

Patient #	Oral Temperature (°F)	Temperature (°F)
1	98.6	98.7
2	99.4	99.3
3	101.2	101.3
4	98.6	98.6
5	100.5	100.7
6	99.7	99.4
7	101.0	101.1
8	98.4	98.6
9	102.9	102.5
10	103.1	102.9

Patient #	Oral Temperature (°F)	Tympanic Temperature (°F)
1	98.6	98.7
2	99.4	99.3
3	101.2	101.3
4	98.6	98.6
5	100.5	100.7
6	99.7	99.4
7	101.0	101.1
8	98.4	98.6
9	102.9	102.5
10	103.1	102.9

1. Is tympanic temperature a similar measure of temperature?

2. Which type of reliability coefficient have you developed with these data?

3. What is the accuracy of tympanic temperature?

4. Is tympanic temperature a valid measure of patient temperature based on the information provided in the second table?

5. Using the example of the pain scale provided in the text, define and develop five additional constructs that might be used to measure pain.

Suggested Readings

Baumgartner, T., & Jackson, A. J. (1999). *Measurement for evaluation in physical education and exercise science* (6th ed.). Dubuque, IA: McGraw-Hill.

Cunningham, G. K. (1986). *Educational and psychological measurement.* New York, NY: Macmillan.

Glass, G. V., & Hopkins, K. D. (1996). *Statistical methods in education and psychology* (3rd ed.). Englewood Cliffs, NJ: Prentice Hall.

Golafshani, N. (2003). Understanding reliability and validity in qualitative research. *Qualitative Report, 8*(4), 597–607.

MedicalBiostatistics.com. (n.d.). Sensitivity-specificity, Bayes' rule and predictivities. Retrieved from http://www.medicalbiostatistics.com /Sensitivity-specificity.pdf

Morrow, J. R., Jackson, A. W., Disch, J. G., & Mood, D. P. (2000). *Measurement and evaluation in human performance* (2nd ed.). Champaign, IL: Human Kinetics.

Thomas, J., & Nelson, J. (2005). *Research methods in physical activity* (5th ed.). Champaign, IL: Human Kinetics.

References

American Psychological Association (APA). (1985). *Standards for educational and psychological testing.* Washington, DC: Author.

Bilkis, S., Loveman, D. M., Eldridge, J. A., Ali, S. A., Kadir, A., & McConathy, W. (2012). Modified Phalen's test as an aid in diagnosing carpal tunnel syndrome. *Arthritis Care & Research, 64*(2), 287–289. doi:10.1002/acr.20664

Hanna, K. M., Weaver, M. T., Slaven, J. E., Fortenberry, J. D., & DiMeglio, L. A. (2014). Diabetes-related quality of life and the demands and burdens of diabetes care among emerging adults with type 1 diabetes in the year after high school graduation. *Research in Nursing & Health, 37,* 339–408. doi:10.1002/nur.21620

Iverson, K. M., Huang, K., Wells, S. Y., Wright, J. D., Gerber, M. R., & Wiltsey-Stirman, S. (2014). Women veterans' preferences for intimate partner violence screening and response procedures within the Veterans Health Administration. *Research in Nursing & Health, 37,* 302–311. doi:10.1002/nurs.21602.

Zou, K. H., O'Malley, A. J., & Mauri, L. (2007). Receiver-operating characteristic analysis for evaluating diagnostic tests and predictive models. *Circulation, 115*(5), 654–657.

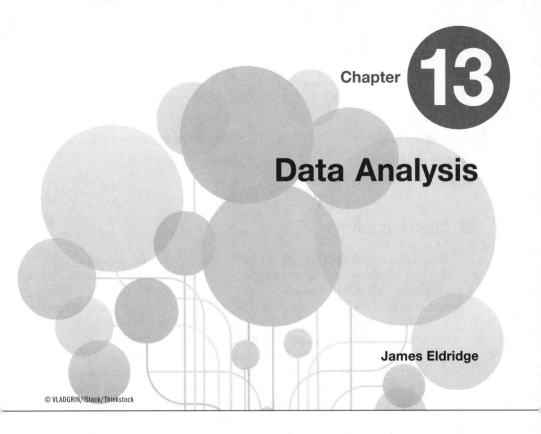

Chapter **13**

Data Analysis

James Eldridge

Chapter Objectives

At the conclusion of this chapter, the learner will be able to:

1. Identify the types of statistics available for analyses in evidence-based practice.
2. Define quantitative analysis, qualitative analysis, and quality assurance.
3. Discuss how research questions define the type of statistics to be used in evidence-based practice research.
4. Choose a data analysis plan and the proper statistics for different research questions raised in evidence-based practice.
5. Interpret data analyses and conclusions from the data analyses.
6. Discuss how quality assurance affects evidence-based practice.

Key Terms

Analysis of variance (ANOVA)	Magnitude
Central tendency	Mean
Chi-square	Median
Interval scale	Mode

Nominal scale

Ordinal scale

Qualitative analysis

Quality assurance

Quality improvement

Quantitative analysis

Ratio scale

Statistical Package for the Social

　Sciences (SPSS)

t-test

■ Introduction

This text methodically explains how to move from the formulation of the hypothesis to the data collection stage of a research project. Data collection in evidence-based practice (EBP) might be considered the easiest part of the whole research experience. The researcher has already formed the hypothesis, developed the data collection methods and instruments, and determined the subject pool characteristics.

Once the EBP researcher has completed data collection, it is time for the researcher to compile and interpret the data so as to explain them in a meaningful context. This compilation and interpretation phase is completed using either quantitative data analysis or qualitative data analysis techniques. **Quantitative analysis** is defined as the numeric representation and manipulation of observations using statistical techniques for the express purpose of describing and explaining the outcomes of research as they pertain to the hypothesis. In other words, quantitative analysis uses numerical values to explain the outcomes of a research project. In contrast, **qualitative analysis** techniques use logical deductions to decipher gathered data dealing with the human element and do not rely on numerical values or mathematical models to explain the results. In other words, qualitative analysis uses words and phrases to explain the outcomes of a research project. Do not confuse qualitative analysis with **quality improvement**, which is a measure of change over time and may use both quantitative and qualitative analyses to develop results and conclusions.

An example of the contrast between quantitative and qualitative analyses would be a research project involving the study of a specific treatment for the reduction of pressure-induced bedsores during convalescent care. To determine if the treatment was effective, data would be collected to compare two groups of individuals who were bedridden. One group would receive the treatment, while the other group would not receive the treatment. Using a scale, such as the Braden Scale, that quantified the number and size of bedsores, the researcher would collect numerical data to determine if differences were apparent between the treatment group and the no treatment group. This custom is a classic example of quantitative analysis. Using the same group of subjects, the researcher could also observe the patients' movement characteristics, attitude, and facial expressions during pre-treatment and post-treatment phases. The nursing staff could chronicle their improvement through the use of a written journal. This process would be an example of qualitative analysis.

In the example using quantitative analysis techniques, the researcher could report significant differences between the end treatment values of the treatment and no treatment groups. For example, a significant difference between the mean post-treatment occurrences of pressure ulcers of the treatment group compared to those of the no treatment group might be the result from the treatment. In the qualitative analysis example, the researcher would state the results in a different way. For example, the treatment group exhibited more positional changes during bed rest, with an observed decline in localized long-term pressure points in a single area of the body, skin blood flow changes, rashes, and blisters; furthermore, the patients had a better attitude and were less likely to complain to the nurse while undergoing the post-test procedures.

Notice that in the qualitative analysis example, no mention of statistical differences occurs. Only a description of the observed differences and changes is included. The only time a researcher can report a significant difference is when he or she has used quantitative analysis techniques to interpret the data. In this chapter, the learner will discover when and how to use these two techniques in the reporting and explanation of a project's results.

Quantitative Analysis

Measurement Scales

As described previously, quantitative analysis requires the use of numeric data to describe and interpret the results. It is often referred to as statistical analysis; in reality, however, statistical analysis is a subunit of quantitative analyses. Before a researcher can understand the nuances of quantitative analysis, he or she must first understand the types of numeric data that are available for analysis. Numeric data are classified into four measurement scales: (1) nominal, (2) ordinal, (3) interval, and (4) ratio. These four scales are listed here in hierarchical order, with the nominal scale being the least precise measurement scale and the ratio scale being the most precise measurement scale in describing results.

The **nominal scale** is the simplest of the measurement scales, because it is used for identification or categorization purposes only. This level of measurement lacks numeric order, magnitude, or size. Examples of nominal scales include race, gender, and patient identification number. A scale for race might collect data in the following way: Anglo equals 1, African American equals 2, Hispanic equals 3, and other race equals 4. In this scale, the number assigned to each race is indicative of group identification only, with no other assumption of magnitude, order, or size. The reason that we use the numerical scale rather than the word terms for race is because most statistical analysis packages have a difficult time interpreting word terms, especially when capitalization and misspellings occur.

The second measurement scale in the hierarchy is the **ordinal scale**. This scale is more precise in measuring items as compared to the nominal scale. It incorporates order or ranking, yet lacks magnitude and size. A researcher using an ordinal scale is unable to make direct comparisons between ranks, because he or she does not know whether the difference between a ranking of 1 and 2 is very small or very large. The only known aspect is that a ranking of 1 is greater or better than a ranking of 2. A medical example of an ordinal scale is the transplant recipient list for a donor heart. A transplant recipient is given a number that identifies his or her order on the list based on symptoms, severity, cross-matching/typing, and time of request. When a donor heart becomes available, the person ranked highest on the list who meets the criteria of proper cross-matching/typing, being symptomatic, with the highest level of illness severity, and the longest time on the donor list receives the heart. Potentially, two patients with the same symptoms, severity, and cross-matching/typing might be separated in the order only by the time (sometimes a few seconds) at which they were placed on the list. Thus, the different aspects have no magnitude or set units of measure between each numeric value. This example illustrates how an ordinal scale represents order but lacks magnitude and size. For both nominal and ordinal scales, mathematical calculations have no meaning, because the scales are unable to represent the magnitude and size of the variable.

The final two scales of measurement in the hierarchy are considered continuous scales, because each incorporates order and magnitude within its description. Continuous scales allow for mathematical calculations to give the results meaning. Researchers can truly describe significant differences because each number in the scale represents a unique place of order within the scale, and there is equal distance between it and the number directly above and below it in the order.

The third scale of measurement is the **interval scale**. This scale is more precise than the nominal and ordinal scales because it incorporates both order and magnitude within the description; at the same time, it lacks a defined size or, for want of a better term, an "absolute" zero point. An example of the interval scale is the Fahrenheit temperature scale. The degrees in the Fahrenheit scale are ordered from high to low. Each degree within the scale has an equal distance from the next degree; however, the point taken as zero in the scale is arbitrary. Using the term "arbitrary zero" in a scale means that the zero point is not defining a complete lack of quantity, but rather just serves as a starting point for the measurement. In the Fahrenheit scale, the point chosen as zero is arbitrary, because you can actually have a score that is below zero. This same consideration also applies when using the Celsius scale for temperature.

The final and most precise scale in the hierarchy is the **ratio scale**. This scale combines the attributes of the interval scale with the addition of an absolute zero point. The best example of a ratio scale is weight, whether measured in pounds or kilograms. The weight scale has order: 1 pound weighs less than 2 pounds. It has magnitude, and the difference between 1 pound and 2 pounds is the same as the difference between 2 pounds and 3 pounds. Finally, it has an absolute zero point, in that 0 pounds means there is a complete absence of weight.

Multiple levels of measurement can be identified in the article by Hanna, Weaver, Slaven, Fortenberry, and DiMeglio (2014). The glycemia control (HbA1c) represents an interval level of measurement. The diabetes-related quality of life tool, emerging adult diabetes management self-report, and independent functioning and decision making in daily and non-daily diabetes management checklist provide examples of ordinal levels of measurement. The final grouping of data collected for this article describes living independently from parents, which represents the nominal level of measurement.

This section of the chapter has opened with the description of the measurement scales, because the measurement scale used determines the type of statistical analysis performed. It is important to understand that the more precise a scale, the more stable the statistic used to calculate the outcome implies. Consider the measure of pain. When determining pain, a physician might use a nominal pain scale that implies only the absence or presence of pain (1 = pain, 0 = no pain), or a physician could use the ratio analog pain scale that implies degrees of pain. If the physician used a nominal scale, no differences between the groups (treatment versus no treatment) could be identified, because all of the patients in both groups still exhibited pain at the end of the study. In the analog pain example, however, the physician used a ratio scale so that the degree of pain could be measured. Although none of the patients completely lacked pain, it is clear that the group receiving the treatment had a lower degree of pain at the end of the study when compared with the no treatment group. Remember, precision not only adds reliability and validity to the study, but it also enhances the statistical power of the results.

❓ THINK OUTSIDE THE BOX

Review the article by Iverson and colleagues (2014) article and determine what types of scales were used to collect the data.

Descriptive Statistics: Nominal and Ordinal Data

The first step and lowest order of any quantitative analysis is the description of the data in numeric terms. As described earlier, the measurement scale used for each item on an instrument determines how the data are presented in a descriptive form. Reporting of data for instrument items that use a nominal or ordinal scale usually takes the form of frequencies or percentages of the response for the item. For example, demographic data for a sample might be reported using variables such as gender, race, marital status, or educational status. Data of this type are presented in the form of percentages, such as the percentage of males and females in the sample (**Figure 13-1**).

Novice researchers often make the mistake of reporting nominal or ordinal data in the form of means; this is absolutely incorrect. Nominal and ordinal data have no **magnitude** or size, measures of central tendency; therefore, a mean and standard deviation are meaningless with these data.

Interval and Ratio Data

Central Tendency

Central tendency is a way to allow the researcher to show the audience how the scores are distributed around a central point. Central tendencies are described in three ways: the mean, the median, and the mode.

The **mean**, or average, of a set of scores is determined by the sum of the scores divided by the total number of scores. An example of the

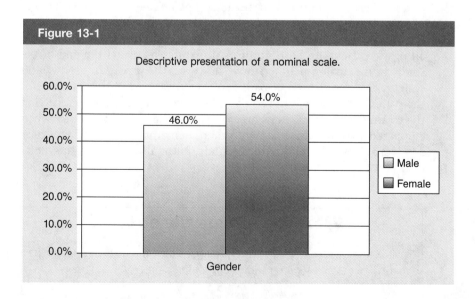

Figure 13-1

Descriptive presentation of a nominal scale.

Figure 13-2

Mathematical representation of the mean.

$$\text{Mean} = \frac{\Sigma x}{n} \text{ where } X \text{ is the observed score and } n \text{ is the number of scores}$$

$$= \frac{\Sigma 125,130,122,128, \text{ and } 130}{5}$$

$$= \frac{635}{5}$$

$$= 127$$

provision of the mean scores can be seen in the Hanna and colleagues (2014) article. Within the first table provided in the article (p. 403), each of the mean scores for the different variables is provided in a column designated with the letter M. Consider also the example of taking a patient's systolic blood pressure five times. The systolic scores are 125, 130, 122, 128, and 130 mmHg. Notice that these scores are ratio scale data, because an absolute zero point (meaning no pressure or the absence of any pressure might be measured) is possible. The calculation of the mean of these scores is shown in **Figure 13-2**. The average (mean) for the systolic pressure scores is 127 mmHg. Notice that 127 mmHg does not appear in the set of original scores. Rarely does the mean actually equal one of the scores in the observed list; rather, it represents a best estimate of the central point of all the measured scores. Measurement error is inherent in all instruments. The mean allows a researcher to develop a central point within the data, incorporating the error within the measure. The process and rationale for doing so are explained in more detail in the discussion of the standard deviation that appears later in this chapter.

The **median** is the second measure of central tendency. The median is the middle score of a set of data. It represents the 50th percentile; thus, it allows the researcher to show the exact point at which half of the scores fall above the median and half of the scores fall below the median. In the previous systolic pressure example, the median of the scores 125, 130, 122, 128, and 130 is 128 mmHg. Notice that in these readings, the score of 128 is the second to the last score. If the median is the middle number, then how can 128 be the median score? A specific point needs to be made when determining the median. The data should always be ordered from lowest to highest when determining the median. In this case, the data for systolic pressure should be ordered as follows: 122, 125, 128, 130, 130. When determining the median, all of the scores are included, even the duplications stand within the listing of the scores.

The final measure of central tendency is the **mode**. The mode is the most frequently observed score within a variable's data. In the previous example, the systolic pressure of 130 mmHg is the mode of the data because it occurs twice, while all other scores appear only once. Whereas the mean is the most stable measure of central tendency (meaning it represents the absolute possible middle score), the mode is the least stable measure of central tendency (meaning it represents only the most frequently occurring score). As a researcher increases the number of observations within a variable, the chances are that the mean, median, and mode will be more representative or equal to each other.

Variability

A second issue when describing interval and ratio data is the variability of the data. Variability describes how the data vary between each score and also from the mean. Two types of variability that the EBP researcher might report are the range of the data and the variance or standard deviation of the data.

The range of the data is calculated by subtracting the lowest score for the variable from the highest score for the variable. In the previous example involving systolic blood pressures, the range of the data is 130 − 122 mmHg, or 8 mmHg. This calculation simply means that the highest score and lowest score vary by only 8 mmHg. When reporting this range, the reader can infer that because the mean of the data was 127 mmHg and the range was 8 mmHg, then the scores ranged from 123 to 131. In such a case, the reader of the report must assume that the variability was uniform. This rating reflects that the scores varied from the mean evenly: In other words, the upper scores varied 4 mmHg from the mean, and the lower scores varied 4 mmHg from the mean. With the aforementioned assumption, the reader infers some error, because the actual scores ranged from 122 to 130 mmHg. When reporting the range of 8 mmHg and the mean of 127 mmHg, however, the range was 123 to 131 mmHg.

One other point to remember is that the range is unstable if the data being used include numerous outliers, either above the mean or below the mean. Again, using the systolic pressure example, assume that the data were 125, 130, 122, 128, and 160 mmHg. The mean for these data is 133 mmHg (approximately 6 mmHg higher than the mean found in the first example), and the range is 38 mmHg. Notice that the inclusion of a single high value increased the range by 30 mmHg. Also notice that when interpreting the data, the reader would assume falsely that with a mean of 133 mmHg, the data would range from 114 to 152 mmHg. In this case, the description of the data is lacking, because the outlier of 160 mmHg negatively affects the description.

The second measure of variability in describing data is the standard deviation, which is the square root of variance. Variance is the measure of the spread of scores around the mean based on the squared deviations

Figure 13-3

Mathematical representation of standard deviation.

$$\sqrt{\frac{\Sigma x^2 - \frac{(\Sigma x)^2}{n}}{n-1}}$$ where X is the observed score and n is the number of scores

of the observed scores from the mean of the data. The concept of a standard deviation allows a researcher to develop a description of the scores' variability from the mean based on a normal distribution. The standard deviation, which can be determined using the formula in **Figure 13-3**, provides the ability to describe the data based on a normal distribution and the percentage of the normal distribution expected to occur between each standard deviation unit.

As shown in **Figure 13-4**, the researcher can more fully describe the pattern of the data by using both the mean and the standard deviation. The standard deviation can be interpreted as meaning that the reader of the data can expect 68.26% of the observed scores to fall plus or minus one standard deviation from the mean. Conversely, the reader can expect less than two-tenths of 1% of the scores to fall plus or minus one standard deviation from the mean. In presenting both the mean and the standard deviation, a researcher describes the data in terms of a normal distribution, allowing the reader of the results to get a mental picture of how the scores compare to the normal distribution. For example, Hanna and colleagues (2014) provide each of the standard deviation calculations along with the range of scores for the different variables noted within their study (p. 403).

Figure 13-4

The normal distribution.

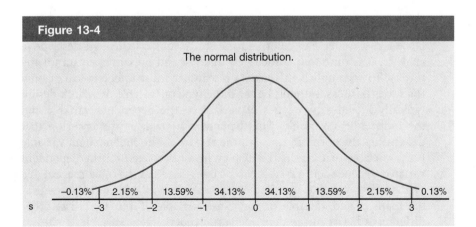

> ### ? THINK OUTSIDE THE BOX
>
> Discuss how statistics can be used in an evidence-based practice and/or quality improvement project.

Consider the systolic pressure example once again. With scores of 122, 125, 128, 130, and 130 mmHg, the mean is 127 mmHg, with a standard deviation of 3.46 mmHg. When data are presented in this form, the reader can visualize that 68.26% of the scores fell between 123.54 and 130.46 mmHg. The reader can also determine from the mean and the standard deviation that less than 0.26% of the scores were less than 116.62 mmHg or greater than 137.38 mmHg. In looking at the data described in this manner, the reader begins to understand that most of the scores from this sample were within the normal range for systolic blood pressure.

This type of analytical presentation emphasizes the verbal descriptions that are made when describing the sample demographics. ("The sample when beginning the study had normal systolic blood pressures.") Some people might shy away from reporting the mean and the standard deviation in their research reports because of math phobia. This fear is unwarranted, because most statistical software packages make the process of computing these values very simple. In the current world of research, most researchers utilize a statistics software package, such as the **Statistical Package for the Social Sciences (SPSS)**, to complete all of the calculations for the data collected.

From this point forward in this chapter, all data analysis is described for the learner. To finish the lesson on the mean and standard deviation, the learner is asked to determine the mean and standard deviation of a set of scores for hemoglobin content (**Table 13-1**). In this example, all of the scores would need to be totaled and divided by 10.

Inferential Statistics

Once a researcher has described the study subjects through descriptive analysis, it is time to quantitatively analyze and present the data for the results. To accomplish this task, a researcher must understand not only the scales of measurement, but also the type of variable. Research design typically includes two types of variables—the dependent variable and the independent variable. The dependent variable is the criterion that determines the entire purpose of the research. The independent variable is the variable that affects the change in, or is related to, the dependent variable. A dependent variable can be categorized as the outcome variable or the effect variable, while the independent variable is categorized as the manipulated variable or the cause variable. **Table 13-2** lists other differences between the dependent and independent variables.

Table 13-1	
Hemoglobin Scores	
Patient ID	**Hemoglobin**
1	14.10
2	12.20
3	11.90
4	14.50
5	13.80
6	13.20
7	13.50
8	14.00
9	11.10
10	9.60

An example of a statement using an independent variable and a dependent variable would involve a researcher attempting to determine if there is a difference between use of a statin drug and use of niacin alone in reducing cholesterol level. The dependent variable in this case is cholesterol level (the outcome measured in mg/dL); the independent variable is the type of treatment (statin or niacin). Determining which variable is the dependent variable and which is the independent variable is only the first step in identifying the statistic to use for data analysis, however. The second step is to determine the scale of measurement for both the dependent variable and the independent variable. The scale of measurement for each of these variables then determines the proper

Table 13-2	
Differences Between Dependent and Independent Variables	
Independent Variable	**Dependent Variable**
Cause	Effect
Manipulated	The consequence
Measured	Outcome
Predicted to	Predicted from
Predictor	Criterion
x	y

Table 13-3

Statistical Choice for Measurement Scales of Dependent and Independent Variables

Independent Variable	Dependent Variable	Statistical Test
1 nominal	1 nominal	Chi-square
1 nominal (2 groups)	1 continuous	t-test
1 nominal (2 groups)	1 continuous	One-way ANOVA
2 nominal	1 continuous	Two-way ANOVA

Note: ANOVA = analysis of variance.

statistic for analysis of the data. General guidelines for choosing the proper statistic based on the measurement scale of the dependent and independent variables are presented in **Table 13-3**.

Chi-Square

Whenever the dependent variable is scaled nominally, the chi-square statistic is typically used for its analysis. The **chi-square** (χ^2) value suggests whether an association exists between nominally scaled variables.

An example of a research design that warrants a chi-square analysis would be the case in which a researcher wants to know if there are differences between men and women in undergoing annual checkups (yes or no). The dependent variable for these data is whether the person underwent an annual checkup, while the independent variable is gender. With the use of a statistical software package, the chi-square value could be calculated quite easily. Once the calculation is completed, the determination of any difference between men and women in terms of whether they underwent an annual checkup could be made by reviewing the chi-square statistic and the significance of the test. Generally, most research studies seek to find statistical differences at the $p < 0.05$ level. Anything greater than 0.05 is considered not significant.

At this time, it is important to point out that in data analysis, the results are either significant or not significant. Statistical significance does not "prove" anything. When a statistical significant result is determined, the understanding is that the independent variable impacts the dependent variable but does not prove that something will occur. The p value does not impose magnitude. Therefore, even if the results have a significance of 0.0001, this finding does not mean that the results are "extremely" significant—just that they are significant.

t-Test

Now that we have described the analysis of a nominally scaled dependent variable, it is time to learn how to determine which test to use for a continuous scaled dependent variable. Review Table 13-3 to refresh your memory. The number of nominal variables and levels within the nominal variables for the independent variable determines which statistic (t-test or analysis of variance [ANOVA]) should be used.

If the independent variable has one nominal variable with two groups (e.g., gender), the researcher would use a **t-test** to determine statistical differences between the groups. Two types of t-tests can be calculated— the independent t-test and the dependent t-test. An independent t-test is used when a single continuous dependent variable is being compared, while a dependent t-test allows a researcher to compare two continuous variables as long as the variables are related.

An example of a dependent t-test would be a comparison of the pre-treatment and post-treatment cholesterol levels of a group of individuals receiving a statin drug as single-agent therapy. Interpretation of the t-test statistic is the same for both variables; the nuance relates to the number of dependent variables and whether they are related.

The independent t-test statistic determines if a difference is present in a single dependent variable between the two groups. An example of a research design that warrants an independent t-test analysis would be a researcher who wants to know if there are differences between men and women in terms of their hemoglobin content. The dependent variable for these data is hemoglobin content, which is a ratio-scaled continuous variable; the independent variable is gender. Data are provided in **Table 13-4** to assist in determining the answer to this question.

Once the results are input and statistics are calculated using a statistical software package, the determination of the difference between men

Table 13-4		
Quantitative Analysis: Data for *t*-Test Analysis		
Patient ID	**Gender**	**Hemoglobin**
1	Male	14.10
2	Female	12.20
3	Male	11.90
4	Female	14.50
5	Female	13.80
6	Female	13.20
7	Male	13.50
8	Male	14.00
9	Male	11.10
10	Female	9.60

> ### ❓ THINK OUTSIDE THE BOX
>
> Describe the different numerical values used in the clinical setting. Discuss which level of measurements each of those types of values represent (i.e., blood pressure readings, fasting blood sugars, weights). Differentiate among the different measurement scales that you use on a daily basis. Does this understanding change the way you think about the values that you use when delivering care?

and women in hemoglobin levels could be identified by assessing the significance of the test. Again, remember that most research studies seek to find statistical differences at the $p < 0.05$ level.

ANOVA

The final statistical analysis to be discussed for interpreting data is the **analysis of variance (ANOVA)**. As described previously in the t-test section, the number of nominal variables and levels within the nominal variables for the independent variable determine which statistic (t-test or ANOVA) should be used. If the independent variable has one nominal variable with more than two groups (e.g., race), an ANOVA test would be used to determine statistical differences.

Two types of ANOVA can be calculated: the one-way ANOVA and the two-way ANOVA. The one-way ANOVA is used when a research study is comparing a single nominal independent variable. The two-way ANOVA allows the researcher to compare two nominal independent variables. An example of a two-way ANOVA would involve comparing men and women (one independent variable) by trial (pre-treatment versus post-treatment; the second independent variable) in terms of their cholesterol levels. This example would be considered a 2×2 design, which is used in many clinical trials.

Interpretation of the ANOVA statistic is the same for both variables; the nuance relates to the number of independent variables. The one-way ANOVA statistic determines whether a difference is present in a single dependent variable among the several groups within a single independent variable.

An example of a research design that warrants an ANOVA analysis would be used by a researcher who wants to know if there are differences among people of various ethnicities in terms of their hemoglobin content. The dependent variable for these data is hemoglobin content, which is a ratio-scaled continuous variable, while the independent variable is race (white, African American, or Hispanic). Data are provided in **Table 13-5** to assist in answering this question. Notice that in the data entry for race, the variables are dummy coded (1 = white, 2 = Hispanic, and 3 = African American). These variables are treated as nominal scale

Table 13-5

ANOVA Model

Patient ID	Race	Hemoglobin
212	1	8.119
172	2	16.029
183	2	14.569
152	2	17.624
153	2	15.242
154	2	19.942
182	2	16.111
186	2	14.230
213	3	16.951
237	1	12.400
105	1	12.350
106	1	12.106
107	1	11.811
149	1	12.972
150	1	13.930
151	1	12.038
181	2	13.703
227	2	16.433
228	2	13.446
128	2	14.953
129	2	12.624
130	2	13.169
142	2	14.987
159	2	12.596
170	3	15.996
171	3	11.476
179	1	11.233
187	1	12.253
222	1	14.090
173	1	14.060

variables. To determine if a difference among people of these races in terms of their hemoglobin levels is present, the significance of the test would need to be calculated using a statistical software package. Again, remember that most research studies seek to find statistical differences at the $p < 0.05$ level.

A final note about ANOVA techniques: When completing either a one-way ANOVA or a two-way ANOVA, the statistical program will require the ANOVA to be defined as a one-tailed or two-tailed test. Defining the number of tails simply means that the researcher must determine whether the differences among the data are expected to occur in a single direction on the normal curve or in both directions on the normal curve. A single-tailed test suggests that the expected differences for all groups will occur in a single direction, either above the mean (an increase) or below the mean (decrease). A two-tailed test assumes that group differences are expected to change in a bidirectional manner, where one group may have a decrease from the mean while another group may have an increase from the mean. An example of a single-tailed test would be the measurement of body temperature with the onset of a disease. The researcher might expect that body temperature will increase from the normal temperature of 98.6°F only with the onset of a disease, so the ANOVA in this study will be a single-tailed test.

An example of a two-tailed test would be the measurement of body weight among a dieting group and a control group. The researcher might expect that body weight will decrease in the dieting group, whereas it will increase with the control group, so the ANOVA will be a two-tailed test.

Repeated Measures ANOVA

A final type of ANOVA not only looks at differences between groups, but also differences between times. This type of analysis is known as a repeated ANOVA. Repeated ANOVA in EBP not only can describe end-point differences but can also describe differences in the change among variables over time. Repeated ANOVA is specifically important in developing quality improvement measures where numerous time points of data may be collected to determine if a quality metric is improving.

An example of a research design that warrants a repeated ANOVA analysis would be similar to the pressure-induced bedsore study described previously. In this example, rather than determining only the treatment effect, the nurse practitioner could also determine if time had an effect on individuals who were bedridden. The study design would be similar so that one group would receive the treatment, while the other group would not receive the treatment; however, in this study data would be collected each week. Using the same group of subjects, the researcher could observe how bedsore numbers, size, and pain level increased over time to determine if changes in the timing of treatment implementation might improve the treatment's effect.

Reporting the Results of Quantitative Analysis

The final step in the quantitative analysis of data is disseminating the results in an intelligible form. Put simply, a researcher must thoroughly describe the sample using the descriptive analysis techniques. Once the sample is described, each inferential statistic needs to be described within the results. The *a priori* probability value (usually $p < 0.05$) must be stated. Finally, the statistical tests need to be reported, including what their probability is and whether these results are significant. These analyses allow a researcher to develop the discussion by comparing the results of the study with the findings from other research and inferring whether these results have substantial implications for practice.

Qualitative Analysis

The second major form of analysis that an EBP researcher may perform is a qualitative analysis. As described previously, qualitative analysis incorporates observation and language to develop an in-depth description of the results. Whereas quantitative analysis describes results and outcomes based on numeric data, inferential statistics, and sample size, qualitative analysis relies on the observational method of the researchers and their ability to describe the in-depth intricacies of the observations to explain outcomes and develop theories for the research. The final outcome of most qualitative analyses is not based on significant differences from the numeric data, but rather consists of a refined conceptual framework of the research that is improved through logical reasoning.

Another way to think about the difference between quantitative and qualitative analysis is to frame it in the terms of the reasoning process. Quantitative analysis uses the deductive reasoning process—that is, a top-down method of analysis. With this approach, the researcher begins with a theory on a topic, then narrows the scope to one or more hypotheses, and finally hones in on conformational results collected from a specific sample. In contrast, qualitative analysis most times uses the inductive reasoning process—a bottom-up analysis that goes in the opposite direction of the deductive process. With this approach, the researcher starts with observations of a specific pattern and, from those observations, develops hypotheses and theories. Once these theories are developed, the quantitative method can be used to test those theories and generalize the results to a population. Many times, the final outcome of a qualitative analysis is not a set of specific results, but rather a set of specific questions or hypotheses in need of quantitative analysis.

Two types of qualitative analysis apply to the EBP provider—the case study and the program evaluation. Each of these types of analysis occurs at some time during a nurse's professional practice. Each has commonalities and distinct characteristics that are based in the foundation of observation. The major skills that all EBP researchers must possess to ensure well-derived products from qualitative analyses are good language skills and keen observational techniques.

Notice that observation is the key element in all qualitative analyses. As a result, most qualitative research plans focus on small groups of individuals to develop the conceptual framework that encompasses the final deductions, unlike quantitative analyses that use large samples to derive the results. For example, Iverson and colleagues (2014) used conventional content analysis for the focus group data; care and thought were given to the determination of specific themes. Also, comparison data are minimal, because qualitative analysis, although not constrained by the assessment of significant differences, lacks the distinct comparable traits that are inherent in the use of quantitative analysis.

The Case Study

The case study is the most commonly practiced type of qualitative analysis occurring in EBP research. Case studies are individualized and personal. Many of the case studies gleaned from EBP eventually lead to larger quantitative analysis trials. In developing a case study, the researcher's initial response is to assume that all aspects of the case are important and to take a broad overview of the topic in an attempt to explain the outcomes.

In any qualitative analysis, focus on the conceptual framework determines the success or failure of the end product. The conceptual framework explains the dimensions of the study, the key factors, the variables, and the relationship among different variables. The EBP researcher must focus on and define the conceptual framework prior to implementing a case study. Effective preparation and focus can help eliminate unnecessary observations and shorten the time for completion of the study.

To develop a conceptual framework for a case study, or any other qualitative analysis, the EBP nurse must be well-versed in the area of study and thoroughly familiar with research previously conducted on the topic (i.e., the literature). The conceptual framework many times starts as a new observation that piques the curiosity of a researcher. In the process of becoming interested, the researcher begins to focus his or her observations, collecting data through a written journal or diary of the observations, and then attempts to develop a coherent framework that explains the novel observations. In nursing practice, patient files may be reviewed and described to develop the conceptual framework for the analysis.

Once a conceptual framework sets the boundaries of the analysis, the research questions must be developed. This is done in the same manner as in any research—through review of the literature and comparison of the case with the previous findings of other research. Case studies, like program evaluations, must be described in depth to improve the impact of their findings. A lack of depth in such descriptions may lead subsequent reviewers of the research to discard it as being poorly substantiated.

Once the conceptual framework is completed and the research questions are defined, it is time to develop the means to explain the observations in the context of the questions. A researcher should focus on and include only those material observations that are relevant. Inclusion of minutiae and irrelevant observations in the report of a study tends to detract from the impact of the overall analysis. The relevant findings should be described in detail and previous research should be used, when available, to help derive the conclusions. The end product of the effective completion of this process is often the identification of questions needing further study.

The Program Evaluation

The program evaluation is another method of qualitative analysis that the EBP researcher may use to evaluate a specific program rather than an individual case. Program evaluation allows the EBP researcher to observe the workings of a specific program, rather than a single case, and develop explanations for the success or failure of the program.

Like the case study, the program evaluation needs a well-defined conceptual framework through which to judge success or failure. Many times the program evaluator will ask the program participants to complete a self-study exercise listing the items that each participant perceives as important to the successful implementation of the program. The evaluator will then review the self-study and compare it with previously successful programs that incorporated the same conceptual framework. The researcher may also review characteristics of the site where the program implementation occurs to determine if site-specific barriers are present that might potentially hamper the successful implementation of the program.

The end product of a program evaluation should include well-defined areas of success within the program and identification of all observed barriers in the program that might increase the likelihood of failure. The final product of a program evaluation should include well-founded conclusions that will improve the likelihood of successful implementation of the program. Many times the end product will either help strengthen the implementation of the program or determine that, in the present state and site reference, the program needs to be reconceptualized.

■ Quality Assurance

Quality assurance analysis is becoming one of the most important analyses required of the EBP researcher in the healthcare setting. Patients, insurance companies, and regulatory agencies demand that programs, hospitals, and clinics provide ever-increasing evidence of the quality of the health care available to the public. Quality assurance analysis is not a recognizable single technique for analyzing data, but is the process that allows the EBP researcher to guide them in developing the necessary outcome measures that will provide the evidence of quality health care.

Quality assurance analyses may include using both quantitative and qualitative statistical techniques. These statistical techniques will define the degree to which quality exists in the healthcare services provided to the patient or the community. The ultimate outcome of a quality assurance analysis is to help the EBP researcher determine strengths and weaknesses associated with the healthcare service and allow for the development of quality improvement practices that may improve the likelihood of desired health outcomes or improve the process of efficiently delivering the healthcare service. The Institute of Medicine (2010) defines healthcare quality as being effective, safe, patient-centered, timely, efficient, and equitable. Two specific elements expected from measuring healthcare quality are the assessment of the effects of the healthcare service on improved health status and the assessment of the degree to which the healthcare services adhere to evidence-based practices and processes as defined by current scientific research, professional body consensus statements, and/or patient preferences.

The ultimate goal of quality assurance is to provide feedback to the EBP researcher for the development of quality improvement initiatives. To this end, the EBP researcher must carefully define the desired measures of quality. To aid in the development of a quality assurance measure, the EBP researcher must first determine if the measure will assess outcomes or processes associated with health care. Advantages and disadvantages to both types of quality measures must be considered. Process measures are easily benchmarked, tend to use readily accessible data, require smaller sample sizes, take less time to accumulate the data, and can provide clear feedback to the provider; however, process measures must have well-defined criteria for patient inclusion and may be difficult to summarize due to lack of available comprehensive data. Outcome measures use easily defined populations, tend to be more specific, produce clearer results concerning patient survival, health changes, and well-being, and they can be compared across conditions; however, outcome measures require much larger sample sizes, tend to be more labor intensive, and require collection of data beyond that which is collected for clinical or billing purposes; additionally, feedback generally cannot be interpreted for changes in processes. Once the type of measurement is defined as an outcome measure or a process measure, the EBP researcher can then decide which of the six measurable characteristics of quality (efficacy, efficiency, safety, timeliness, equity, and/or patient-centeredness) will be incorporated into the measure. Finally, the EBP researcher must ensure that the defined measure has adequate validity and reliability. Well-defined and developed quality assurance measures will result in effective treatments and policies, thereby improving healthcare services and healthcare delivery.

■ Conclusion

Data analysis is one of the most stressful aspects of the research process because of the complexity of the endeavor. Table 13-3 is designed to help address some of the confusion related to which tests to use. Care must be taken to select the appropriate data analysis test, thereby ensuring the broad applicability of the study's findings. For quantitative data, focusing on the level of measurements for the different variables is of paramount importance. Consideration of the appropriate central tendency measurement has application when determining which statistical test to use. For most researchers, the statistical tests are calculated using statistical software. The researcher must then make sense of the results that are provided.

Summary Points

1. Quantitative analysis uses numeric values to explain the outcome of a research project.
2. Qualitative analysis uses words or phrases to explain the outcomes of a research project.
3. Nominal scales use only group identification or categories to organize data.
4. Ordinal scales use ranking to organize data.
5. Interval scales have an arbitrary zero point.
6. Ratio scales have an absolute zero point.
7. Measures of central tendency include the mean, median, and mode.
8. Variability of the data describes how data vary between each score and from the mean.
9. The standard deviation statistic provides the ability to describe data based on a normal distribution and the percentage of the normal distribution expected to occur between each standard deviation unit.
10. A chi-square test is used to analyze data when the dependent variable is scaled nominally to determine if an association exists between the variables.
11. A t-test is used to analyze data that include one nominal variable with two groups.

12. ANOVA is used to analyze data that include one nominal variable with more than two groups.
13. Case studies often lead to larger quantitative analysis trials.
14. Quality assurance is a means of assessing the outcomes and processes of health care in terms of efficacy, efficiency, safety, timeliness, equity, and patient-centeredness.

RED FLAGS

- Means are not calculated for nominal data.
- Large standard deviations imply a wide range within the individual scores. This result suggests there is greater variability and less consistency within the resulting data.
- Outliers within the data set can skew the results of analysis of those data.
- If the data consist of a nominal level of measurement for the variable, the chi-square (χ^2) statistic would be the statistical test of choice.
- Chi-square (χ^2) tests reflect association between variables.

Multiple-Choice Questions

1. Which statistic is often used for nominally scaled variables?
   A. t-test
   B. ANOVA
   C. Chi-square
   D. Pearson product moment

2. What level of measurement is most often associated with categorical data such as gender?
   A. Nominal
   B. Ordinal
   C. Interval
   D. Ratio

3. Which inferential procedure is appropriate when there is one nominal-scale dependent variable and one nominal-scale independent variable?
   A. Chi-square
   B. t-test
   C. One-way ANOVA
   D. Factor analysis

4. Inferential statistics are used to decide if differences among treatment groups are due to the:
   A. Significance.
   B. Dependent variable.
   C. Confounding variable.
   D. Independent variable.

5. Selection of the appropriate statistical technique is based on:
   A. The research question.
   B. The level of measurement of the independent variable or variables.
   C. The level of measurement of the dependent variable or variables.
   D. All of the above.

6. What do statistically significant findings imply?
   A. The results are very important.
   B. The results are not very important.
   C. The results are likely due to chance differences among groups.
   D. The results are likely due to real differences among groups.

7. A researcher investigated the relationship between vitamin C supplements (none, 500 mg, 1,000 mg) and workers (office, outdoors) in terms of the frequency of colds. Which of the following is (are) the dependent variable(s)?

A. Colds
B. Vitamin C
C. Colds and workers
D. Vitamin C and workers

8. Which of the following is an inferential statistic?

A. Mode
B. t-test
C. Standard deviation
D. Range

9. Which statistical test has a dependent variable that is nominal in nature?

A. Chi-square
B. t-test
C. ANOVA
D. Two-way ANOVA

10. What is standard deviation?

A. The square of the mean deviation
B. The square of the variance
C. The square root of the variance
D. The square root of the sum of squares

11. The t-test is used to:

A. Adjust for initial differences within the groups.
B. Estimate the error of prediction.
C. Test whether two groups differ significantly.
D. Test whether more than two groups differ significantly.

12. Use of a one-tailed versus a two-tailed test of significance of the difference between two samples is determined by:

A. Whether there is expected overlap between the error curves of the two sample distributions.
B. Whether the difference is expected to be in one direction only.
C. The size of the samples relative to population size.
D. Whether the subjects were matched or chosen randomly.

Discussion Questions

1. A nurse has decided to research the following PICOT question: "Adult clients who are admitted to the cardiac unit with congestive heart failure are more likely to develop nosocomial infections than other cardiac clients admitted to the cardiac unit." A quantitative research design is planned for this project. From the PICOT question, determine the variables, the levels of measurement of each variable, and the statistical test to be used.

2. A research study assessing vital signs for 15 clients has the following results. Calculate the mean, median, mode, range limits, range, and presence of outliers for each of the vital sign indices.

Client Number	Oral Temperature (°F)	Pulse (Beats/Minute)	Respirations (Breaths/Minute)	Blood Pressure
1	97.6	80	12	160/80
2	98.6	60	20	154/90
3	98.6	54	32	132/60
4	99.0	92	16	90/62
5	98.0	86	18	200/140
6	98.4	84	22	116/76
7	99.2	74	28	132/80
8	100.0	72	18	124/78
9	98.6	90	20	140/90
10	98.6	88	32	160/90
11	98.6	64	30	100/50
12	98.8	68	20	118/84
13	98.4	74	18	120/88
14	98.2	50	14	132/74
15	97.6	100	32	190/110

3. A research project is envisioned to analyze preintervention and postintervention cholesterol levels for a group of high school students participating in an after-school athletic program. Which type of statistical test could be used for this study and why?

Suggested Readings

American Psychological Association (APA). (2001). *Standards for educational and psychological testing* (5th ed., pp. 8–9). Washington, DC: Author.

Baumgartner, T., & Jackson, A. J. (1999). *Measurement for evaluation in physical education and exercise science* (6th ed., pp. 57–109). Dubuque, IA: McGraw-Hill.

Colling, J. (2004). Coding, analysis, and dissemination of study results. *Urology Nursing*, *24*(3), 215–216.

Cunningham, G. K. (1986). *Educational and psychological measurement*. New York, NY: Macmillan.

Glass, G. V., & Hopkins, K. D. (1996). *Statistical methods in education and psychology* (3rd ed., pp. 31–77). Englewood Cliffs, NJ: Prentice Hall.

Happ, M. B., Dabbs, A. D., Tate, J., Hricik, A., & Erlen, J. (2006). Exemplars of mixed methods data combination and analysis. *Nursing Research*, *55*(2), S43–S49.

Institute of Medicine. (2010). *The future of nursing: Leading change, advancing health*. Washington, DC: National Academies Press.

Magee, T., Lee, S., Giuliano, K., & Munro, B. (2006). Generating new knowledge from existing data: the use of large data sets for nursing research. *Nursing Research*, *55*(2S), S50–S56.

Morrow, J. R., Jackson, A. W., Disch, J. G., & Mood, D. P. (2000). *Measurement and evaluation in human performance* (2nd ed., pp. 65–70). Champaign, IL: Human Kinetics.

Owen, S., & Froman, R. (2005). Focus on research methods. Why carve up your continuous data? *Research in Nursing & Health*, *28*(6), 496–503.

Priest, H., Roberts, P., & Woods, L. (2002). An overview of three different approaches to the interpretation of qualitative data. Part 1: Theoretical Issues. *Nurse Researcher*, *10*(1), 30–42.

Rubin, H. R., Pronovost, P., & Diette, G. B. (2001). The advantages and disadvantages of process-based measures of health care quality. *International Journal for Quality in Health Care*, *13*(6), 469–474.

Seibers, R. (2002). Data in abstracts of research articles: Are they consistent with those reported in the article? *British Journal of Biomedical Science*, *59*(2), 67–68.

Thomas, J., & Nelson J. (2005). *Research methods in physical activity* (5th ed., pp. 110–212). Champaign, IL: Human Kinetics.

References

Hanna, K. M., Weaver, M. T., Slaven, J. E., Fortenberry, J. D., & DiMeglio, L. A. (2014). Diabetes-related quality of life and the demands and burdens of diabetes care among emerging adults with type 1 diabetes in the year after high school graduation. *Research in Nursing & Health, 37*, 399–408. doi:10.1002 /nur.21620

Institute of Medicine (IOM). (2010). *The future of nursing: Leading change, advancing health.* Washington, DC: National Academies Press.

Iverson, K. M., Huang, K., Wells, S. Y., Wright, J. D., Gerber, M. R., & Wiltsey-Stirman, S. (2014). Women veterans' preferences for intimate partner violence screening and response procedures within the Veterans Health Administration. *Research in Nursing & Health, 37*, 302–311. doi:10.1002/nur.21602

Chapter

14

The Research Critique Process and the Evidence-Based Appraisal Process

Carol Boswell and Sharon Cannon

Chapter Objectives

At the conclusion of this chapter, the learner will be able to:

1. Provide a rationale for completing a research critique.
2. List the necessary elements in a research critique.
3. Examine the evidence-based appraisal.
4. Evaluate evidence needed for clinical decision making.
5. Use evidence-based practice guidelines to manage holistic nursing practice.

Key Terms

Critique

Hypothesis

Qualitative research

Quantitative research

■ Rationale for Doing a Research Critique

When a critical question in nursing practice has been posed, the immediate reaction is often itself a question: What's in the literature? A common assumption made by most people is that the printed words are absolute or true. This assumption is even more commonplace when the literature is a researched study. Unfortunately, not all published research is scientifically sound. As a result, it is imperative that a nurse be able to critically assess a report.

According to Burns and Grove (2009), in the 1940s and 1950s nursing research generated critiques that were less than pleasant. Consequently, little nursing research was undertaken until the 1980s and 1990s. No studies are without some imperfections, but fearing imperfect studies is not a valid excuse for failure to conduct research. The basic concept of research management is that the researcher makes decisions about the research plan and justifies those decisions. According to Glasofer (2014), "quality is the extent to which a study has minimized biases in the selection of subjects and measurement of outcomes, as well as minimized influence of anything outside of the factors being studied on the results" (p. 19). If the researcher has done a good job with the justifications, then the strength of the results is supported. When poor justifications for the research decisions are evident, the strength of the results must be questioned. As a result of this realization, scrutiny focusing on the limitations and strengths of studies is now commonplace. This shift from criticism to analysis provides a more positive approach to examining the usefulness of the scientific data generated. Nurses must critically contemplate and evaluate studies, particularly research studies, to determine the appropriate application to practice. Melnyk and Fineout-Overholt (2015) support this sentiment in relation to research and evidence-based practice (EBP). In EBP, research provides the evidence that guides clinical practice in making decisions about the care nurses provide.

According to Polit and Beck (2008), a research critique is a mechanism to provide feedback for improvement. They suggest that nurses who can critically review a study make valuable contributions to the body of nursing knowledge. Individuals conducting critiques need to be aware of biases that they could insert into their review. Care needs to be given

 THINK OUTSIDE THE BOX

Looking critically at the evidence required of nurses today, how could you start the process of gaining confidence in doing research critiques? What are some of the reasons for doing research critiques?

when looking at sources to determine the effectiveness of the material for practice, so that changes in practice are based on material that has minimal biases within the review of the material.

Finally, considering a rationale for a research critique can be found in the definition of the word "critique" as offered by the Merriam-Webster (2015) *Learner's Dictionary*: "a careful judgment in which you give your opinion about the good and bad parts of something (such as a piece of writing or a work of art)" (p. 1). If one thinks of nursing as both an art and a science, then a critical review of nursing research can be seen as a work of art. Studies withstanding the test of time through careful exploration of findings and implementation allow nurses to practice the art and science of the profession. Each nurse is asked to regularly and consistently examine how and what they are doing in light of the evidence to ensure that the care provided is current. By examining the different articles for positive and negative items within the discussion, gaps and consistencies can be determined. Research is a significant aspect of EBP; therefore, this chapter discusses the research critique first.

Elements of a Research Critique

Before considering the elements of a research critique, let's discuss the types of critiques. Burns and Grove (2009) have identified nine types of critiques, ranging from student critiques to critiques of research proposals:

- Students learn to critique in their nursing education programs.
- Practicing nurses analyze studies for evidence on which to base the care provided.
- Educators approach critiques from the aspect of improving instruction.
- Nurse researchers focus on building a program of research emphasizing the review of studies in one specific area.
- Abstracts are frequently reviewed for use in presenting research findings.
- Presenting research at meetings, conferences, and workshops allows participants to verbally critique studies.
- Several nursing journals publish critiques of published articles, with the authors of the original article subsequently responding to concerns raised with the critique. These types of critiques often take the form of letters to the editor.
- An article submitted for publication in a peer-reviewed journal undergoes a review by peers who assess the quality of the study.
- Requests for funding for research studies from agencies such as the National Institute of Nursing Research (NINR) are subjected to scrutiny.

Critiques are essential to EBP and are expressed in the various forms just discussed. Regardless of the type of critique, each critique includes certain elements. Brink and Wood (2001) have suggested that the rationale for a research critique is to ascertain whether the conclusions are serviceable within the setting in which you are functioning. Some general questions can be associated with the elements of a critique.

Study Purpose

The first element of a research critique generally involves determining the purpose of a study. For example, this material is found in the introduction of the study by Iverson and colleagues (2014), although it is not labeled as such. Questions to be asked about this element include the following:

- Is the purpose understandable?
- Is it appropriate to your practice?
- Is a need for the study clearly stated?
- Will the study improve nursing practice and add to the body of nursing knowledge?

In the Hanna, Weaver, Slaven, Fortenberry, and DiMeglio (2014) article, these questions would be assessed by reading the untitled introduction along with the correlation of diabetes-related quality of life section. Answers to these questions guide the critique. If the responses are negative, then the notion of applying the study to practice is questionable. The purpose section should clearly and effectively present the importance of the need to complete this study on this topic. When the goal of the study is not evident with the initial information, the article may be overlooked as not connected to the material being sought. This determination is based on that key, preliminary clarification of the "why" statement. The reasons for the study must be unmistakably declared within the first few paragraphs of the article.

Research Design

A second element involves the design of the research. In the Iverson and colleagues (2014) manuscript, this material is found in the section labeled as methods, particularly the data collection component. Questions to ask about this element include the following:

- Is there a framework/theory to guide the study?
- If there is no framework/theory, are you able to identify how data will be evaluated?
- Do the authors provide a clear discussion of how data will be collected and maintained?

- Who will be studied?
- What is the plan for conducting the study?
- Are the research plan decisions adequately justified?

In the Hanna and colleagues (2014) manuscript, these questions would be assessed by reading the conceptual framework along with the methods in the design section. Each question provides a nuance related to the different components of a study.

Constructing the different components for a research study with the rationales for the decisions made along with the generating of the research project is a multifaceted and intricate enterprise. Adequate planning is important to allow the use of the best evidence for incorporation in nursing practice. A well-thought-out design allows for assurance that the evidence has practicality. The research design can be likened to a set of instructions allowing the builder to put together the pieces of a puzzle resulting in a usable product. The determination of the rationales as to how and why decisions within the research process were made is imperative to the successful development of a sound and reasonable research application. The justification for the decisions made provides the foundation for users of the research to determine the reasonableness of the results and outcomes recommended.

Literature Review

Another element to consider is whether the literature review focuses on the problem presented. The literature review should speak to the gaps and consistencies found within the evidence. This material is found laced throughout the Iverson and colleagues (2014) manuscript. A resourceful and constructive literature review provides clarity as to what has been done and what continues to be needed.

Questions to ask about this element include the following:

- Is the literature review thorough and detailed?
- Is the literature review current—that is, has the literature been published within the last 5 years?
- Are there benchmark publications?
- Are the majority of sources primary or secondary?
- Is the literature review well organized, including an introduction and a summary?
- Does the literature review include a section for a model/theory?

 THINK OUTSIDE THE BOX

Which aspects of a research article do you perceive as important, and why? Which aspects of the article seem to be the hardest to locate, and why?

These questions would be assessed in multiple areas within the Hanna and colleagues (2014) manuscript. Care should be given to the clarity of the literature discussion when the different aspects are laced throughout the discussion.

A thorough literature review allows for assessment of the credibility of the present study. Of major importance in beginning a research study is the need to ask, "What has been written about the problem?" The literature review provides the foundation for the study's significance and relationship to practice. Benchmark publications are valuable because they serve as the foundation for the ongoing investigation on the topic of interest. Publications that have been deemed as underpinning and supporting of the ongoing work are paramount to successful progression to the next level of knowledge concerning a topic of interest.

Research Question/Hypothesis

The next element of a research critique is the research question(s) or **hypothesis**(es). This element of the critique is of extreme importance, as it should reflect the purpose of the study. Within the Iverson and colleagues (2014) manuscript, this material is denoted as the purpose statement that comes at the end of the introduction. Research questions in EBP are the "who, what, when, where, why, and how" guiding the nursing care provided to patients. Thus, it is essential to assess the following issues:

- Is the research question clearly stated?
- Does it match the purpose of the study?
- Are the decisions made about the research question adequately justified?
- Is there a theory/framework/model discussed that establishes a relationship with the question?

In the Hanna and colleagues (2014) manuscript, these questions would be assessed by noting the purpose statement provided at the end of the introduction section.

A study can contain a hypothesis rather than a research question. In some studies, the research purpose may be the only statement provided. Whether it is a research purpose, research question, and/or hypothesis, it is important that the connection to the study purpose is evident. The expectation that the study purpose is evident in all aspects of the development of the study is crucial. Polit and Beck (2008) define a hypothesis as "a prediction about the relationship between two or more variables" (p. 755). Simply put, a hypothesis may predict, propose, suppose, explain, or test a quality, property, or characteristic of people, things, or settings. People often talk about or discuss "hypothetical situations." A hypothesis proposes a solution. Questions to ask about a hypothesis and/or research questions include the following:

- Are the independent and dependent variables described?
- Is the hypothesis clearly stated?
- Does the hypothesis reflect the purpose of the study?
- Are the decisions made regarding the hypothesis adequately justified?
- Is there a theory/framework/model discussed that establishes a relationship with the hypothesis?

The establishment of the research question or hypothesis is paramount to the focus of the study. Each aspect of the wording within the questions or hypotheses needs to be clear and concise to allow for the effective concentration of the research endeavor. The PICOT (population, intervention, comparison, outcome, time) statement should play a part toward the development of the research question or hypothesis. The PICOT process drives the literature review and can evolve into the research question or hypothesis, based on the outcomes of the literature review. From the gaps and consistencies identified during the literature review within the EBP process, the research question/hypothesis can be structured to advance toward the next level the body of knowledge concerning the topic under investigation.

Study Sample

Another element of the research critique focuses on the sample. Sampling questions address the different aspects of the population. Within the Iverson and colleagues (2014) manuscript, the section to read and consider is labeled "Setting and recruitment." Each aspect within the clarification of the sampling design should be supported by rationales within the dissemination of the study. Questions regarding the sample should include the following:

- Who is identified as the target population?
- How were the subjects chosen (e.g., randomly, conveniently)?
- Who is included (e.g., males, females, children, adults)?
- Who is excluded (e.g., elderly, pregnant women, minorities)?
- How large is the sample?
- Are the decisions made regarding the sampling plan adequately justified?
- Were ethical considerations clearly addressed within the sampling process?

In the Hanna and colleagues (2014) manuscript, these questions are located in the area entitled "Sampling Procedure." Answers to these questions can help the nurse decide if decisions about patients and clinical problems are practical for their unique setting. By looking at these aspects of the sampling plan, generalization to a population can be supported. Clarification of the sample population must be denoted. Each aspect of the sampling process should be carefully and thoroughly described within the discussion of the project.

Data Collection

Data collection embraces many aspects that are critical to the success of the research study. Essential to the critique is a description of how the data were collected. Within the Iverson and colleagues (2014) manuscript, this material is found in the section labeled "Data Collection Component." Questions about this element include the following:

- What steps were taken to collect the data?
- How often were data collected and for how long?
- Which instruments or tools were used?
- Who designed the tools?
- Are the tools valid and reliable?
- Are the tools adequately described so that readers can understand what the scores mean?
- Were data analysis procedures appropriate?
- Are the plans for data collection and analysis decisions adequately justified?
- Were ethical considerations adequately addressed within the data collection process?

In the Hanna and colleagues (2014) manuscript, these questions would be assessed by reading the data collection section. Justification for the data collection processes should be evident within the discussion of the data.

Data collection gives information about the research question or hypothesis. Quantitative data, for example, are often collected by a survey mechanism that provides a score for analysis. In such a case, a clear understanding of how and where the data were collected, the description of the instrument (tool) that was used, and how the results were statistically analyzed are essential. In contrast, the data collected for a qualitative study are presented in narrative format. Qualitative data utilize collection methods that must include a discussion of how potential biases were addressed.

Study Results

Clear discussion of the results from a study is essential. Results must be placed within the context of where and when they were collected. Within the Iverson and colleagues (2014) manuscript, this material is found in the

> ### ❓ THINK OUTSIDE THE BOX
>
> Frequently, the theoretical foundation for a study seems to be omitted in research articles due to page restrictions imposed by the journal. Debate the importance of including the theoretical foundation for a study in the report of its findings.

two sections labeled as data analysis and results. A critique should provide the results of the study. Questions about results include the following:

- Is the research question answered or the hypothesis supported?
- Were limitations listed and explained?
- Can generalizations to a wider population be made?
- Did the results support what was reported in the literature?
- Were there any unexpected findings?
- Did the outcomes affirm the theory used as the basis of the study?

In the Hanna and colleagues (2014) manuscript, these questions would be assessed by reading measures, covariates, data analyses, and results.

The elements of the critique summarize the study, including what was found and how the findings might be applied to similar situations. The summary of the findings needs to be carefully presented to allow for generalization to other settings and populations. Care must be given to this aspect within the report of the study outcomes to provide an understanding for where and how the results can be used within the practical world of health care.

Study Recommendations

The final element of the research critique is the section presenting the author's recommendations. The author understands what the study means and has the responsibility for providing guidance as to where the next steps should be directed. In the Iverson and colleagues (2014) manuscript, this material is found in the discussion section. With the in-depth work pivotal to the study completion, avenues that were identified but not addressed and/or unexpected outcomes are key areas that should be recommended for further study. Questions for this element include the following:

- Are suggestions for further use in practice included?
- Is there an identified need for further research?
- Could you make a change in your practice based on the results of this study?
- What are the benefits to using the information learned?

In the Hanna and colleagues (2014) manuscript, these questions would also be assessed by reading the discussion section.

The necessary elements of a research critique can be organized as answers to a series of questions. Utilizing a logical format for reporting the decisions made as the study was planned, along with the results that were obtained, provides a foundation for moving healthcare research forward. This process of carefully and thoroughly considering all aspects within a reported study demonstrates accountability for advancing health care and patient safety. Those questions then form the basis for the process of conducting a research critique. As the individual investigates the quality of a study, these questions can provide a beginning place for the critique. A validated study should successfully address the majority of these questions in a positive and constructive manner. The purpose of reporting the results of a study is to allow colleagues to carefully assess the outcomes to identify ways to improve patient care.

Process for Conducting a Research Critique

The word **critique** can be defined as "an article or essay criticizing a literary or other work; detailed evaluation; review, a criticism or critical comment on some problem, subject, etc., the art or practice of criticism to review or analyze critically" (Dictionary.com, 2015). Although *research critique* is the term frequently used, several other terms—such as *critical analysis, review, evaluation,* and *appraisal*—can also be associated with the process. Any of these terms could be, and are, used as the method for assessing a published research article.

To gain a true understanding and appreciation of the process of a research critique, one must recognize the expectations for conducting the process. As the definition implies, it is undertaken to allow individuals to carefully and thoroughly examine a research endeavor. The outcome is not anticipated to be a negative grilling of the project to identify all of its shortcomings. Wood and Ross-Kerr (2006) affirm this point: "In your best judgment, you decide if what you have read will serve your purpose" (p. 65). The materials should be practical and applicable to your individual practice setting and the patient situation.

Studies should be scrutinized for their merits, limitations, implications, and consequences. Each and every report should be assessed with a critical eye toward each unique setting. The resulting critique should be impartial, presenting both strengths and challenges. Any review should have a goal of providing constructive recommendations related to how the study might be improved, along with where the results/outcomes could be used within health care. It is envisioned as a review or analysis of the research undertaking. Both the strengths and challenges within the process of conducting the research study are judiciously

THINK OUTSIDE THE BOX

If nurses do not value research, their engagement with the critique process and their participation in research studies are decreased. Identify steps and incentives that might be used to get you and your peers involved in doing research critiques or research projects.

examined to verify that the ending results can truly be generalized to the target population.

By completing an effective research critique, a reviewer becomes aware of both the strengths and the shortcomings of the research project. As a consequence of identifying these concerns, the assessor can efficiently incorporate the results into practice based on this in-depth knowledge of the study findings. Thus, the incorporation of the results into nursing practice is based on an understanding of the comprehensiveness of the study.

Every study has limitations, because researchers must inevitably make multiple methodological judgments that influence the significance, integrity, and value of the resulting research outcomes (San Jose State University, 2005). No study in humans is ever perfectly conducted, and even nonhuman studies frequently have limitations and weaknesses. It is true that research conducted on laboratory animals can be controlled with greater success than projects in which humans are the subjects. Put simply, when working with laboratory animals, the variables can be manipulated. If the same project were envisioned using human subjects, however, the ethical ramifications could be increased, because manipulation of the variables for human subjects might result in damages. Thus, the ethical nuances of human research must be considered when the results are proposed to be incorporated into practice.

Another factor—the austere style of journal articles—also triggers some concerns. The amount of space allocated to articles within journals is prescribed by the companies that publish those journals. As a result of these restrictions regarding page length and word count limits, key elements within the research process must be succinctly presented. Depth of discussion about the basic research principles must, therefore, be limited or even omitted. Unfortunately, discussions of the operational

 THINK OUTSIDE THE BOX

Look at some research articles. Can you identify within them any discussion related to patient preferences that is part of evidence-based practice? Discuss your thoughts about your findings.

definitions for key variables; models, plans, and systems; and conceptual or theoretical frameworks are often omitted due to space restrictions. Classic research studies include a description of the theory/framework and concepts underlying the study, but many other studies use a model, plan, or system for the research.

Another aspect of the process that deters nurses from participating in research critiques is the unfamiliar jargon. Statistical aspects are quite intimidating to many practicing nurses. The definitions used within research to discuss sampling, variables, hypotheses, and quantitative and qualitative methods are typically foreign to the practicing nurse. Although many of these are common terms, such as "independent," "dependent," "convenience," and "variable," they take on new meanings within a research project. This specificity of the terms within research leads to conflict and misunderstanding for novice evaluators of research. In the future, nurses will be increasingly confronted with the expectation that they will center their practice on evidence. Nurses must become proficient at reading and understanding research reports to incorporate their findings into EBP. They need to take a deep breath now and plunge into the critiquing process.

The most valuable advice for developing expertise in this process is to continue doing research critiques, because practice does diminish the confusion and overwhelming nature of the process. By reading research articles, nurses become increasingly accustomed to the format and terminology. Evidence-based nursing practice mandates that nurses begin to build a knowledge base by the "steady diet" approach—specifically, by digesting at least one research report each week. By accepting the challenge to become comfortable with research reports, nurses will find that the different aspects of the report become more familiar, even commonplace—and, therefore, less threatening. Not all nurses will strive to carry out research activities, but it is imperative that all nurses become comfortable with the use of research results to advance the discipline of nursing and ultimately improve nursing care.

Initially, some general areas of the research study must be considered. The author(s) of the study needs to be evaluated. Precisely who is completing the research, including those persons' job titles and qualifications to conduct the project, needs to be carefully contemplated. After the author information is pondered, an assessment of the study title provides valuable information. The title of the project should provide a clear, concise description of the project. It should stimulate a prompt perception of the fundamental nature of the paper.

At this point, the abstract is examined to further clarify the focus for the research endeavor. The abstract should condense the main points from the research project. A quick read of the abstract and discussion sections should provide valuable insight into the complexity of the study and its applicability to a unique practice setting.

Four key aspects to carefully address when initiating a research critique are:

- Recognizing the purpose and problem, while resolving if the design and methodology are consistent with the study intent
- Verifying that the methodology is utilized appropriately
- Contemplating if the outcomes and conclusions are credible and confirmed by the findings
- Reflecting on the report's overall quality, strengths, and challenges, and whether they contribute to the knowledge base and offer suggestions for improvement

Research critiques can take many different pathways. The principal idea is to make sure that, regardless of the tool or process used, each aspect of the research process is carefully examined for appropriateness. An example of the research critique process should involve the following steps:

1. Read the entire study carefully and with purpose.
2. Examine the organization and presentation of the different components for logical flow.
3. Identify any term you don't understand by seeking clarification as to the meaning of the term.
4. Highlight and examine each step of the research process.
5. Identify the strengths and challenges without bias.
6. Consider modifications for future studies.
7. Determine how well the study followed the expectations for an ideal study.

Table 14-1 provides an example of a critique worksheet. Some worksheets provide areas for comments while others may have checkboxes to complete. Any format that addresses the different areas that need to be included in a critique can be used to help the individual develop confidence in completing a review of a scholarly article.

These guidelines are fairly general, but they do provide a place to start. A careful, general reading of the entire study must be the beginning point for any critique. The examiner initially should read the complete research report to gain an awareness of the study and its contribution to knowledge improvement. A second reading of the document allows the focus to be directed toward the questions appropriate to each stage of the critiquing process. The use of a photocopy of the article may facilitate the research critique process, because areas can be highlighted, questions can be added to the margin, and key points can be circled. For individuals just beginning the process of critiquing articles, the use of note-taking and comment-making in the margin allows for the questions to be directed to the correct place within the article.

Table 14-1

Critique Worksheet

Areas for Consideration	Comments Concerning Completeness of the Information Provided
Title of the study	
Author credentials	
Purpose of the study	
Timeliness of literature used	
Literature review addressed each of the variables	
Theory/framework, concepts, and the relationship to nursing	
Research question or hypothesis	
Dependent and independent variables listed	
Definitions given	
Tools and their reliability and validity information (quantitative)	
Data collection methods and triangulation of process (qualitative)	
Sample description	
Study ethics description (i.e., institutional review board [IRB] information)	
Data collection procedures	
Data analysis	
Results, recommendations, and implications for practice	

As the reader begins this initial review of the research project, he or she will develop a feel for the organization of the article, along with the manner of presentation for the entire research process. At this point, the examiner will become aware of the complexity of the identified material. To become somewhat relaxed with the content, he or she should expect to read the article several times. Each time the article is read, the examiner comes to terms with a different aspect of the article. Frequently, an initial question relates to the researcher's ability to verbalize the process in a manner that nurses can understand and be able to utilize in practice. The reader may also find that some of the initial questions raised in the introductory section are answered in other sections within the article. After this general overview of the article, a more critical examination of the document can then be completed.

Each aspect within a research article is examined to identify areas of concerns and assets (**Table 14-2**). The evaluator will benefit from taking the time to highlight each of the steps of the research process, spotlighting the hypothesis(es), literature review, sample, ethical considerations, and research design. During this focused examination, any limitations

Table 14-2	

Rules for an Ideal Study	
Areas for Consideration	**Comments Concerning Completeness of the Information Provided**
Research problem	• Significance of problem noted • Clarification of aim of study • Practicality of study • Clarity, significance, and documentation
Review of literature	• Organization of literature • Progression toward study question through previous research reports • Rationale and direction for the study presented
Study conceptual framework/theory	• Clear link between conceptual framework/theory and research question/purpose • Any maps/models logically presented
Research questions or hypotheses	• Expressed appropriately and clearly • Logically related to the research purpose/aim and framework/theory
Variables	• Concepts identified within the framework/theory used • Variables operationally defined • Conceptual definition consistent with operational definition of each variable
Research design	• Design appears appropriate • Clearly defined protocol for conducting research project • Any treatment closely scrutinized to guarantee consistency • Threats to internal validity minimized • Logically connected to the sampling method and statistics used
Sampling method	• Method appropriate to result in representative sample • Biases identified • Human rights protected • Setting described and appropriate for target population
Measurements	• Instruments sufficient for measuring the study variables • Instrument validity and reliability levels • Instrument scoring techniques clearly described
Data collection	• techniques for using observation clearly described • Methods for recording measures clearly described • Interrater reliability described when appropriate • Process clearly, consistently, and ethically described
Data analysis	• Procedures suitable for the type of data collected • Analysis procedures clearly portrayed • Outcomes offered in a comprehensible way

Source: Data from San Jose State University. (2005). Reading and critiquing research. Retrieved from http://www.sjsu.edu/upload/course/course_969/Reading_and_CritiquingResearch.ppt

identified by the researchers should be noted. Another area to recognize explicitly is the operational definitions, which reflect the standards used within the research project to clarify the specific variables. After noting the operational definition for each variable, a reviewer should not have many additional terms that require explanation. The evaluator should define any term that continues to be unfamiliar to enable him or her to better understand the entire process. Every reader should develop a habit of looking up unfamiliar terms instead of skipping over them, which simply causes those terms to remain unfamiliar. The objective of critiquing any research report is to become familiar with the language and procedures used regularly within the scheme.

At this point in the research critique, the reviewer attempts to identify the strengths and limitations of the research process described in the report. The reviewer should be aware that the limitations so identified might actually be a consequence of the lack of space allowed within the documentation of the research endeavor rather than representing the intended omission of the aspect. All journal articles have space limitations, which can result in some items being cut because of space considerations rather than because they were lacking in the study.

One major challenge for novice research readers is the evaluation of statistics. In considering this aspect of any research process, the key point is to ask for help. To better understand the material presented in articles, it could be suggested that reviewers either find someone to provide help in this area or obtain an introductory book to statistics to aid in the assessment of the statistical data. Nurses who practice evidence-based nursing are not expected to become statisticians. Nurses are, however, expected to acknowledge their limitations and seek help from statisticians and others as needed to improve their evaluation of research results for incorporation into everyday nursing practice.

One means of utilizing the expertise of peers and colleagues is through establishment of a journal club. The journal club members can select a different article on a regular basis. The group then completes the review/critique. By using the group to complete the work, each participant grows in their own knowledge and confidence to be able to complete a review individually.

As nurses are asked to become involved with the critiquing of research articles for EBP, several formidable factors emerge and must be dealt with. Several Internet sites are available to use as resources for exploring the development of research critiques geared toward EBP.

◼ Critically Assessing Knowledge for Clinical Decision Making

The various aspects of EBP are of fundamental importance in considering the assessment of knowledge related to clinical decision making. As nurses, the evidence required to steer a competent and effective practice does not occur after reviewing a single independent study. Changes within best practices are based upon a sound foundation of evidence, not just the results from a single study. Gray, Bliss, and Klem (2015) provide an example of a level of evidence ranking system along with a taxonomy for strength of recommendation for treatment (SORT) statement. While the level of evidence ranking mirrors most other ranking tools, the SORT statement provides clear guidance on how to use the level of evidence ranking to determine the level of recommendation. Within this discussion, the idea moves from the strength of the evidence to the level of recommendation related to implementing the results into day-to-day practice. The practicing nurse comes to the research critique process with a foundation of clinical experience. Thus, the critique of the research endeavor is tempered by this clinical expertise. Yoder (2005) suggests, "clinical decisions require that one use a problem-solving approach to clinical practice that integrates a systematic search for and critical appraisal of the relevant evidence to answer the clinical questions" (p. 91). Every nurse has been taught a problem-solving methodology. During the review of research, it becomes essential for nurses to utilize this critical thinking framework, which has already been incorporated into practice, to validate and conceptualize the research critique process. The idea behind a research critique is to provide a systematic process for critically appraising research projects. Within this process, nurses must become comfortable with looking at all aspects of the various studies to assess any strengths and limitations that might be apparent. Carefully considering these different aspects of the report facilitates critical thinking concerning the results reported and the applicability of those results to the workplace.

One aspect of paramount importance to be considered within any research critique is the determination of the sampling process. According to Pajares (2007), "The key word in sampling is representative" (Section VI.E.4). Determining the appropriateness of the sampling method is critical in any study appraisal. Whatever sampling method is used, the rationale and limitations related to this methodology must be meticulously discussed. While all aspects of the research decision-making process are important, the inclusion of an effective sample (representative of the population) is critical.

Evaluating Quantitative Research Evidence

Quantitative research reports tend to be slightly easier to critique because of the concreteness of the quantitative research design. The various aspects of quantitative research reports document the expectations for all of the various elements of the article—that is, the introduction, literature review, hypothesis(es), sampling, research design, statistical testing, and discussion.

Although each of these areas includes considerable levels and components, the clarity of the descriptions of these aspects is more distinct than in qualitative methodologies.

According to Carter (2006), the critiquing of quantitative research reports should address four basic areas: comprehension, comparison, analysis, and evaluation. Each of these four levels of review adds a different dimension to the resulting scrutiny. Comprehension and comparison provide the overall appraisal of the report. Analysis then takes the investigation of the report to the level of reflecting on the continuity among the different parts (Carter, 2006). At this point of assessing the report, the principal concern is whether the hypothesis flows into decisions made about the sample, and whether that sample is appropriately managed by the research design. The final aspect of the review carefully considers the meaning and significance of the study process for implementation into nursing practice. The focus is to determine whether the findings, implications, and recommendations presented in the study report are truly supported and presented.

A key aspect of this review process unique to the quantitative research appraisal is the use of a conceptual or theoretical framework (Pajares, 2007). Although it can be provided in any of the research methodologies, this framework is essential in all quantitative research endeavors. Having said this, within printed articles documenting quantitative research, the discussion of the conceptual/theoretical framework is frequently omitted to satisfy the journal's page length requirements. Of course, the omission could also reflect the researcher's failure to include a conceptual/theoretical framework as part of the study design. The total omission of this framework would be a marked limitation within a quantitative research methodology. When a lack of theoretical foundation for a study is determined (yet the study outcomes appear to be applicable to your setting), sending a query to the authors about the issue may be helpful to determine the status of the theoretical foundation.

Evaluating Qualitative Research Evidence

When evaluating **qualitative research** efforts, the examination of the entire process assumes a slightly different perspective from that employed with a quantitative research undertaking. Assessment of the clarity of the purpose and statement of the phenomenon remains consistent with that of any other methodology critique. These components must be presented up front. From that point onward, the specificity of the qualitative design must be considered. Broad research questions, instead of hypotheses, are employed within this type of research design. The literature review may follow the data collection process rather than driving the research attempt from its inception. A framework may or may not be clearly presented as part of the study report. Qualitative research reviews must carefully discuss the researcher–participant relationship, because this aspect is a critical component of the data collection process. Ethical considerations also play significant roles in determining the appropriateness of this methodology.

Carter (2006) has detailed five standards to keep in mind when conducting a qualitative research critique. First, the research report must present a comprehensible depiction of the research environment, data collection process, sampling process, and the researcher's thought process. A second standard relates to the importance of congruence among the methodological aspects. According to Carter (2006), this section should indicate "rigor in documentation, procedural rigor, ethical rigor, and auditability" (Critique of qualitative research, 2). The third standard is the analytical preciseness: The researcher's thoughts and decisions related to the data should be evident in the report. The fourth standard stresses the importance of addressing the theoretical connectedness presented within the report. The fifth standard identified suggests that the relevance (value of the study) needs to be apparent within the documentation of the research project. Appropriate examination of each of these facets within a research report should yield a strong, valid depiction of the research project.

The data collection aspect of the study is a crucial component of the presentation of qualitative research projects. The reader must be walked through the entire process, from identification of the participants to the management of the data collected from them. The congruence of these data with the research purpose, question, and tradition needs to be assessed. The researcher is obliged to discuss how the field engagements and observations ought to build trust and ensure validity of the data collected. Another aspect that should be identifiable within the report is the ongoing and concurrent nature of data collection and analysis. Because data collection and analysis occur in tandem in qualitative research, the codes used as categories and the process utilized to determine data saturation must be explicitly discussed in the report. The research report should also address triangulation, peer review of the research process, articulation of researcher biases, member checking, and external audit by expert consultants.

A final aspect that must be noted within qualitative research reports is the sampling data. Because the sample population in such studies is usually small and focused, a description of this population is critical to allowing the reader to determine if the study findings are generalizable to other populations.

Qualitative research often employs additional terminology that must be defined and clarified, which can cause further confusion and frustration. As a result, the critique of qualitative research tends to be an area that is best entered into after learning how to conduct critiques of quantitative research. Put simply, qualitative research tends to be less structured than quantitative research.

Evaluating Mixed Methods Evidence

Mixed methods research embraces both quantitative and qualitative design aspects. According to Creswell (2003), the mixed methods approach takes advantage of the strengths of both quantitative and qualitative research by employing sequential, concurrent, and transformative strategies of inquiry. As a critique of a mixed methods research study is undertaken, the reader must, therefore, consider the presentation of both methodologies within the discussion. A unique aspect of a mixed methods research critique is the expectation of a stated rationale for the use of this method.

The quantitative and qualitative data in a mixed methods research report are frequently presented separately, which allows the reader to concentrate on one type of data prior to considering the other type. Within mixed methods research, one type of research design usually drives the second research design process. The reporting of the data and results must reflect this research progression of data collection. The discussion section should integrate the two types of data, thereby strengthening the study's findings. When a transformative study design is employed, this section should address the advancement of the agenda for change or reform that has developed as a result of the research.

■ Employing EBP Guidelines: Instruments for Holistic Practice

EBP requires that multiple related articles be correlated to provide a sum of evidence rather than a single data set. Contradictory evidence must be reconciled through the evaluation and association of data from multiple quality research projects. Of course, this process of reconciling contradictory evidence and multiple research discussions generates additional questions that need to be investigated at some point in time. According to the Oncology Nursing Society (2005), the EBP process comprises six steps:

1. Identify the problem.
2. Find the evidence.
3. Critique the merit, feasibility, and utility of the evidence.

 THINK OUTSIDE THE BOX

Can you think of any data other than research that can be used as evidence for nursing practice? Identify data that nurses provide in their practice.

4. Summarize the evidence.
5. Apply the ideas to practice.
6. Evaluate the results.

Each of these steps, with the exception of the application to practice (Step 5), can be visualized within the research critique process. Research critiques require the identification of the problem; an examination of the literature review; a critique of the merits, feasibility, and use of the research process; summarization of the research process; consideration of the applicability of the research results to practice; and evaluation of the results.

The Evidence-Based Appraisal

Evidence comes from many different sources. The first part of this chapter examined the research critique process, which is part of EBP. Now let's examine other important elements for nurses to use in their nursing practice. According to Vincent, Hastings-Tolsma, Gephart, and Alfonzo (2015), "many clinical decisions are undergirded by value judgments, tradition or habits, and a mixture of evidence from a variety of sources that may or may not include robust research" (p. 48). By including evidence-based appraisals, the inconsistencies identified by the challenge of assessing evidence can be managed in an increasingly positive and beneficial manner. Asserting the strength of each component of evidence used to support a healthcare practice should be a penetrating and significant expectation from each healthcare discipline. By carefully and thoroughly considering the biases and implications from research projects, quality improvement activities, and EBP investigations, the optimal health care can be determined and implemented. Melnyk, Gallagher-Ford, Long, and Fineout-Overholt (2014) employ three categories as strategies for integrating EBP competencies into health practices. The three categories are: "1. Promote a culture and context or environment that supports EBP, 2. Establish EBP performance expectations for all nurse leaders and clinicians, and 3. Sustain EBP activities and culture" (p. 13). As an assessment is done on EBP projects, these three categories should be considered and supported. As the health community becomes increasingly comfortable with EBP integration, the health practices provided will further move toward being based on the best evidence available.

Expert Opinion

When no definitive data are available, nurses often turn to experts with knowledge needed about a specific aspect of nursing care. A body of thought exists that implies that expert opinion is not valuable. However, when no valid answers or data are available, expert opinion is considered a viable alternative. Expert opinion may be expressed in books, conferences, forums, reports, or even from expert clinicians in practice. Most often, textbooks and expert clinicians are the only valid resources when scientific data are not readily obtained.

Hopp and Rittenmeyer (2012) suggest the use of the term *local data*. This type of data may be internal to an organization such as patient/employee satisfaction surveys, audits, or employee performance evaluations. Of particular interest to local data is quality improvement (QI)/quality assurance (QA). Hospitals and clinics, accredited by the Joint Commission and other accreditation agencies, compile QI/QA data. These data are often reported to national agencies, which allows for comparisons of how a local hospital clinic is doing compared to other agencies of like size and function. For example, the Agency for Healthcare Research and Quality (AHRQ) looks at access to care, costs, and patient outcomes. The Area Health Resource Files (AHRF) examine data specific to a county. The Hospital Consumer Assessment of Healthcare Providers and Systems (HCAHPS) is a national survey of patients about the quality of hospital care they receive (Mason, Leavitt, & Chaffee, 2012). The Joint Commission is particularly interested in sentinel events. Sentinel events may be medication errors, wrong-site surgery, suicide, operative and postoperative complications, or even nurse staffing issues (Sorbello, 2008). Sentinel events require healthcare organizations to conduct a root cause analysis, which is a structured process to examine why an adverse event occurred. A plan is then developed to ensure that the event does not occur again.

Each of the items discussed in this section demonstrates a variety of ways to obtain data that may not be the result of scientific research. The evidence-based appraisal is necessary to provide nurses with knowledge to improve their nursing practice through expert opinion and internal data. The evidence-based appraisal is an important aspect in the daily practice of nurses, whether it applies to patient/nurse satisfaction, cost, or patient safety.

Summary Points

1. Critiques of research are essential to EBP and allow nurses to practice the art and science of the profession.
2. There are nine types of critiques.
3. The necessary elements in a research critique can be compiled in a series of questions for the process of critiquing research.
4. Critiques should be balanced, identifying both strengths and limitations in the study report examined.

5. Journal articles have restrictions on page limits and word limits, which sometimes result in information being omitted.

6. Jargon in research reports often deters nurses from doing research critiques.

7. The critical appraisal of research is a skill to be developed through repeated practice.

8. General areas of the research study include author qualifications, study purpose, study design, sample, research methodology, outcomes, limitations and strengths of the research, and recommendations.

9. Nurses in EBP do not need to be statisticians, but they do need to be comfortable asking for help when evaluating the statistical analysis portion of a research report.

10. Quantitative research studies are concrete in nature and should include a theoretical framework.

11. Qualitative research studies contain broad research questions and are unstructured.

12. Mixed methods research embraces both quantitative and qualitative aspects of study design.

13. Research critiques should consider the applicability of the research results to practice.

14. Evidence-based appraisals may include evidence from sources other than research.

RED FLAGS

- A critique is not a negative process, but rather should entail a careful examination of all aspects of the research process.
- A research critique should identify gaps within the study's research process.
- Future research possibilities should be identified as part of the original study and the critique of that study.
- Recommendations for advancement of the nursing profession should be documented in transformative research.
- For EBP, multiple related articles need to provide a sum of evidence rather than a single data set.
- Evidence-based appraisals are critical to patient safety and quality of patient care.

Multiple-Choice Questions

1. Nurses must critically assess research studies to:

    A. Understand that all research is scientifically sound.

    B. Determine the applicability of their findings to practice.

    C. Know that all studies are perfect.

    D. Identify a negative approach to research utilization.

2. Of the nine types of critiques, which of the following are considered essential to EBP?

    A. Student, practicing nurse, and peer review critiques

    B. Abstracts, presentations, and email critiques

    C. Program of research, letters to the editors, and lay-journal critiques

    D. National Institute of Nursing Research, educator groups, and newspaper critiques

3. The purpose of a study applies to EBP when it:

    A. Adds to the body of nursing knowledge.

    B. Is complete and requires multiple readings.

    C. Is relevant to the authors.

    D. Is hard to find in the literature.

4. A hypothesis may be described by which of the following terms?

    A. Results, introduces, criticizes, reviews

    B. Findings, improvements, collections, sets

    C. Studies, plans, appreciates, concerns

    D. Proposes, predicts, supposes, tests

5. An essential component of a critique is a description of how the data were collected. Which of the following statements provides the best data collection description?

    A. Data collection was timely and used a tool developed by the researcher.

    B. Multiple tools were used to collect the data.

    C. The data was collected at 2-week intervals using a pre-test/post-test procedure.

    D. The score for the tool is easily understood and needs little description.

6. Results of the study should include:

    A. Unexpected findings.

    B. Unanswered questions.

    C. Pictures of subjects.

    D. Endorsements of peers.

7. A research study recommendation should include:
   A. No further need for research.
   B. No benefits for use in practice.
   C. Ways to change practice based on results.
   D. Ways to avoid using the results in other studies.

8. What is the definition of a research critique understood to imply?
   A. Analytical examination or commentary of a research report.
   B. A negative assessment related to the weaknesses of a research report.
   C. An analytical evaluation of the literature review.
   D. A positive assessment of the research design.

9. Although many aspects are discussed within a research critique, the basic aspects that the critique is attempting to identify are:
   A. Hypothesis(es) and literature review.
   B. Strengths and limitations.
   C. Research design and sampling methodology.
   D. Shortcomings and critical problems.

10. Evidence-based nursing practice requires that nurses initiate a pattern to facilitate effective utilization of research results. The best method for improving a nurse's ability to incorporate research results into practice is:
    A. Planning a monthly session to complete a literature review.
    B. Completing a critique of a single research project.
    C. Assessing at least one research report on a weekly basis.
    D. Reviewing abstracts from selected research projects.

11. Several basic guidelines can be used to make the research critiquing procedure less threatening. Which of the following reflects the utilization of these guidelines?
    A. The nurse reads the entire discussion section carefully to gain an overview of the research report.
    B. The nurse identifies shortcomings that are unfamiliar to clarify the limitations within the study.
    C. The nurse reads the entire study meticulously to acquire a general understanding of the research report.
    D. The nurse identifies modifications for the selected research report.

12. Quantitative research design tends to be easier to critique due to the:
    A. Length of the research reports.
    B. Incorporation of triangulation into the process.
    C. Use of convenient sampling methodology.
    D. Concreteness of the research design.

13. When attempting to critique a qualitative research endeavor, what must individuals be able to do?

    A. Easily identify the hypothesis(es).
    B. Carefully assess the data collection and management processes.
    C. Quickly determine the conceptual framework utilized.
    D. Effectively understand the statistical results.

14. One unique aspect present in reports of mixed methods research projects is a(an):

    A. Rationale for the utilization of the method.
    B. Clear delineation of the sampling method.
    C. In-depth discussion of the methodology.
    D. Listing of the strengths and limitations.

15. What do sentinel events require?

    A. The nurse to be fired.
    B. The hospital to ignore it.
    C. A root cause analysis.
    D. The doctor to be present.

Discussion Questions

1. You and your peers, as staff nurses, have found a research article that has the potential to change the way you practice. List questions about the report elements that could guide your critique of the study.

2. Select an article on a research topic for your practice area and complete the critique worksheet in Table 14-1. After completing the critique of the article, give the article a "level of evidence" rating and a "strength of evidence" score. Would you change your practice based on the information in this article?

3. You are a manager on a medical–surgical acute care unit. Your facility is moving toward an EBP format. Each unit has been charged with establishing a process for involving the staff nurses in this transformation. You have decided to implement a journal club for staff nurses to review and critique research articles for potential inclusion in evidence-based policies. What would you set as the ground rules for the implementation of this journal club activity?

4. You are a circulating nurse when a patient is to have his left leg amputated, but the scrub nurse is preparing the right leg. You realize this could be a wrong-site surgical procedure. During your operating room orientation, you were given the hospital policy/procedure for making sure this does not occur. How would you proceed?

Suggested Readings

Daggett, L., Harbaugh, B. L., & Collum, L. A. (2005). A worksheet for critiquing quantitative nursing research. *Nurse Educator, 30*(6), 255–258.

Pellechia, G. L. (1999). Dissemination of research findings: Conference presentations and journal publications. *Topics in Geriatric Rehabilitation, 14*(3), 67–79.

Riley, J. (2002). Understanding research articles. *Tar Heel Nurse, 64*(3), 15.

Valente, S. (2003). Critical analysis of research papers. *Journal for Nurses in Staff Development, 196*(3), 130–142.

References

Brink, P. J., & Wood, M. J. (2001). *Basic steps in planning nursing research: From question to proposal* (5th ed.). Sudbury, MA: Jones and Bartlett.

Burns, N., & Grove, S. K. (2009). *The practice of nursing research: Appraisal, synthesis, and generation of evidence* (8th ed.). St. Louis, MO: Saunders Elsevier.

Carter, K. (2006). *How to critique research.* Retrieved from http://www.runet .edu/~kcarter/Course_Info/nurs442/chapter12.htm

Creswell, J. W. (2003). *Research design: Qualitative, quantitative, and mixed methods approaches* (2nd ed.). Thousand Oaks, CA: Sage.

Dictionary.com. (2015). Critique. Retrieved from http://dictionary.reference.com /browse/critique

Glasofer, A. (2014). Searching with critical appraisal tools. *Nursing Critical Care, 9*(2), 18–22. doi:10.1087/01.CCN.0000444001.15811.a2

Gray, M., Bliss, D., & Klem, M. L. (2015). Methods, levels of evidence, strength of recommendations for treatment statements for evidence-based practice cards: A new beginning. *Journal of Wound, Ostomy, and Continence Nursing, 42*(1), 16–18. doi:10.1097/WON.0000000000000104

Hanna, K. M., Weaver, M. T., Slaven, J. E., Fortenberry, J. D., & DiMeglio, L. A. (2014). Diabetes-related quality of life and the demands and burdens of diabetes care among emerging adults with type 1 diabetes in the year after high school graduation. *Research in Nursing & Health, 37*, 399–408. doi:10.1002/nur.21620

Hopp, L., & Rittenmeyer, L. (2012). *Introduction to evidence-based practice: A practical guide for nursing.* Philadelphia, PA: F. A. Davis.

Iverson, K. M., Huang, K., Wells, Y. S., Wright, J. D, Gerber, M. R., & Wiltsey-Sterman, S. (2014). Women veterans' preferences for intimate partner violence screening and response procedures within the Veterans Health Administration. *Research in Nursing and Health, 37*, 302–311. doi:10.1002/nur.21602

Mason, D. J., Leavitt, J. K., & Chaffee, M. W. (2012). *Policy & politics in nursing and health care* (6th ed.). St. Louis, MO: Elsevier Saunders.

Melnyk, B. M., & Fineout-Overholt, E. (2015). *Evidence-based practice in nursing and health-care: A guide to best practice* (3th ed.). Philadelphia, PA: Lippincott Williams & Wilkins.

Melnyk, B. M., Gallagher-Ford, L. Long, L. E., & Fineout-Overholt, E. (2014). The establishment of evidence-based practice competencies for practicing registered nurses and advanced practice nurses in real-world clinical settings: Proficiencies to improve healthcare quality, reliability, patient outcomes, and costs. *Worldview on Evidence-Based Nursing, 11*(1), 5–15. doi:10.1111/WBN.12021

Merriam-Webster. (2015). Critique. Retrieved from http://www.learnersdictionary .com/search/critique

Oncology Nursing Society. (2005). *Evidence-based process.* Retrieved from http://onsop content.ons.org/toolkits/evidence/Process/index.shtml

Pajares, F. (2007). The elements of a proposal. Retrieved from http://www.des .emory.edu/mfp/proposal.html

Polit, D. F., & Beck, C. T. (2008). *Nursing research: Generating and assessing evidence for nursing practice* (8th ed.). Philadelphia, PA: Lippincott Williams & Wilkins.

San Jose State University. (2005). *Reading and critiquing research*. Retrieved from http:// www.sjsu.edu/upload/course/course_969/Reading_and_Critiquing Research.ppt

Sorbello, B. C. (2008). Responding to a sentinel event. *American Nurse Today, 3*(10), 30–32. Retrieved from http://www.americannursetoday.com/assets/0/434/436/440 /5426/5428/5442/5446/5b587e3d-6b56-4558-b2f7-05ab3738549b.pdf

Vincent, D., Hastings-Tolsma, M., Gephart, S., & Alfonzo, P. M. (2015). Nurse practitioner clinical decision-making and evidence-based practice. *The Nurse Practitioner, 40*(8), 47–54. doi:10.1097/01.NPR.0000463783.42721.ef

Wood, M. J., & Ross-Kerr, J. C. (2006). *Basic steps in planning nursing research: From question to proposal* (6th ed.). Sudbury, MA: Jones and Bartlett.

Yoder, L. H. (2005). Evidence-based practice: The time is now! *Medsurg Nursing, 14*(2), 91–92.

Chapter 15

Translational Research, Improvement Science, and Evaluation Research with Practical Applications

Carol Boswell

Chapter Objectives

At the conclusion of this chapter, the learner will be able to:

1. Discuss the use of translational research principles within the process of systematic decision making.
2. Construct a basic logic model for an identified project of individual choice.

Key Terms

Applied research

Basic research

Impact

Logic model

Outcomes

Outputs

Patient-oriented research

Population-based research

Translational research

◼ Introduction

Many different concepts and ideas come together as investigators struggle with the idea of appreciating systematic decision making. Evidence-based practice, research, and quality improvement are all aspects that play a part in the development of critical decision making and the validation of successful and competent healthcare practices. These processes take diverse paths based upon the outcomes desired. Full experimental, basic research is the process required to get to the results being sought. At other times, a quality improvement exercise is the way to gain the information essential for the advancement of quality practice. With each encounter of questions, the type and depth of evidence needed must be carefully and consciously considered. According to O'Brien (1998), individuals within the focus of structured inquiry are embracing the phrase, "If you want it done right, you may as well do it yourself." This idea, while interesting, does not hold with the current health environment of interprofessional engagement. The inclusion of strategic individuals to respond to the questions and challenges identified requires different individuals to appreciate the multifaceted nature of systematic decision making.

◼ Translational Research

Woolf (2008) describes **translational research** as a "'bench-to-bedside' enterprise of harnessing knowledge from basic sciences to produce new drugs, devices, and treatment options for patients" (p. 211). The idea of moving basic research from laboratory facilities to the frontline to aid in the day-to-day care of patients is critical for the healthcare community. The National Institutes of Health (NIH) embraced the idea of translational research in 2006 with the formation of centers to manage the process, and with the unveiling of the Clinical and Translational Science Award (CTSA) program (Rubio et al., 2010; Woolf, 2008). While translational research has been discussed since 2006, it continues to be complicated and obscure. Rubio and colleagues (2010) define translational research as fostering a long-term ambition of assimilating basic research, patient-oriented research, and population-based research using multiple routes with involvement from a variety of disciplines to improve the health of the public. Within the process of implementing translational research, diverse components are integrated to focus the attention of the decision-making process toward the patient and populations.

Several types of research methodologies can be incorporated into this delivery idea. **Patient-oriented research** strives to provide knowledge advancement through the use of inclusion of groups of patients or healthy individuals to determine the patients' perceptions related to health care. When employing patient-oriented research, the patient and stakeholders are embraced from the beginning. They are not just the subjects but serve as part of the research team from pre-planning to dissemination. For this methodology, the patient is the center for the entire process. Each aspect within the study focuses on the manner in which the patient will be impacted. From a different focus, **population-based research** seeks to mesh epidemiology, social and behavioral sciences, public health, quality evaluation, and cost-effectiveness into the research process to allow for a holistic outcome when answering critical questions. While the population of individuals is important within the study, the holistic nature of the research is a driving force. The problem tends to be examined from multiple fronts, instead of a single vantage point. **Basic research** embraces the research conducted within a laboratory setting to advance the knowledge on a topic for the sake of knowledge, without any focus on clinical practice at that point. Basic research is a foundation for the examination of questions. The process does not have to be linked to a group of people or a situation. It is research to discover information. All research that is not basic research is placed into the category of applied research. **Applied research** encompasses translational research, patient-oriented research, population-based research, and any other research that strives to utilize research results in a practical application.

Translational research has two areas of focus. The initial area relates to basic research. During this phase of investigation, the preclinical studies along with human trials are used to establish the foundation for further development of the information. The second focus within translational research strives to move the outcomes determined through basic research to actual adoption at the bedside, or frontline of health care, as examples of best practices for the community. The process of moving the basic research to the frontline encompasses nurses at all levels. As basic research is completed, the frontline nurse takes on the challenge of implementing the process with patients in unique settings. As new medications, procedures, and equipment are developed and studied using basic research strategies, the frontline nurse becomes the tool for implementing those innovations into clinical practice in an operational and methodical manner. With the assimilation of each new skill and/or instrument, the translational aspect of research becomes significant. The process for making it serviceable in the clinical setting requires the proficiency of the nurse working in cooperation with the patient for the optimum outcome. Each component of the process is crucial and imperative. The first phase provides the foundation of evidence on which to structure the best practices for the day-to-day delivery of health care. The central and noteworthy consequences from the totality of the translational research process address the "cost-effectiveness of prevention and treatment strategies" (Rubio et al., 2010, p. 472). By embracing a focus toward prevention and treatment that is cost-effective, the ultimate outcome is improved health for the public.

When reading about translational research, the initial stage that incorporates the basic research and patient-oriented research is identified as T1. This process undertakes the challenge to move new knowledge and understanding about disease processes identified within the laboratory setting into new areas. Those unique areas include the diagnosis, treatment, and prevention of the disease progression within patients. The timely movement of identified strategies for the management of diseases is needed within the healthcare arena to support the prevention and aid in the supervision of the disease within individuals.

The second phase (T2) assimilates the identified results from laboratory research into the practical management at the bedside. This transformation of results from the clinical, laboratory setting into the judicious guidance of healthcare delivery allows for the up-to-date harnessing of knowledge to advance health care. Woolf (2008) notes that this process supports the involvement of disciplines that utilize clinical epidemiology, evidence synthesis, communication theory, behavioral science, public policy, finances, organizational theory, system redesign, and informatics. Each of these different applications necessitates that the investigator carefully considers the implications within the human world of change and conflict. The uniqueness of the individual patient comes into the picture as the laboratory results are moved into the practical world.

Action research is a term identified along with patient-oriented research that integrates the ideas of best practices, patient inclusion, inclusion into practice, and evidence-based practice. O'Brien (1998) speaks about action research as assimilating interested individuals into the process of identifying a problem, ascertaining a method for confirming it, and testing the outcomes. Action research is the practical application of systematic inquiry that reflects the evolution of solutions toward the bedside and/or frontline of health care for quality management of disease processes.

Within the process of translational research, basic research, population-based research, and patient-oriented research play a part toward the goal of moving research outcomes to frontline implementation for the advancement of disease prevention and management. Basic research and population-based research are not totally translational in nature (see **Figure 15-1**). As a result, these two types of research do not reside completely within the realm of translational research. On the other hand, patient-oriented research essentially tackles those areas and issues foundational for utilization in the clinical setting, which eventually impact health care (Rubio et al., 2010). All aspects of patient-oriented research support and advance the concept of translational research.

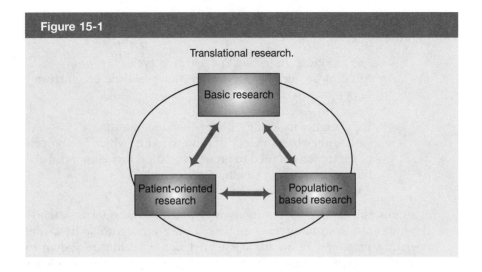

Figure 15-1

Translational research.

Improvement Science

In 2003, the idea for *improvement science* was introduced. Its beginning resulted from work initiated by Don Berwick, who sought to challenge health care to embrace the idea of continuous improvement as a foundation for the health community (Improvement Science, 2010). The term *improvement* was defined as the collective efficiency when system changes were viewed within uncertain situations (Improvement Science, 2010). The general question related to the process of improving the work to be done. Improvement science moved this definition to the point of viewing uncertainty related to systems changes in the direction of using the shared learning to advance the knowledge (Improvement Science, 2010). Thus, the general question associated with improvement sciences speaks to the manner by which the improvement will work within the healthcare environment. The maximizing of the learning to advance the improvement of healthcare provision is the foundation resulting from improvement science. Systems thinking and statistical thinking components are essential within the implementation of improvement science research. The process of improvement sciences moves from knowledge-based change (improvement) to knowledge about change (improvement science). Improvement science strongly embraces the Plan-Do-Study-Act (PDSA) process developed in association with quality improvement efforts (Institute for Healthcare Improvement, n.d.). Within this process, a team approach is enthusiastically and passionately embraced. Having the right people working to improve care delivery by accelerating improvements is paramount within this process. According to Perla,

Provost, and Parry (2013), the seven propositions of the science of improvement:

- Are grounded in testing and learning cycles
- Are philosophically founded on conceptualistic pragmatism
- Adopt an amalgamation of psychology and logic
- Respect the perspectives of justification and discovery
- Stipulate the inclusion of operational definitions
- Utilize Shewhart's theory of cause systems, which is a process of control charts used to present statistical process control and link with systems thinking (Wilcox, 2003)
- Enlighten by systems theory

By using these seven assumptions related to improvement science, the healthcare community has embarked on a process to address core operating principles in an attempt to redesign a healthcare system to meet the growing demands for improved care, lower costs, and safer health care for the population. Change is not easy. With the mounting pressure to transform healthcare delivery, healthcare providers must use every opportunity to uncover innovative ways to meet the challenges presented within the healthcare environment.

■ Logic Modeling

With the advancement of translational research, the innovative application of planning, implementation, and evaluation has been advocated and sponsored. One decisive concept incorporated within the movement toward best practice and evidence-based practice has been the logic modeling process. Different terms may be used for this process, such as program theory, logical framework, theory of change, or program matrix. A **logic model** is a step-by-step roadmap for getting to the desired result. According to Erwin and colleagues (2015), logic models "help identify underlying assumptions, focus on the processes and systems of change, and clarify desired outcomes" (p. 1). **Table 15-1** lists the multiple definitions provided for this process. Each of the definitions speaks to the idea that the logic model is utilized to advance a project in a focused, organized manner. Whether the modeling is used for a research endeavor, quality improvement project, or evidence-based practice venture, the aspects included within the model help to pull the needed components together to provide a clear and concise visual of the steps within the planned activity. **Figure 15-2** provides a simple version of a logic model framework. Erwin and colleagues (2015) denote the benefit of using a logic model to graphically depict the activities within the project along with the processes that lead to the outcomes attained. Each aspect builds upon the previous components to provide a template for planning,

Table 15-1	
Definitions for Logic Modeling	
Source	**Definition**
University of Wisconsin-Extension (2003, section 1, p. 2)	• Simplified picture of the projected program • Logical relationships found within the process • Program theory of action that reflects the different activities within the project • Denotes the underlying rationales for the activities selected to advance the project • Provides core for the planning, implementation, management, communication, and evaluation of the project
California Living 2.0. (2009, p. 1)	• Process used to create a graphic picture for how you think your work will lead to a collective vision for your community • Shows relationships among resources, strategies, and changes
Innovation Network, Inc. (n.d., p. 2)	• Commonly used tool to clarify and depict a program within an organization • Logical framework • Theory of change • Program matrix
W. K. Kellogg Foundation (2004, p. III)	• Defines a picture of how your organization does its work—the theory and assumptions underlying the program • Links outcomes with program activities • Facilitates thinking, planning, and communications about program objectives and actual accomplishments

implementation, and evaluation. The model encourages the connection of strategies to the results. It also advocates timely and knowledgeable communication regarding the project and/or task. The sequencing of events related to the resources needed for a project, activities involved in a project, and the changes/benefits resulting from a project should be depicted within the tool. According to the W. K. Kellogg Foundation (2004), the declaration of the resources and activities reflects the planned work while the **outputs**, **outcomes**, and **impact** demonstrate the intended results. Each aspect endorses and promotes the next step.

Three categories of logic modeling are available for agencies to use (W. K. Kellogg Foundation, 2004). Each of the unique types emphasizes discrete strengths. The theory approach model spotlights change theory that influences the designing and planning of a program. This model strives to provide a vivid justification for the development of a new program. Its intent is to "make a case" for the program through the use of the different components found within the model. This model type is frequently utilized by grant funders and individuals involved with grants. A second category is the outcome approach model. This type is also utilized early in the planning phase but grapples with the connections between the resources and the activities. Within this model, short-term

Figure 15-2 Logic model template.

Inputs	Outputs		Outcomes–Impact		
	Activities	Participation	Outcomes	Outcomes	Outcomes
What we invest	What we do	Whom we reach	Short-term	Long-term	Impact
(To achieve this set of activities, the following resources are needed.)	(To address the identified challenge, the following activities will be conducted.)	(To be successful at addressing this challenge, the following individuals should be engaged.)	(Once the activities are completed, the following short-term [1–3 years] outcomes will be realized.)	(Once the activities are completed, the following long-term [4–6 years] outcomes will be achieved.)	(Once the activities are completed, the following impact [7–10 years] outcomes will be achieved.)

Sources: Data from University of Wisconsin-Extension. (2003). Enhancing program performance with logic models. Retrieved from http://www.uwex.edu/ces/lmcourse; W. K. Kellogg Foundation. (2004). Logic model development guide. Battle Creek, MI: Author. Retrieved from http://www.wkkf.org/knowledge-center/resources/2006/02/WK-Kellogg-Foundation-Logic-Model-Development-Guide

(1–3 years), long-term (4–6 years), and impact (7–10 years) outcomes are provided for the set of activities. This category is most effective when designing effective evaluations. The third type of logic modeling is called activities approach models. This modeling process concentrates on the implementation strategies needed to accomplish the project. This model is used for program supervision and administration.

The initial step in this process of establishing a logic model is the analysis of the challenge identified or the problem. The Pell Institute (2010) lists several key steps to use when creating a logic model, including the following:

1. Assembling a self-motivated and energetic team
2. Disseminating strategic and significant details before the initial meeting
3. Clarifying a process for keeping effective annotations
4. Establishing a timetable for managing progress within the process
5. Determining a method for staying on topic to ensure the momentum for the project

The University of Wisconsin-Extension (2003) identifies six questions to use during this process of problem/challenge analysis:

- What is the problem?
- Why is this a problem? (What causes the problem?)
- For whom (individual, households, group, community, society in general) does this problem exist?
- Who is involved in the problem?
- Who has a stake in the problem? (Who cares whether it is resolved or not?)
- What do existing research and experience say? What do we know about the problem? (p. 10)

Each of these questions provides essential information as the problem/challenge is conceptualized. As bedside/frontline nurses are asked to implement innovative strategies to advance healthcare delivery, these questions are key to ensuring that the process is organized and timely. By using a tool such as the logic model, implementation of change within a clinical setting can be accomplished successfully. Significant progress, such as introducing a new instrument (e.g., an intravenous pump), can be organized and managed to ensure that the optimum result can be reached through the use of the new information. While this tool can be time consuming, it is crucial for the management of large projects addressing multiple sites and components. By addressing these questions, the focus for the project can be distinctly established and presented. Once the problem is determined clearly, a goal for the project can be formulated. The problem statements can also be classified as issue statements or situations. The problem statement usually addresses the ideas of who, what, why, where, when, and how.

These components are also used in the PICOT (population, intervention, comparison, outcome, time) and/or hypothesis statements. The problem statement and goal should be narrow in focus, while objectives used within the process can reflect the scope of the project. Each component should drive the subsequent aspects within the model. The goal statements should address the intended results and target populations in general terms.

The following steps within the framework are driven by "if–then" statements. Regarding resources, certain means and/or assets are needed to activate the project. Resources identify currently available assets and opportunities. Resources can also be viewed as inputs or program investments. Some of the common areas of resources are people, budgetary items, space, technology, equipment, and materials. From this idea, the framework moves to the idea of if these means and/or assets are used, then specific activities can be utilized to advance the project. Thus, activities that support and utilize the resources are listed within the plan. The determination of activities is not the "to-do" list, but should be the processes, strategies, methods, and/or action steps. The "to-do" list is provided within an action plan tool.

In relation to the activities, the statement is depicted: If the activities are successful, then certain outputs such as products or services will be completed. These outputs should be measurable, perceptible, and ensuing from the activities. The outputs reflect the deliverables, units of services, or products resulting from the project. Usually within the outputs, quantity is addressed but quality is not.

Once the outputs are determined, the outcome declaration demonstrates: If the deliverables are obtained, then the participants will be rewarded with certain benefits. The outcomes are the results, impacts, and/or objectives for the project. Outcomes should be measurable and reflect the change that occurs from the project process. Outcomes can reflect who or what will undergo the expected change. The focus can embrace the individual (client-focused), family/community, systemic, or organizational level. Olney and Barnes (2006) include within the individual level a focus toward cognitive, affective, skills, and quality-of-care outcomes. At the community level of the outcomes, environmental and social aspects need to be carefully considered and included as appropriate (Olney & Barnes, 2006).

The final aspect within the model is the impact. The statement that depicts the process is: If the benefits are achieved, then the resulting change to the organization, community, or system can be expected. The output, outcome, and impact aspects manifest the intended results of the project. The outcomes and impact fall into three categories. Outcomes can be viewed as short-term (1–3 years) and intermediate (4–6 years) results while the impact (7–10 years) is understood to represent the long-term results. The W. K. Kellogg Foundation (2004) utilized the acronym SMART for the outcomes and impact statements, which represents specific, measurable, action-oriented, realistic, and timed. When short-term outcomes, long-term outcomes, and impact statements are developed, these five aspects should be integrated into the record. Short-term outcomes address the individual, while the long-term outcomes and impact statements tackle the idea of the community and/or populations. Both the short-term and long-term outcomes endeavor to change "attitudes, behaviors, knowledge, skills, status, or level of functioning expected to result from program activities" (W. K. Kellogg Foundation, 2004, p. 18). Impacts work to affect organization-, community-, or system-level modifications.

With some formats of the logic model, assumptions and external factors are provided. Assumptions consider how and why the change activities will work with the identified community/population. Frequently, the assumptions are viewed in a box directly below the input and output sections of the model to reflect the link between the sections. External factors are viewed as rationales, existing policy environments, risk factors, successful strategies, and other factors that can affect the outcomes and impacts recognized for the project.

Logic models are becoming an integral part within grants, research, quality improvement, and evidence-based practice projects. The models allow for concise and organized planning, implementation, communication, and evaluation to provide an effective decision-making path for projects. For each and every project that necessitates multiple applications, the utilization of a logic model framework endeavors to organize and structure the process for success. By using this type of framework on large projects, each component needed within the implementation can be planned and controlled. One example of using this type of framework on a large project would be when an acute care setting is planning a move into a new construction area. The many different aspects that must be planned and organized to allow for a successful, smooth transition can be laid out within a logic model. This model provides a framework on which to clearly and distinctly address the different components required for effective and efficient planning, implementation, and evaluation. With all of the elements in one tool, the entire process moves with one voice toward success. Each member of the team can easily and productively identify the components needed within each phase of a project. Evaluation becomes increasingly operational, since the objectives and activities are organized within the framework. Strategic planning for the next steps can be openly developed on the foundation provided within the logic model management.

❓ THINK OUTSIDE THE BOX

Consider the idea that a new catheter kit is being introduced within the acute care setting. Try to complete an action plan for this change from one type of catheter kit to the new one.

■ Action Plans

Once the logic model is carefully constructed, it can be used to formulate the action plan for the day-to-day management of the project. The action plan (**Figure 15-3**) specifies the means to obtain concrete measurements of the objectives/outcomes. According to Sajdyk and colleagues (2015), "teams of experienced investigators with a wide variety of expertise are now critical for developing and maintaining a successful, productive research program" (p. 40). Action plans provide the structure needed by these teams to pull the different aspects of the projects together in an organized, progressive manner. The action plan takes the form of the "to-do" list for the logic model. At this level of development, the clearly worded objectives are supported by measurable indicators, target levels, and timeframes. Also within the process, the key individuals who are responsible for each level are denoted. By thoroughly and painstakingly completing this level of clarity, the progression toward the goal is visibly noted. According to Community Toolbox (n.d.), an effective action plan should be complete, clear, and current. Pulling the activities from the logic model will help to determine the step-by-step process needed to advance the project. Taking the time and energy to effectively plan in an organized manner allows for successful management of the project. Carefully and thoroughly considering the different aspects of the program and putting the results into an action plan enables:

- The development of credibility for the organization, group, or project
- The group to be sure that all aspects are addressed
- Improved understanding of the magnitude of the organization's potential
- Efficiency related to time, energy, and resources
- Accountability for the project being considered and implemented

The action plan should be viewed as a working document. Leedy and Ormrod (2013) suggest that breaking full projects down into manageable pieces allows for several beneficial outcomes. By dissecting the project into small activities, the ordering of the activities can be determined. For projects of small to moderate size, the use of an action plan provides the structure needed to move the project forward. As frontline nurses look to institute a quality improvement plan, the use of a planning tool ensures that each of the steps is in place and that all aspects are carefully and thoroughly considered. A project development team can be functional for mentoring other team members, providing a single point for accessing resources, being responsive to requests, breaking down institutional barriers, and managing the data accumulated (Sajdyk et al., 2015). For example, one medical–surgical unit elected to use the action plan format

Figure 15-3

Action plan worksheet.

Target Completion Date	Action Step	Accountable Person(s)	Assigned Person(s)	Actual Completion Date

when the decision was made to convert from routine checking to hourly rounding on patients. For each of the different aspects used in the conversion to hourly rounding, specific target completion time periods, action steps, the accountable individual, and assigned personnel were laid out on an action plan worksheet. By establishing this plan, the process over the following months was organized and calculated. When the manager for the unit changed during the implementation of the quality improvement project, the plan provided structure and organization for the new manager to use.

In addition, small successes as each activity is completed can be acknowledged. The division of the project into a series of actions provides the opportunity to establish multiple target dates to strive toward instead of just one huge hurdle to confront. Self-confidence can be developed as the project is viewed by the group as moving forward. The communication of the completion of the smaller tasks toward the large project reflects the evolution toward the goal.

While attempting to be as clear and complete as possible with the initial design, changes and situations may develop requiring a change within the action plan. The columns used in an action plan (Figure 15-3) need to address the key areas identified within the unique project. Each column and elements provides the structure for the advancement of the project by providing support and enhancement of the group's mission and goal. The action plan can also be used to present opportunities for communication across the group. Communication of the successes and challenges is paramount for the progression of the project. A final benefit

---

❓ THINK OUTSIDE THE BOX

What types of projects are occurring within the facility you are connected with that could benefit from completing an action plan?

---

of the use of an action plan relates to its ability to keep the project on track. Columns are provided for timeline and accountability so that the supervision of the project becomes visible and to the point.

◼ Conclusion

Evidence-based practice, research, and quality improvement must be organized and directed in an appropriate manner to facilitate the success of the process. Care must be given to the creation or selection of tools and processes that can be used to advance the achievements of the selected challenges. Translational research, with two components of basic and applied research process, is established to move knowledge from the laboratory to the bedside. By moving the results of the different projects to actual implementation for the patients, quality and best practice become standards in the practice arena. Tools such as logic modeling and action plans are crucial and strategic instruments to advance the science of nursing and health care. These tools can be used to support and coordinate the different venues within the decision-making process. By using each and every tool and resource available, the evidence will become second nature in the practice sites.

Summary Points

1. Evidence-based practice, research, and quality improvement are all aspects that play a part in the development of critical decision making and the validation of successful and competent healthcare practices.
2. The inclusion of strategic individuals to respond to the questions and challenges identified requires the different people to appreciate the multifaceted nature of systematic decision making.
3. Translational research has two areas of focus. The initial area relates to basic research. The second focus strives to move the outcomes determined through basic research to actual adoption at the bedside/ on the frontline as examples of best practices for the community.
4. Within the process of translational research, basic research, population-based research, and patient-oriented research each play a part toward the goal of moving research outcomes to bedside/

frontline implementation for the advancement of disease prevention and management.

5. Each aspect of a logic model builds upon the previous components to provide a template for planning, implementation, and evaluation.

6. Three categories of logic modeling are available for agencies to use—theory approach model, outcome approach model, and activities approach model.

7. The outputs reflect the deliverables, units of services, or products resulting from the project. Usually within the outputs, quantity is addressed but quality is not.

8. The outcomes are the results, impacts, and/or objectives for the project. Outcomes should be measurable and reflect the change that occurs from the project process.

9. Logic models are becoming an integral part as a means for grants, research, quality improvement, and evidence-based practice projects.

10. Once the logic model is carefully constructed, it can be used to formulate the action plan for the day-to-day management of the project. The action plan specifies the means to obtain concrete measurements of the objectives/outcomes.

11. Improvement science moved the process of improving health care to the position of viewing vagueness associated to changing systems toward the focus of applying shared learning for the enhancement of knowledge.

RED FLAGS

- Each aspect within a logic model should build upon the prior pieces. No part stands alone.
- Within any decision-making process, attention to the entire process should be evident within the materials provided.

Multiple-Choice Questions

1. Translational research strives to use a decision-making process to:

    A. Move the results from the bench to the bedside.
    B. Identify selected topics for research.
    C. Restrict who can complete research to individuals understanding the entire process.
    D. Focus only on the use of basic research.

2. The focus of attention for the implementation of translational research is:

    A. Patients only.
    B. Populations only.
    C. Patients and populations.
    D. Patients, animals, and populations.

3. The type of research conducted in a laboratory setting to advance the understanding of knowledge is:

    A. Translational research.
    B. Patient-oriented research.
    C. Population-based research.
    D. Basic research.

4. What are the two areas of focus for translational research?

    A. Basic research and moving the outcomes to the best practices
    B. Basic and patient-oriented research
    C. Cost-effectiveness and communication
    D. Understanding prevention and treatment options

5. Terms used for logic modeling are:

    A. Basic research, patient-oriented research, or program theory.
    B. Program theory, logical framework, or action plan.
    C. Logical framework, theory of change, or program matrix.
    D. Theory of change, action plan, or program matrix.

6. The logic modeling approach that underscores the use of change theory to transform the design and plan for a program reflects which approach?

    A. Theory approach
    B. Outcome approach
    C. Activities approach
    D. Action plan approach

7. The logic modeling approach that concentrates on the implementation strategies to transform the program reflects which approach?
   A. Theory approach
   B. Outcome approach
   C. Activities approach
   D. Action plan approach

8. The preliminary action taken for a logic model development is:
   A. Determining the challenge/problem.
   B. Setting up the resources and activities to be done.
   C. Clarifying the impact of the process.
   D. Developing the action plan.

9. The outputs as used within a logic model depict the:
   A. Action plan.
   B. Translational research.
   C. Deliverables and/or units of services.
   D. Activities.

10. What do impact statements within a logic model tend to address?
    A. Individuals
    B. Clients
    C. Action plan statements
    D. Communities

Discussion Questions

1. A medical–surgical unit at your hospital wants to change from using a team nursing model to a primary care nursing model. The unit director asks the group to develop a logic model tool to show the problem, goal, resources, activities, and short-term goals involved in making this type of change. You are one of the staff members charged with preparing these aspects for the logic model. Discuss the details of the logic model you prepared.

    Items to consider when completing this request include the following: The initial step in this process of establishing a logic model is the analysis of the challenge identified or the problem. Once the problem is determined clearly, a goal for the project can be worded. The problem statements can also be classified as issue statements or situations. Usually the problem statement addresses the ideas of who, what, why, where, when, and how. The problem statement and goal should be narrow in focus, while objectives used within the process can reflect the scope of the project. From the activities, the statement is depicted: If the activities are successful, then certain outputs such as products or services will be completed. These outputs should be measurable, perceptible, and ensuing from the activities. Once the outputs are determined, the outcome declaration demonstrates: If the deliverables are obtained, then the participants will be rewarded with certain benefits. The outcomes are the results, impacts, and/or objectives for the project. Outcomes should be measurable and reflect the change that occurs from the project process. Outcomes can be viewed as short-term (1–3 years).

2. Using the SMART acronym, change the following outcome and impact statements to include the needed information.

    Outcome statement: Registered nurses will enjoy 12-hour shifts.
    Impact statement: Having 12-hour shifts will improve the retention rate of registered nurses.

    Items to consider when completing this request: W. K. Kellogg Foundation (2004) utilized the acronym SMART for the outcomes and impact statements. SMART represents specific, measurable, action-oriented, realistic, and timed.

Suggested Readings

Dillon, K. A., Barga, K. N., & Goodin, H. J. (2012). Use of the logic model framework to develop and implement a preceptor recognition program. *Journal for Nurses in Staff Development, 28*(1), 36–40.

Olney, C. A., & Barnes, S. (2006). *Collecting and analyzing evaluation data*. Seattle, WA: National Network of Libraries of Medicine Outreach Evaluation Resource Center.

Olney, C. A., & Barnes, S. (2006). *Getting started with community-based outreach*. Seattle, WA: National Network of Libraries of Medicine Outreach Evaluation Resource Center.

University of Wisconsin-Extension. (2003). Enhancing program performance with logic models. Retrieved from http://www.uwex.edu/ces/lmcourse

W. K. Kellogg Foundation. (2004). Logic model development guide. Battle Creek, MI: Author. Retrieved from http://www.wkkf.org/knowledge-center/resources/2006/02/WK-Kellogg-Foundation-Logic-Model-Development-Guide

References

California Living 2.0. (2009). Logic modeling & frequently asked questions. Building Healthy Communities: The California Endowment. Retrieved from http://www.calendow.org/healthycommunities/pdfs/EvaluationLogicModeling_FAQs_9_11_09.pdf

Community Toolbox. (n.d.). Developing an action plan. Retrieved from http://ctb.ku.edu/en/tablecontents/sub_section_main_1089.aspx

Erwin, P. C., McNeely, C. S., Grubaugh, J. H., Valentine, J., Miller, M. D., & Buchanan, M. (2015). A logic model for evaluating the academic health department. *Journal of Public Health Management Practice.* Advance online publication. doi:10.1097/PHH.0000000000000236

Improvement Science. (2010). Defining improvement science: A means to a beginning. Retrieved from http://improvementscience.org/?p=263

Innovation Network, Inc. (n.d.). *Logic model workbook.* Washington, DC: Author. Retrieved from http://www.innonet.org/client_docs/File/logic_model_workbook.pdf

Institute for Healthcare Improvement. (n.d.). Science of improvement: How to improve. Retrieved from http://www.ihi.org/resources/Pages/HowtoImprove/ScienceofImprovementHowtoImprove.aspx

Leedy, P. D., & Ormrod, J. E. (2013). *Practical research: Planning and design* (10th ed.). Boston, MA: Pearson.

O'Brien, R. (1998). An overview of the methodological approach of action research. Retrieved from http://www.web.ca/robrien/papers/arfinal.html

Olney, C. A., & Barnes, S. (2006). *Including evaluation in outreach project planning.* Seattle, WA: National Network of Libraries of Medicine Outreach Evaluation Resource Center.

Pell Institute. (2010). How to create a logic model. Retrieved from http://toolkit.pellinstitute.org/evaluation-guide/plan-budget/use-a-log

Perla, R. J., Provost, L. P., & Parry, G. J. (2013). Seven propositions of the science of improvement: Exploring foundations. *Quality Management in Health Care, 22*(3), 170–186. doi:10.1097/QMH.0b013e31829a6a15

Rubio, D. M., Schoenbaum, E. E., Lee, L. S., Schteingart, D. E., Marantz, P. R., Anderson, K.E., ... Esposito, K. (2010). Defining translational research: Implications for training. *Academic Medicine, 85*(3), 470–475.

Sajdyk, T. J., Sors, T. G., Hunt, J. D., Murray, M. E., Doford, M. E., Shekhar, A., & Denne, S. C. (2015). Project development teams: A novel mechanism for accelerating translational research. *Academic Medicine, 90*(1), 40–46. doi:10.1097/ACM.0000000000000528

University of Wisconsin-Extension. (2003). Enhancing program performance with logic models. Retrieved from http://www.uwex.edu/ces/lmcourse

Wilcox, M. (2003). The philosophy of Shewhart's theory of prediction. Modified version of the author's presentation to the Proceedings of the 9th Research Seminar Deming Scholar's Program, Fordham University, New York.

W. K. Kellogg Foundation. (2004). *Logic model development guide.* Battle Creek, MI: Author. Retrieved from http://www.wkkf.org/knowledge-center/resources/2006/02/WK-Kellogg-Foundation-Logic-Model-Development-Guide

Woolf, S. H. (2008). Commentary: The meaning of translational research and why it matters. *Journal of the American Medical Association, 299*(2), 211–213.

Chapter 16

Application of Evidence-Based Nursing Practice with Research

Sharon Cannon and Carol Boswell

Chapter Objectives

At the conclusion of this chapter, the learner will be able to:

1. Synthesize key components from evidence-based nursing practice and research utilization to drive the provision of quality nursing care.
2. Demonstrate proficiency in one component of evidence-based practice using the principles of the research process and evidence-based appraisal.

Key Terms

Evidence-based practice (EBP)

Integrative review

Meta-analysis

Research utilization

Systematic review

◼ Introduction

Evidence-based practice (EBP) is defined as a process of utilizing confirmed evidence (research and quality improvement), decision making, and nursing expertise to guide the delivery of holistic patient care. The recent need for and acceptance of EBP is apparent in the literature. Cost-effective, high-quality care based on evidence is essential today. Results of a 2006 survey conducted by Sigma Theta Tau International (STTI, 2006) suggest that a majority of the nurses surveyed needed evidence on a weekly basis to guide practice. Approximately 90% of the participants indicated a moderate to high level of confidence in EBP. The results of this survey again support the premise that EBP is a driving force for the use of scientific data in the decision-making process in the provision of nursing care. In addition, Finkelman and Kenner (2009) recommend nurses be actively engaged with patient safety issues and concerned about quality research. They also stated that nurses must participate in the evaluation of nursing care, because it is connected to safety and quality (Finkelman & Kenner, 2009). Their pronouncement is a direct result of the Institute of Medicine's imperative to ensure patient safety. Nurses' involvement in gathering evidence to support safe, quality nursing care is essential for the future growth of the profession and, most importantly, to the patients receiving the care they deserve.

As the United States moves forward with the implementation of the recommendations from the Institute of Medicine (1999) and the requirements included in the Patient Protection and Affordable Care Act (PPACA), attention to how best to address these recommendations and requirements is vital. EBP is a problem-solving process that mandates the use of current evidence to ensure safe and appropriate health care for patients. Melnyk (2012) states that the "ultimate purpose of EBP is to improve healthcare quality and patient outcomes and reduce hospital costs" (p. 130). Combining the ideas of research and quality improvement to address areas of concern within healthcare delivery allows for optimal use of the information currently available. Care must be given to the incorporation of scientific inquiry concepts as a mainstay for nurses. Bator, Taylor, and Catalano (2015) state, "it takes approximately 20 years to fully embed research findings into facility-wide client care" (p. 582). They further indicate that EBP is a compelling movement to today's nursing issues. Nurses should and must be willing to challenge the status quo as health care moves forward to address the problems and opportunities facing us. Nurses are the underpinning for addressing clinically relevant questions and solving the problems that are identified in a systematic and efficient manner.

Understanding the research process is the first step in using evidence in everyday nursing practice. It is also important to have some historical background knowledge about research in nursing (as provided in this text) to better comprehend the research process. According to Gawlinski and Miller (2011), "research is one of the most powerful tools for advancing the science of nursing and improving the quality of patient care and outcomes" (p. 190). Examples of EBP have been given elsewhere to demonstrate how EBP is applied in specific components of the research process.

Difficulty in analyzing the evidence has been identified as a major obstacle to **research utilization**. The modern-day nurse can use this text in the analysis of research findings, with their subsequent application to nursing care. This text is designed to "pull the pieces together" by suggesting a practical approach for research utilization in evidence-based nursing practice. Evidence-based practice and research utilization must become commonplace for the frontline staff nurse. Only when it develops into a practical and everyday part of health care will evidence truly become a mainstay of healthcare practice.

EBP and research are interconnected. As a dilemma is acknowledged, a PICOT (population, intervention, comparison, outcome, time) statement should be created. This PICOT statement propels the literature review. Each element in the PICOT statement provides strategic words to limit the search for applicable articles. Gaps and consistencies within the literature need to be determined to provide the pathway to the next phase of the process. These gaps and consistencies direct the process toward either a research study or a quality improvement project. If the evidence reveals that a policy, procedure, or protocol needs to be scrutinized, a quality improvement process would be commended for that intent. If the gaps and consistencies indicate that supplementary research should be needed to achieve an answer for the recognized problem, a full research project would need to be designed and executed.

If a research project is the trajectory, the principal process for conducting a thorough project would need to be ascertained. As a research venture is considered, the methodology for best addressing the challenge would need to be selected. Certain steps are generally followed when performing quantitative or qualitative research.

■ Process for Evidence-Based Practice

According to Myers and Meccariello (2006), "Outdated practices are barriers to decreased length of stay, favorable patient outcomes, and lowered costs" (p. 24). To move evidence-based nursing practice forward, a realistic approach for allowing frontline nurses to actively engage in the process must be determined and used. At each stage of providing holistic care, nurses have to be confident in asking the questions and seeking the best practices to advance the provision of effective nursing care. Nurses must seek the best evidence to make sure that the care

---

⁇ THINK OUTSIDE THE BOX

Prior to a surgical procedure, patients are instructed not to take anything by mouth (NPO) after midnight on the preceding day. Due to surgical schedules, some patients can go as long as 10–12 hours without any liquids.

1. Based on the evidence, what time limit is the best choice to manage this health challenge for the patient scheduled to have a surgical procedure?
2. List PICOT questions that could be generated from this scenario.
3. Which ethical considerations would need to be addressed prior to conducting a research study on this topic?
4. How would you incorporate patient preferences into the evidence-based practice?

---

provided represents the optimal health care available for the specified treatment plan. By determining a functional method for documenting an EBP search, nurses can then gain confidence in the overall process of conducting and implementing EBP.

The process for EBP determination is different from the process for research utilization. Research assessment involves completing a research critique. The research utilization process involves carefully examining a distinct study to determine the strengths and limitations assumed within that one study and deciding whether to apply its findings to nursing practice. Research utilization becomes a key aspect within the overall process of EBP, but it is only one piece of the EBP puzzle. For a nurse to be able to effectively utilize EBP, it is clear that he or she must be able to perform research critiques. The idea that nurses need to be able to use research, while acknowledging that not everyone has to be able to conduct research, is imperative. To facilitate implementation of EBP, frontline nurses need to understand how to recognize those elements of a particular research process that either strengthen or limit the use of its results.

Armed with this understanding of the applicability of the research results to practice, a nurse can then determine which study results might be used to sustain best practices in EBP. Clearly, to make this determination, nurses need to appreciate the intricacies of the research process. Frontline nurses should be able to identify the justifications that a researcher provides for selecting a specific method of sampling, data collection, research design, and data analysis. If a researcher has a valid explanation for the choices employed within a study, the results can be assigned a higher value and incorporated into practice. Having begun the work with research critiques, the nurse can then move to the next step of development to use those skills within the EBP process.

Melnyk and Fineout-Overholt (2015) suggest that the process of EBP involves five critical steps:

1. Raise the urgent clinical question using a format that includes the key aspects of the issue.
2. Assemble the most appropriate evidence that addresses the issue identified.
3. Evaluate the evidence critically to determine its validity, relevance, and applicability.
4. Assimilate the evidence into clinical practice.
5. Assess the changes resulting from the use of the best evidence.

Each of these steps must be conscientiously finished to come to a conclusion about the best practices for a nursing setting. If an EBP process does not include all of the five steps, the result does not take into consideration all of the available evidence related to the clinical question.

Although many models for EBP are currently being evaluated and modified, **Table 16-1** summarizes the key points in a quick and easy organizational design for evidence consideration. This format allows the individual to pull the needed aspects from any group of articles to reflect the current knowledge available regarding the topic under consideration. Within this format, the initial step is to refine the question confronting

---

 THINK OUTSIDE THE BOX

In recent years, more parents have begun seeking alternative birthing options. Some individuals elect to deliver at home due to the burden placed on them by rising healthcare costs. Others make this decision based on a desire to have a more natural birthing process. When complications occur during the birthing process, however, the baby may have to be admitted to an acute care setting. For newborn infants, the standard initial treatment process includes erythromycin eye ointment, application of triple dye onto the umbilical cord, and a vitamin K injection. If the parents voice concerns about these procedures, which steps would a nurse need to take to provide evidence-based information to alleviate their fears?

1. List PICOT questions that could be generated from this scenario.
2. Which ethical considerations would need to be addressed prior to conducting a research study on this topic?
3. Which key words would be used in a literature search to locate evidence related to this EBP question?
4. Which type of research project could be developed to further study this concern?
5. How would you incorporate patient preferences into the evidence-based practice?

Table 16-1 Format for Documenting Aspects of Evidence-Based Practice

Questions to Consider Within the Evidence-Based Practice Process

P (Population of Interest): _____

I (Intervention of Interest): _____

C (Comparison of Interest): _____

O (Outcome of Interest): _____

T (Time): _____

Articles (Level of Evidence/ Evaluation of Strength of the Evidence)	Who Is Involved (Sample Size, Sampling Method, Population)	What Occurred (Qualitative, Quantitative)	Where Completed (Type of Agency, State, Country)	When (Year Research Done)	Why (Research Question)	How (Data Collection, Tool Used with Validity and Reliability, Statistical Tests, Qualitative Control)	Consistencies (How It Addresses the PICOT Question, How Similar to Other Studies Reviewed)	Gaps (How It Does Not Address the PICOT Question, What Did the Researchers State Still Needed to Be Studied)

Summary of Findings

Application of Findings to Evidence-Based Practice That Validates or Changes Policies and Procedures

the nurse. Careful time and attention should be given to clarifying the five aspects driving the EBP question. As discussed previously, the question should consider the following aspects of the research issue (PICOT):

P Population of interest (required aspect)
I Intervention of interest (required aspect)
C Comparison of interest (recommended aspect)
O Outcome of interest (required aspect)
T Time (recommended aspect)

The development of a clear and concise clinical question is of vital significance because the question guides the comprehensive EBP and/or research process. Once the question is clarified, the nurse needs to work with a librarian to establish strategic words and terms to employ in accomplishing the literature review. Using appropriate terms for the diverse search engines facilitates the search results to ensure the appropriate materials are located for the subsequent analysis of the best practices. As Melnyk (2003) has stated, "Evidence-based practice is a problem-solving approach to clinical decision making that incorporates a search for the best and latest evidence, clinical expertise, and assessment, and patient preference and values within a context of caring" (p. 149). Concerns are being raised at this time as to what are "best practices." Proehl and Hoyt (2012) contend that the term *best practices* is an indistinct phrase that indicates that the practice is founded on data but not necessarily research. The data on which best practices are constructed tend to be based on data utilized by respected and highly valued organizations and/or practitioners.

Malloch and Porter-O'Grady (2010) have classified investigations of practices as meta-analyses, systematic reviews, or integrative reviews. The combining of these different study types identified through the literature review and search engine inquiry process provides the foundation for determining whether there is a need to change practice patterns. **Meta-analysis** incorporates a statistical technique to determine the rigorousness of the findings from multiple studies dealing with a focused question. A **systematic review** summarizes all quantitative evidence found through the literature search that is correlated to an identifiable research or clinical issue, employing a rigorous format to ensure completeness of the assessment. An **integrative review** also summarizes prior research studies on a selected topic but, in addition, draws conclusions from the summary concerning the studies examined.

Evidence can be evaluated using two different formats. One method is to use the levels of evidence. The levels of evidence are based upon the research method design. If an article or information is not research, the classification of that data into the levels of evidence becomes complex. To determine the level of evidence, the available literature is ranked. For example, Level 1 evidence (meta-analysis) is considered to be the highest level, most important evidence that can be gathered. While Level 1 evidence is the most desirable, the researcher should not toss out evidence classified as being at the other levels. Sometimes the only evidence that is available is a case study (Level 5). A case study can still provide evidence for clinical decision-making purposes, though it is not the strongest form of support. The depth of the justification for using this level of evidence provided by the researcher aids in the determination of the value of the results documented.

The second method for classifying evidence is based upon the perceived strength of the evidence. Evaluating the strength of evidence classification involves looking into the risks and benefits of using the information for the client population. Healthcare agencies tend to focus more on this aspect of a procedure than what type of research design was used. Risks and benefits can allow increased bias to be used in the determination of the level. Once the level of evidence is established, the researcher needs to evaluate the strength of the evidence. A simple rating system for this aspect of evidence can be used. Depending on the study, the evidence may be very strong or insufficient. The rating tool provides the researcher with a means for further discriminating which studies have significance for the project being considered.

The form provided in Table 16-1 allows for either a systematic review or an integrative review. Once the PICOT question has been determined and the literature review is completed, each of the identified articles/studies is carefully assessed. For each article (citation, level of evidence, and evaluation of strength of the evidence), who is involved (sample size, sampling method, population), what occurred (qualitative, quantitative, level of evidence), where completed (type of agency, state, country), when (year research was done), why (research question), and

---

❷ THINK OUTSIDE THE BOX

Evidence-based practice should cause members of the nursing profession to query their normal activities. A simple skill such as catheterizing an individual can result in an EBP question such as, "How much urine should a nurse drain off the bladder at one time following a catheterization of a client?"

1. List PICOT questions that could be generated from this scenario.
2. Which ethical considerations would need to be addressed prior to conducting a research study on this topic?
3. Which key words would be used in a literature search to locate evidence related to this EBP question?
4. Which type of research project could be developed to further study this concern?
5. How would you incorporate patient preferences into the evidence-based practice?

how (data collection, validity and reliability of any tool used, statistical tests, qualitative control [trustworthiness, confirmability, transferability]) are determined and documented. As these aspects of a research critique are completed on the different studies, consistencies (how the study addresses the PICOT question, how similar it is to other studies reviewed) and gaps (how the study does not address the PICOT question, what the researchers stated still needs to be studied) within the different studies begin to surface. The identification of consistencies within the various studies may either support the proposed changes in practice or confirm that best practices are currently being used. The detection of gaps within the studies suggests the need for further or more in-depth research into the topic under consideration. The idea of identifying consistencies and gaps within the different articles and research reports also incorporates the concept of similarities and omissions that may be present.

During the EBP process, as a clinical problem is identified, individuals are directed to develop that problem concern into a PICOT format. The PICOT question drives the EBP literature search and the subsequent review of the literature discovered. Following the completion of the literature review, the PICOT question can evolve into a research question/hypothesis or a quality improvement focus. The gaps and consistencies found within the review process help to clarify the question to be used for the research or quality improvement process. From the literature review, the focus for the management of the problem is confirmed. When consistencies are identified in the literature, the nurse can elect to repeat the research concentration to strengthen the evidence related to the clinical challenge. Conversely, when gaps in the literature are recognized, additional research projects will be needed to address the gaps found. The third potential outcome is that the literature review might result in either a confirmation or a change in the agency's policies and procedures. In such a case, a quality initiative project may be needed to validate the practices, though further research might not be necessary.

Thus, within an EBP-focused endeavor, the outcomes could be either research projects (to replicate prior work or to address gaps) or quality initiatives (to validate clinical practice). Should the outcome lead to a research study, the research must be conducted in compliance with sound research design. By comparison, for quality initiative projects, any of the many quality initiative models—for example, Six Sigma, plan–do–check–act (PDCA), define–measure–analyze–improve–control (DMAIC), Lean, and root cause analysis—can be utilized. The development of these models has been largely driven by manufacturing businesses, with the models subsequently being adapted to many quality improvement efforts and used in the healthcare arena to improve performance. Some methodologies, such as Six Sigma, rely heavily on statistics and research as their underpinnings. The Lean philosophy relies on standardization to improve both the process and the organization from a consumer approach.

Associations established from the results of the various studies need to be collected to add strength to the rationale for making any changes in policies and procedures related to the selected clinical question. If several studies produce equivalent results, then nursing practice should embrace the behavior as supported by evidence. Conversely, if multiple studies reflect a gap in knowledge related to the selected clinical question, then further research should be directed toward the identified segment of nursing practice. According to Pravikoff, Tanner, and Pierce (2005), "The finding that a lack of value for research in practice was the most frequently selected barrier to the use of research in practice is of greatest concern" (p. 48). When practicing nurses cannot or do not use research results to strengthen and sustain holistic nursing practice, the implementation of EBP at the bedside/frontline falls short of its potential.

After completing the grid portion of Table 16-1, time must be allocated to summarizing the findings. The nurse should pay careful attention to, and critically consider, the meaning ensuing from the consistencies and gaps identified. This painstaking contemplation of the discovered omissions and similarities serves to narrow the focus of the next steps within the process. By taking the time and energy to summarize and synthesize the information collected, the nurse becomes well versed in the current state of the clinical problem. Obtaining this clearer viewpoint related to the clinical problem allows the nurse to make an informed decision about what is needed next in dealing with this challenge.

The final section of Table 16-1 relates to the application aspect of EBP-related research. After completing each of these prior steps, the nurse has a basis for making recommendations for maintaining or changing a

---

❓ THINK OUTSIDE THE BOX

Frequently, an insulin drip protocol will seek to maintain a serum blood sugar level between 70 and 110 mg/dL. At one healthcare agency, a pilot research project revealed that the mean blood sugar for patients dismissed from a cardiac intensive care unit after 3 months was 148 mg/dL. The nurses questioned the protocol ranges as a result of this pilot study result.

1. List PICOT questions that could be generated from this scenario.
2. Which ethical considerations would need to be addressed prior to conducting a research study on this topic?
3. Which key words would be used in a literature search to locate evidence related to this EBP question?
4. Which type of research project could be developed to further study this concern?
5. How would you incorporate patient preferences into the evidence-based practice?

policy or procedure. The time taken to complete this exercise allows for any recommendations to be based on sound, factual data. The suggestions can then be effectively supported by a wealth of tested research endeavors. At this point, the nurse would take this review of the evidence and combine it with the decision-making method employed, personal expertise, and holistic client focus to drive quality, sound nursing care.

◼ Conclusion

According to Yoder (2005), "Both EBP and QI initiatives require ongoing evaluation of the practice environment, the appropriate use of data collection and evaluation, and the dissemination of the information learned through excellent communication process both from the top down and the bottom up" (p. 92). A variety of resources are available to help the nurse in strengthening the healthcare organization's EBP foundations and activities. The current healthcare community requires nurses and other healthcare providers to be diligent in the determination and provision of holistic health care. Whitmer, Auer, Beerman, and Weishaupt (2011) clearly identified that the utilization of a core group of individuals knowledgeable on EBP generates a foundation for the advancement of EBP within an organization. These champions for EBP must be given the time, educational opportunities, and resources to be able to effectively conduct EBP inquiries. The different treatments and plans of care put forth for clients must be based on factual, tested data. Each nurse must take responsibility for ensuring that the care provided is based on firm, accurate research data. These research data are then used to provide individualized health care to clients based on factual data, patient preferences, and nursing expertise.

 THINK OUTSIDE THE BOX

Gather at least three of your peers and form a journal club. Select a topic of your choice and identify a PICOT question. Conduct an integrative review for the selected topic. What conclusions can you draw from the review? How will this new understanding change your practice?

Summary Points

1. Evidence-based practice (EBP) is the process of utilizing confirmed evidence (research and quality improvement), decision making, and nursing expertise to guide the delivery of holistic patient care.

2. Understanding the research process is the first step in using evidence in everyday nursing practice.

3. To move evidence-based nursing practice forward, a realistic approach for allowing frontline nurses to actively engage in the research process must be determined and used.

4. The process for research utilization carefully examines a distinct study to determine the strengths and limitations assumed within that one study.

5. Armed with an understanding of the applicability of the results to practice, a nurse can determine which studies can be used to sustain best practices in EBP.

6. The development of a clear and concise clinical question is of paramount importance, because this question directs the entire research process.

7. Meta-analysis uses a statistical technique to determine the rigorousness of the findings from multiple studies conducted to answer a focused question.

8. A systematic review summarizes all quantitative evidence found in a literature search that is correlated to an identifiable research or clinical issue, employing a rigorous format to ensure completeness of the assessment.

9. An integrative review summarizes prior research studies on a selected topic but, in addition, draws conclusions from the summary concerning the studies examined.

10. For each article (citation, level of evidence, and evaluation of strength of the evidence), the who involved (sample size, sampling method, population), what occurred (qualitative, quantitative), where completed (type of agency, state, country), when (year research was done), why (research question), and how (data collection, validity and reliability of tools used, statistical analysis, qualitative control) are determined and documented as part of the evaluation process.

11. The identification of consistencies (how the research addresses the PICOT question; how similar the research is to other studies reviewed) within the various studies evaluated may either support potential changes in practice or confirm that best practices are currently being used.

12. The detection of gaps (how the research does not address the PICOT question; what the researchers stated still needed to be studied) within the studies evaluated suggests the need for further or more in-depth research endeavors on the topic under consideration.

13. Obtaining a clearer viewpoint related to the clinical problem allows the nurse to make an informed decision about what is needed next in this challenge.

14. Quality improvement activities are designed to incorporate research into the healthcare environment from a consumer approach.

RED FLAGS

- Research utilization and evidence-based practice are not the same thing.
- The recommendation for changing nursing practice must be based on sound evidence, not on the results from a single study.

Case Scenario 1

A Hispanic woman presents to the emergency room complaining of epigastric pain in atypical form, nausea, diaphoresis, and neck pain. The initial assessment reveals a 60-year-old, Hispanic female with a history of diabetes and hypertension. The client reports being a smoker with a family history of cardiac problems. She is 5 feet, 3 inches tall and weighs 185 pounds. She is a homemaker with no outside employment. For the most part, she reports a sedentary lifestyle and denies alcohol consumption.

The emergency department (ED) physician orders an electrocardiogram (ECG) and cardiac panel to rule out an acute myocardial infarction. Other tests ordered include a chest X-ray, urinalysis, and standard chemistry (complete blood count [CBC], troponins, creatinine protein). The tests reveal elevated troponin and ECG changes with an elevation in the ST segment. The client is diagnosed with a full-blown myocardial infarction. The ED physician mobilizes the cath lab team and orders a cardiology consultation. The client is transported to the cath lab for an angiogram, which reveals two blocked cardiac vessels.

After a double angioplasty is performed, the client is transferred to the cardiac care unit (CCU). After she arrives in the CCU, the nursing staff member assesses the client and determines that the angioplasty versus manual compression was completed with Perclose. The use of this closure for angioplasty has been a topic of debate in the CCU.

As a result of this case and others, the nursing staff elects to engage in an EBP activity to determine if the policies and procedures currently used on the unit reflect the best practices for this type of client and medical treatment plan. The PICOT question shown in **Table 16-2** was identified, and the EBP process was initiated.

As can be seen from the case study analysis in Table 16-2, there are gaps in the literature—specifically, a lack of actual research projects on the use of Perclose versus manual pressure. All of the literature reviewed consisted of case studies with reference to recommendations from the manufacturer of Perclose. However, the case study illustrates how EBP and research can lead to specific actions to improve nursing care, thereby improving patient outcomes.

Table 16-2

Documenting Aspects of Evidence-Based Practice: Use of Perclose for Angioplasty

Questions to Consider Within the Evidence-Based Practice Process

P (Population of Interest): Hispanic Adult 50 Years or Older

I (Intervention of Interest): Perclose Usage for Percutaneous Arterial Closure

C (Comparison of Interest): Manual Pressure

O (Outcome of Interest): Decreased Length of Stay, Decreased Hematoma, Decreased Discomfort, Decreased Infection Rate

T (Time): Within 2 Weeks From Discharge From Hospital

Articles (Level of Evidence/Evaluation of Strength of the Evidence)	Who Is Involved (Sample Size, Sampling Method, Population)	What Occurred (Qualitative, Quantitative)	Where Completed (Type of Agency, State, Country)	When (Year Research Done)	Why (Research Question)	How (Data Collection, Tool Used with Validity and Reliability, Statistical Tests, Qualitative Control)	Consistencies (How It Addresses the PICOT Question, How Similar to Other Studies Reviewed)	Gaps (How It Does Not Address the PICOT Question, What Did the Researchers State Still Needed to Be Studied)
Geary, K., Landers, J. T., Fiore, W., & Riggs, P. (2002). Management of infected femoral closure devices. *Cardiovascular Surgery, 10*(2), 161–163. Level of evidence: 5 Strength of evidence: B	4 males, 1 female, age range 63–73, purposive sampling	Qualitative, case study	New York, acute care unit, outpatient general hospital	2002	Examined Perclose	Case study; no indication of prophylactic antibiotic use, Staphylococcus infection	Population correct for age; all had infections, suture placement, antibiotics	Little research; recommendations came from manufacturer; no indication of ethnicity or manual pressure

(continues)

Table 16-2   Documenting Aspects of Evidence-Based Practice: Use of Perclose for Angioplasty *(continued)*

Articles (Level of Evidence/Evaluation of Strength of the Evidence)	Who Is Involved (Sample Size, Sampling Method, Population)	What Occurred (Qualitative, Quantitative)	Where Completed (Type of Agency, State, Country)	When (Year Research Done)	Why (Research Question)	How (Data Collection, Tool Used with Validity and Reliability, Statistical Tests, Qualitative Control)	Consistencies (How It Addresses the PICOT Question, How Similar to Other Studies Reviewed)	Gaps (How It Does Not Address the PICOT Question, What Did the Researchers State Still Needed to Be Studied)
Heck, D. V., Muldowney, S., & McPherson, S. H. (2002). Infectious complications of Perclose for closure of femoral artery puncture. *Journal of Vascular and Interventional Radiology, 13*(4), 430–431. Level of evidence: 5 Strength of evidence: B	2 females, 1 male, age range 40–76, purposive sampling	Qualitative, case study	Three different institutions	2002	No specific question documented; report of cases, 3 days postop	Case studies	Age range exceeds PICOT range; 2 cases had staphylococcal infection, one from bacterial source; concerns about suture placement	Neither manual pressure nor ethnicity noted in this study; refers to published trials

Citation	Sample	Design	Setting	Year	Research Question	Data/Findings	Relation to PICOT	Ethnicity/Pressure
Tiesenhausen, K., Tomka, M., Allmayer, T., Baumann, A., Hessinger, M., Portugaller, H., & Mahler, E. (2004). Femoral artery infection associated with a percutaneous arterial suture device. *VASA: European Journal for Vascular Medicine, 33*(2), 83–85. Level of evidence: 5 Strength of evidence: B	77-year-old male, purposive sampling	Qualitative, case study	Austria	2004	No specific question documented; single case	Add to data; infection identified 4 weeks post hospitalization; seen in ED prior to final admission to hospital with sepsis; Perclose carries risk of femoral artery infections	Age complies with PICOT; sterile field must be maintained	Neither manual pressure nor ethnicity noted in this study; refers to research
Dumont, C. J. (2007). Blood pressure and risks of vascular complications after percutaneous coronary intervention. *Dimensions of Critical Care Nursing, 26*(3), 121–127. Level of evidence: 4 Strength of evidence: B	Convenience sampling, 150 subjects, mean age 62.4, 45% women, 92% white	Case-matched control design	South Atlantic state, tertiary care teaching facility	2006	Determine which variables are significant individual predictors of vascular complications post-PCI—1), comorbidities: 2), physician-sensitive procedural factors (hemostasis method [Perclose compared with manual compression for hemostasis]), and 3), nurse-sensitive procedural factors	Specific details not provided; data collected—body mass index, comorbidity, physician-sensitive procedurals, and nurse-sensitive procedural factors	Mean age within PICOT level; use of Perclose compared to manual pressure included; outcomes of interest addressed	Ethnicity not addressed

(continues)

Table 16-2 Documenting Aspects of Evidence-Based Practice: Use of Perclose for Angioplasty (continued)

Articles (Level of Evidence/Evaluation of Strength of the Evidence)	Who Is Involved (Sample Size, Sampling Method, Population)	What Occurred (Qualitative, Quantitative)	Where Completed (Type of Agency, State, Country)	When (Year Research Done)	Why (Research Question)	How (Data Collection, Tool Used with Validity and Reliability, Statistical Tests, Qualitative Control)	Consistencies (How It Addresses the PICOT Question, How Similar to Other Studies Reviewed)	Gaps (How It Does Not Address the PICOT Question, What Did the Researchers State Still Needed to Be Studied)
Lasic, Z., Nikolsky, E., Kesanakurthy, S., & Dangas, G. (2005). Vascular closure devices: A review of their use after invasive procedures. *American Journal of Cardiovascular Drugs,* 5(3), 185–200. Level of evidence: 5 Strength of evidence: B	Not a research article, so no sampling done	In-depth review of vascular closure devices	Not a research article	2005	Meta-analysis data related to complications and success rates; research reports discussed within the summary of the different closure devices	Not a research article	Outcomes related to Perclose usage provided	Not a research article, so no sampling done

Summary of Findings

Perclose can reduce length of stay and improve outcomes. Proper use of Perclose and consideration of prophylactic antibiotic therapy should be implemented. All of the reviewed articles were case studies; no quantitative research was found, and no nurse-directed research was located. The length of time before infections were identified ranged from 3 days to 4 weeks. Use of sterile technique during the procedure is paramount.

Application of Findings to Evidence-Based Practice That Validates or Changes Policies and Procedures
(Which policies and procedures does this information directly address and why?)

• All articles suggest prophylactic antibiotic use and strict adherence to the manufacturer's recommendations for ensuring a sterile surgical site.
• Emergency departments should review their policies concerning the assessment of post-angioplasty clients who present with vague symptoms, because the infection may be masked until it develops into a sepsis-type infection even as late as 4 weeks post procedure.
• Patient education should be addressed within policies to ensure that clients are taught to maintain a clean site at the incision area, to complete all antibiotic treatment ordered, and to report vague symptoms reflective of infections even up to 4 weeks post procedure.

Case Scenario 2

A school nurse wanted to determine if the placement of alcohol hand sanitizers within the elementary school buildings would decrease the incidence of illnesses. Illnesses for this project were based upon children's absentee patterns. The school nurse has to carefully consider the cost and instructional process that would be required as a result of the placement of these hand sanitizer units.

The case study analysis in **Table 16-3** reflects that research has not been adequately carried out within the elementary school population. Research is available for acute care settings and other healthcare settings but not successfully within this setting. A foundation is established that the use of hand sanitizers is effective for the management of illnesses. Gaps are evident within this case study. A foundation for the use of hand sanitizers can be established with the understanding that application to this setting would need to be verified.

Table 16-3

Documenting Aspects of Evidence-Based Practice: Handwashing in Elementary Schools

Questions to Consider Within the Evidence-Based Practice Process
P (Population of Interest):
I (Intervention of Interest):
C (Comparison of Interest):
O (Outcome of Interest):
T (Time):

Articles (Level of Evidence/Evaluation of Strength of the Evidence)	Who Is Involved (Sample Size, Sampling Method, Population)	What Occurred (Qualitative, Quantitative)	Where Completed (Type of Agency, State, Country)	When (Year Research Done)	Why (Research Question)	How (Data Collection, Tool Used with Validity and Reliability, Statistical Tests, Qualitative Control)	Consistencies (How It Addresses the PICOT Question, How Similar to Other Studies Reviewed)	Gaps (How It Does Not Address the PICOT Question, What Did the Researchers State Still Needed to Be Studied)
Vessey, J. A., Sherwood, J. J., Warner, D., & Clark, D. (2007). Comparing hand washing to hand sanitizers in reducing elementary school students' absenteeism. *Pediatric Nursing, 33*(4), 368–372. Level of evidence: 3 Strength of evidence: B	Sample size— Part I: 383, Part II: 13; Sampling method—Part I: randomized cross-over, Part II: convenient; Population— Part I: 2nd and 3rd graders, Part II: teachers, school nurses, and office personnel	Randomized cross-over design; mixed methods	Elementary schools in Butte, Montana	Not stated; published in 2007	Compare the efficacy of a hand sanitizer to standard hand washing in reducing illness and subsequent absenteeism in school-age children	Part 1: Data collected—absentee rates, two groups: cohort 1/phase 2—hand washing, cohort 2/phase 1—hand sanitizer; cohort switched in second phase; Part 2: focus group No tools were used, so no validity and reliability; Statistical test for part 1—t-test; Control for part 2—audit trail, audio-taped	Population correct for age; intervention and comparison included in this article	The outcome was not directly associated with this one; article looked at absenteeism

Citation				Published	Purpose		Intervention and comparison	Population and outcome
Foster, K. M., & Clark, A. P. (2008). Increasing hand hygiene compliance: A mystery? *Clinical Nurse Specialist*, 22(6), 263–267. Level of evidence: 1 Strength of evidence: B	6 articles Topic—hand hygiene compliance strategies	Meta-analysis	Literature review	Published 2008	The purpose of this article is to investigate some of the evidence-based strategies for increasing hand hygiene compliance, focusing on system-wide solutions to see if they might offer insight to the CNS and other organizational leaders	Articles were reviewed for study design/procedures, sample size/population, findings, and conclusions	Intervention and comparison aspects were present in the articles	Population and outcome not addressed
Fuller, C., Savage, J., Besser, S., Hayward, A., Cookson, B., Cooper, B., & Stone, S. (2011). "The dirty hand in the latex glove": A study of hand hygiene compliance when gloves are worn. *Infection Control and Hospital Epidemiology*, 32(12), 1194–1199. Level of evidence: 5 Strength of evidence: B	n = 56 Healthcare workers in medical or care of the elderly ward and ICUs	Observational study	15 hospitals across England and Wales	October 2006–November 2009	Carried out a study of glove use and associated hand hygiene behaviors	Observed hand hygiene and glove usage during 249 1-hour sessions Tool—hand hygiene observation tool, rigorously standardized and validated; Statistical test—proportions of moments and adjusted odds ratios used	Intervention, comparison, and outcome aspects addressed	Age group not addressed by this article

Table 16-3

Documenting Aspects of Evidence-Based Practice: Handwashing in Elementary Schools (continued)

Articles (Level of Evidence/Evaluation of Strength of the Evidence)	Who Is Involved (Sample Size, Sampling Method, Population)	What Occurred (Qualitative, Quantitative)	Where Completed (Type of Agency, State, Country)	When (Year Research Done)	Why (Research Question)	How (Data Collection, Tool Used with Validity and Reliability, Statistical Tests, Qualitative Control)	Consistencies (How It Addresses the PICOT Question, How Similar to Other Studies Reviewed)	Gaps (How It Does Not Address the PICOT Question, What Did the Researchers State Still Needed to Be Studied)
Haessler, S., Connelly, N. R., Kanter, G., Fitzgerald, J., Scales, M. E., Golubchik, A., Albert, M., & Gibson, C. (2010). A surgical site infection cluster: The process and outcome of an investigation—The impact of an alcohol-based surgical antisepsis product and human behavior. *Anesthesia Analgesia, 110*(4), 1044–1048. Level of evidence: 4 Strength of evidence: B	Sampling—convenience sampling; Sample size—77; Population—patients having an SSI according to National Healthcare Safety Network SSI criteria	Quality improvement methodology	Academic tertiary care medical and level 1 trauma center in New England	2007	The process by which quality improvement methodology was used to investigate and manage the surgical site infection cluster	Specific details not provided; data collected—body mass index, comorbidity, physician-sensitive procedurals, and nurse-sensitive procedural factors	Outcome addressed	Age, intervention and comparison not addressed

Summary of Findings (Consistencies and Gaps from All Articles)

The use of hand sanitizer can affect the number of illnesses reported by individuals. Research reports directed toward the use of these care items within an elementary school age population are not effectively documented at this time.

Application of Findings to Evidence-Based Practice That Validates or Changes Policies and Procedures

(Which policies and procedures does this information directly address and why?)

Policies within an elementary school setting that might need to be reviewed include:

- Instructions to provide to children regarding the proper way to use hand sanitizer systems
- Infection control measures that can be started
- Effective handwashing procedures

Note: CNS = clinical nurse specialist; ICUs = intensive care units; SSI = surgical site infection.

Critical Thinking Exercise

Multiple ideas related to potential clinical questions are provided for your consideration here. Select one of these situations to use in working through the process outlined in Table 16-1. The situations are presented in a brief manner in the following list. Take the chosen idea and develop a PICOT question to best meet the needs at a selected healthcare agency of your choice.

1. One possible clinical question relates to whether a relationship between adequate pain control and length of stay in a community hospital setting could be determined.

2. Another clinical situation for investigation involves the determination of any relationship between glucose control during the operative period and length of stay in an acute care setting.

3. An alternative clinical circumstance relates to the effect of a one-on-one diabetic education course on the patient's HbA1C level.

4. When a medication error occurs, the value of full disclosure to patients and/or family members in building trust and restoring confidence, as opposed to nondisclosure, with a look at the impact on perceived quality of care, could be investigated.

5. An additional idea involves determining whether the length of time and frequency of visits to patients' rooms by nursing staff affect the number of calls and the perception of quality of care by the patient and/or family members.

6. Maternal/child nurses understand that certain treatments (prophylactic eye treatments, vitamin K injections, phenylketonuria [PKU] tests) are provided for all newborn children. What happens to children born outside of an acute care setting (e.g., home births)? What rationales do we have to support these treatments?

7. Childhood immunization is a state-directed process that applies to all school-age children. Certain immunizations (measles–mumps–rubella [MMR], polio–diptheria–pertussis–tetanus [DPT]) are designated at key times prior to and during the school-age years. What is happening with the growing number of home-schooled children? Are they receiving these immunizations? What happens when these children come into acute care settings without having received the expected childhood immunization series?

Suggested Readings

Brody, A. A., Barnes, K., Ruble, C., & Sakowski, J. (2012). Evidence-based practice councils: Potential path to staff nurse empowerment and leadership growth. *Journal of Nursing Administration, 42*(1), 28–33.

Coopey, M., & Clancy, C. M. (2006). Translating research into evidence-based nursing practice and evaluating effectiveness. *Journal of Nursing Care Quality, 21*(3), 195–202.

Marchiondo, K. (2006). Planning and implementing an evidence-based project. *Nurse Educator, 31*(1), 4–6.

Newhouse, R. P. (2006). Examining the support for evidence-based nursing practice. *Journal of Nursing Administration, 36*(7–8), 337–340.

References

Bator, S., Taylor, S., & Catalano, J. T. (2015). Nursing research and evidence based practice. In J. Catalano (Ed.), *Nursing now! Today's issues, tomorrow's trends* (7th ed., pp. 581–674). Philadelphia, PA: F.A. Davis.

Dumont, C. J. (2007). Blood pressure and risks of vascular complications after percutaneous coronary intervention. *Dimensions of Critical Care Nursing, 26*(3), 121–127.

Finkelman, A., & Kenner, C. (2009). *Teaching IOM: Implications of the IOM reports for nursing education* (2nd ed.). Silver Spring, MD: American Nurses Association.

Foster, K. M., & Clark, A. P. (2008). Increasing hand hygiene compliance: A mystery? *Clinical Nurse Specialist, 22*(6), 263–267.

Fuller, C., Savage, J., Besser, S., Hayward, A., Cookson, B., Cooper, B., & Stone, S. (2011). "The dirty hand in the latex glove": A study of hand hygiene compliance when gloves are worn. *Infection Control and Hospital Epidemiology, 32*(12), 1194–1199.

Gawlinski, A., & Miller, P. S. (2011). Advancing nursing research through a mentorship program for staff nurses. *AACN Advanced Critical Care, 22*(3), 190–200.

Geary, K., Landers, J. T., Fiore, W., & Riggs, P. (2002). Management of infected femoral closure devices. *Cardiovascular Surgery, 10*(2), 161–163.

Haessler, S., Connelly, N. R., Kanter, G., Fitzgerald, J., Scales, M. E., Golubchik, A., Albert, M., & Gibson, C. (2010). A surgical site infection cluster: The process and outcome of an investigation—The impact of an alcohol-based surgical antisepsis product and human behavior. *Anesthesia Analgesia, 110*(4), 1044–1048.

Heck, D. V., Muldowney, S., & McPherson, S. H. (2002). Infectious complications of Perclose for closure of femoral artery punctures. *Journal of Vascular and Interventional Radiology, 13*(4), 430–431.

Institute of Medicine. (1999). *To err is human: Building a safer health system and the future of nursing.* Washington, DC: National Academy Press.

Lasic, Z., Nikolsky, E., Kesanakurthy, S., & Dangas, G. (2005). Vascular closure devices: A review of their use after invasive procedures. *American Journal of Cardiovascular Drugs, 5*(3), 185–200.

Malloch, K., & Porter-O'Grady, T. (2010). *Introduction to evidence-based practice in nursing and health care* (2nd ed.). Sudbury, MA: Jones and Bartlett.

Melnyk, B. M. (2003). Finding and appraising systematic reviews of clinical interventions: Critical skills for evidence-based practice. *Journal of Pediatric Nursing, 29*(2), *125*, 147–149.

Melnyk, B. M. (2012). Achieving a high-reliability organization through implementation of the ARCC model for systemwide sustainability of evidence-based practice. *Nursing Administration Quarterly, 36*(2), 127–135.

Melnyk, B. M., & Fineout-Overholt, E. (2015). *Evidence-based practice in nursing and healthcare: A guide to best practice* (3th ed.). Philadelphia, PA: Wolters Kluwer.

Myers, G., & Meccariello, M. (2006). From pet rock to rock-solid: Implementing unit-based research. *Nursing Management, 37*(1), 24–29.

Pravikoff, D. S., Tanner, A. B., & Pierce, S. T. (2005). Readiness of U.S. nurses for evidence-based practice. *American Journal of Nursing, 105*(9), 40–51.

Proehl, J. A., & Hoyt, K. S. (2012). Evidence versus standard versus best practice: Show me the data! *Advanced Emergency Nursing Journal, 34*(1), 1–2.

Sigma Theta Tau International (STTI). (2006). Results of EBN survey. Retrieved from an email dated June 12, 2006, from Sigma Theta Tau International Honor Society of Nursing. NurseAdvance: Knowledge Solutions.

Tiesenhausen, K., Tomka, M., Allmayer, T., Baumann, A., Hessinger, M., Portugaller, H., & Mahler, E. (2004). Femoral artery infection associated with a percutaneous arterial suture device. *VASA: European Journal for Vascular Medicine, 33*(2), 83–85.

Vessey, J. A., Sherwood, J. J., Warner, D., & Clark, D. (2007). Comparing hand washing to hand sanitizers in reducing elementary school students' absenteeism. *Pediatric Nursing, 33*(4), 368–372.

Whitmer, K., Auer, C., Beerman, L., & Weishaupt, L. (2011). Launching evidence-based nursing practice. *Journal for Nurses in Staff Development, 27*(2), E5–E7.

Yoder, L. (2005). Evidence-based practice: The time is now! *Medsurg Nursing, 14*(2), 91–92.

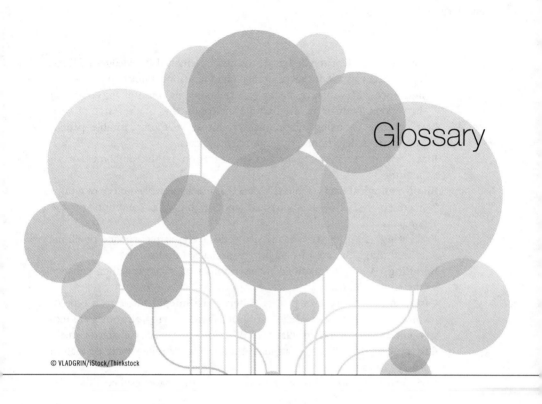

Glossary

© VLADGRIN/iStock/Thinkstock

Accessible data Data that can be linked into for use within a research study.

Accessible population Individuals and/or groups accessible for a specific participation study; frequently a nonrandom division of the target population.

Accuracy The correctness of the information used within the process.

Action research Applied research that is attentive to the resolution of nursing personnel's identified challenges.

Analysis of variance (ANOVA) Parametric statistical test used to determine the statistical differences between the means among two or more groups; another name for it is F-test; computed as either one-way or two-way.

Annotated bibliography A listing that summarizes the research and published information related to a given topic; presents a concise and succinct synopsis of the knowledge known on a topic.

Applied research Research that concentrates on resolving functional questions to supply reasonably direct solutions.

Associative hypothesis A hypothesis stated in a way that indicates that the variables exist side by side and that a change in one variable is accomplished by a change in another variable.

Autonomy The state of being free from influence; the ability to make informed decisions.

Basic research   Research designed to generate elemental knowledge and theoretic agreement about crucial human and foundational innate processes.

Beneficence   Maximizing possible benefits while minimizing potential harm to individuals involved within the conducting of a research project.

Best practice   Nursing action that produces the most desirable patient outcome, as determined through scientific data.

Bias   Any pressure that generates an alteration in the outcomes of an inquiry.

Biophysiological data   Objective data that use a specialized piece of equipment to establish the physical and/or biologic condition of the subjects.

Bracketing   To categorize or classify collectively; to incorporate or eliminate through the use of established specialized limitations.

Bundling   Multiple identified interventions that, taken together, enhance the clinical outcomes.

Case-controlled   Type of project pattern used in epidemiology; a type of observational analysis where two groups with varying outcomes are recognized and contrasted related to differing contributory characteristics.

Case report   The documentation of the aspects identified with a situation such as a case study.

Case series   Incorporates several case studies that have resulted in similar outcomes.

Case study   A qualitative research method that concentrates on supplying a comprehensive description and scrutiny of an identified case situation.

Categorical variable   A variable that diverges in type or kind but that has distinct values instead of values spaced along a continuum.

Causal hypothesis   A hypothesis stated in a way that indicates that one variable causes or brings about a change in another variable or variables.

Central tendency   Statistical qualities associated with quantitative data classified as the mean, median, or mode.

Chi-square   Statistical test employed to establish if an association recognized in a contingency table is statistically significant.

CINAHL   Cumulative Index to Nursing and Allied Health Literature; a database supplying reliable reporting of the literature associated with nursing and allied health.

Clinical decision making   The course of action by which a person resolves who needs what and when it is needed.

Clinical research   Research calculated to produce knowledge to direct nursing practice.

Closed-ended question   A question that is set up to force specific responses through the options provided within the question.

Cluster sampling   A method of sampling in which a sizable group is divided into consecutive subsampling of smaller units; a style of sampling in which groups are randomly selected.

Code of ethics   Underlying ethical assumptions that are recognized by a discipline or organization to direct researchers; management of the research related to the safe handling of human subjects.

Comparative design   A design that does not entail any manipulation or control of the independent variable, such that the dependent variable is the only variable measured in two or more groups.

Comparison group   A company of participants whose results related to a dependent variable classification are used as a foundation for appraising the results of the grouping of designated significance; phrase employed in place of "control group" for studies not applying an exact experimental plan.

Complex hypothesis   A statement that specifies the relationships between and among more than two variables.

Conceptual definition   Characterization of the identified word, variable, or activity from the dictionary-specific explanation of the term.

Concurrent validity   Verification that is based on the correlation between the calculated scores and criterion scores acquired at the same time.

Concurrently   Occurring at the same time (data or processes).

Confidence interval   A range of numbers assessed from the sample that has a specific likelihood or probability of containing the population limitation.

Confidentiality   Protection of study participants that results in the individuals' identities not being linked to the information they provided, meaning that the information can be provided only in the aggregate; not revealing the data collected from study participants to any person except the researcher and designated staff.

Confounding variable   A type of extraneous variable that is not controlled for; it regularly fluctuates with the independent variable and affects the dependent variable.

Consensus   Individuals involved in a process come to a common understanding about the topic; the majority of individuals reach an agreed upon resolution or understanding.

Consistency   The extent to which the equivalent outcome can be anticipated when measuring a variable more than a single time.

Construct validity   The degree to which a higher-order concept is characterized in a specific inquiry.

Content analysis   The practice of categorizing and combining qualitative results to establish the materializing premises and perceptions.

Content-related validity   The extent to which the details in a tool effectively characterize the totality of the content that needs to be included.

Contingency table   A table that places data in cells produced by the juncture of two or more categorical variables.

Continuous variable   A term that can take on a wide range of values, such as from 0 to 100, or larger.

Control   The procedure for managing the extraneous influences that could affect the dependent variable.

Control group Participants in an experiment who provide the baseline for the study, in contrast to the treatment group. Members of the control group do not receive the experimental treatment.

Convenience sampling The process of selecting individuals to be in the sample who are accessible and/or who volunteer; also called accidental sampling.

Convergent validity A type of construct validity.

Correlation coefficient The outcome of the calculation of the relationship between two or more observed scores.

Correlational design Any of a variety of nonexperimental research designs in which the primary independent variable of interest is a quantitative variable.

Covert Covered up, hidden. Covert data are collected without the subject having knowledge of the collection of the information.

Criterion The yardstick or benchmark used for predicting the accuracy of test scores.

Criterion-related validity Based on the comparison of the tests being used with some known criterion.

Critique An impartial, analytic, and reasonable appraisal of a research report.

Cross-validation A method for triangulating qualitative data by confirming the results through some other process.

Data collection The compilation and assembling of information related to concepts and variables in a reputable manner that facilitates answers for PICOT questions, research questions, and hypotheses leading to establishing outcomes.

Database An organized body of related information arranged for speed of access and retrieval.

Demographic variable A term that refers to characteristics of the subjects in the study.

Deontology Ethical theory connected with duties and rights; intrinsic nature or "rightness" of an action itself.

Dependent variable The outcome variable that is alleged to be influenced by one or more independent variables; the presumed outcome of the study.

Descriptive design A research study whose foremost intention is providing the truthful depiction of the distinctiveness of persons, situations, or groups and/or an accurate explanation or representation of the condition of a state of affairs or phenomenon.

Dichotomous variable A characteristic that can be measured only in the sense that it is present or not present; often assigned a number for identification purposes, rather than to represent a quantity.

Directional hypothesis A statement that predicts the path or direction that the relationship between variables will take.

Discrete variable A term that can take on only a finite number of values, usually restricted to whole numbers.

Discursive prose   Summary of material provided in a manner organized by themes or identified trend, not as a summary of different reports.

Editorials   Statements of the opinions of an owner, manager, or the like. Weight of the evidence is based on the perceived biases associated with the thoughts and statements.

Effect size   The expected strength of the relationship between the research variables; used in the calculation of desired sample size through power analysis.

Eligibility criteria   The conditions employed by a researcher to indicate the detailed characteristics of the target population that are used to select participants for a study.

Emic term   The point of view provided by the individuals directly involved in a situation.

Empiric   Established by inspection, experiment, or practice (data and/or results).

Equivalency reliability   A measure of reliability that is calculated in the same manner as the consistency and stability coefficients, except, instead of a single variable over two trials, the test is between two forms of a single test.

Ethical theories   A collection of ideology and philosophy of right behavior; a system of moral principles and ideals.

Ethics   The main beliefs, ideology, and guidelines that facilitate the maintenance of an issue that we appreciate and respect.

Ethnography   A type of qualitative research that conscientiously illustrates the customs of a grouping of individuals.

Evidence   Foundation on which beliefs and proofs are established; a pathway to clear and organized proof on a given topic.

Evidence-based practice (EBP)   A process of utilizing confirmed evidence (research and quality improvement), decision making, and nursing expertise to guide the delivery of holistic patient care.

Exclusion criteria   Characteristics that, if present, would make persons ineligible for participation in a study, even if they meet all of the other inclusion criteria.

Experimental design   Research in which the independent variable is manipulated, a control group is established, and randomized selection of the participants is employed to select who does and does not receive the treatment or intervention.

Expert opinion   Information provided by an individual who is viewed as an authority, based upon a set of criteria related to information applicable and/or significant to a designated problem or situation.

External validity   The degree to which the analysis outcomes can be generalized to a specific group of persons, settings, times, outcomes, and treatment variations.

Extraneous variable   A variable that confuses the association between the independent and dependent variables; for this reason, it needs to be restricted either within the research design or through statistical procedures.

Fidelity   Demonstration of loyalty and defense for a person, cause, or belief.

Focus group   A small group of people assembled to participate in a moderator-facilitated discussion geared toward the designated topic being researched.

Forensic science   The study of evidence; the process of utilizing data to formulate judgments and decisions.

Formative evaluation   An appraisal conducted to improve the evaluation process.

Framework   The conceptual foundation of a study; sometimes classified as a theoretic framework, for projects centered on a theory, and as a conceptual framework, for projects with a connection to a definite conceptual model.

Generalizability   The extent to which findings from a study can be extended from a sample of a population to the population at large.

Grounded theory   A general methodology for developing new theory that is based on data that are systematically gathered and analyzed.

Hawthorne effect   A change in a dependent variable that occurs as a result of the participants' recognition that they are engaged in a study.

Honesty   Integrity, truthfulness, and straightforwardness.

Hospital Care Quality Information from the Consumer Perspective (HCAHPS)   Nationwide, standardized, publicly reported appraisal of patients' perceptions of healthcare delivery.

Human experimentation   Medical testing performed on human beings with the expectation of gaining new knowledge to improve a situation or manage a health-related problem.

Hypothesis   A prediction or educated guess about the relationships among variables; the recognized proclamation of the researcher's prediction of the affiliation that exists among the variables under investigation.

Ideas   Thoughts, convictions, and/or principles based upon a potential or actual existing foundation, considered to be individual work.

Impact   The consequence or influence resulting from the use of a logic model.

In vitro   Requiring the extraction of physiologic materials from a participant in a research study, frequently via a laboratory analysis.

In vivo   Requiring the use of some apparatus to evaluate one or more elements of a participant in a research study.

Inclusion criteria   Characteristics that must be met to be considered for participation in a study; also known as eligibility criteria.

Independent variable   The variable in experimental research that is established as the cause or influence on the dependent variable; it may be identified as the manipulated (treatment) variable.

Informed consent   The decision of an individual to participate in a research study based on an understanding of the project's purpose, procedures, risks, benefits, alternative procedures, and limits of confidentiality.

Institutional review board (IRB)   A council of individuals representing an institution who assemble to evaluate the ethical considerations related to proposed and ongoing research studies.

Instrument   A tool that a researcher uses to accumulate information.

Integrative review   Summarization of prior research studies on a selected topic with a summation provided as a conclusion.

Interclass reliability   The reliability between two measures that are presented in the data as either variables or trials.

Internal validity   The capacity to conclude that a contributory affiliation exists between two or more variables.

Interval scale   Scale of measurement used in statistical analysis that incorporates both order and magnitude within the description but lacks a defined zero point.

Intervention   The experimental treatment or manipulation employed during a research endeavor.

Interview   A data collection technique in which an interviewer poses questions to the interviewee.

Intraclass reliability   A type of reliability that allows a person to develop a reliability coefficient for more than one variable.

Justice   The standard of decent rightness; agreement with truth, fact, or sensible intention.

Literature review   A rigorous examination of research related to a topic of interest that is documented to categorize a research problem or as the beginning of a research use project.

Logic model   A plan that denotes how an intervention produces distinct consequences using four aspects in a linear cycle: inputs, activities, outputs, and outcomes.

Longitudinal design   A study design in which information is accumulated at various times for use in comparisons.

Magnitude   The degree of size of a result or outcome.

Manipulation   An intervention or treatment initiated in an experimental or quasi-experimental study to assess the independent variable's impact on the dependent variable.

Mean   The mathematical average of a data set.

Median   The 50th percentile.

Medical Subject Heading (MeSH)   A glossary for finding the terms that correctly identify or agree with the search terms or concepts in the MEDLINE database; the controlled vocabulary for MEDLINE.

MEDLINE   Medical Literature Analysis and Retrieval System Online; the leading bibliographic database for retrieval of North American biomedical literature.

Meta-analysis   A process of quantitatively comparing the results from multiple research studies on a selected subject.

Meta-synthesis   The process for analyzing information to determine a conclusion from the facts.

Mixed methods research Also called multimethod research; a type of study in which a researcher uses qualitative research methodology for one phase of the study and quantitative research methodology for another phase of the study.

Mode The most frequently occurring number in a data set.

Morality What a person believes to be right and wrong and is shaped by what a person has been taught within society and their own culture.

National Center for Nursing Research (NCNR) A division within the National Institutes of Health that directs research efforts within the profession of nursing.

National Institute of Nursing Research (NINR) A division of the National Institutes of Health that focuses on funding nursing research projects and conducting studies to advance the professional of nursing.

National Institutes of Health (NIH) Biomedical research facility that oversees federally funded research projects directed toward health care.

Nesting A collection of comparable ideas and processes related to the management of research projects.

Nominal scale A level of measurement that applies symbols, such as numbers, to describe, categorize, or recognize people or objects.

Nondirectional hypothesis A statement that predicts a relationship between variables but not the path or direction of that relationship.

Nonequivalent control group A research sampling method where random selection is not used to determine the membership of the control group.

Nonexperimental design A research study in which data are collected without introducing any treatment, and no random assignment of participants to groups occurs.

Nonmaleficence A bioethics principle directed toward the expectation of not inflicting intentional harm when dealing with individuals.

Nonprobability sampling A sampling strategy that does not include random selection of elements.

Nonsignificant results The outcome of a statistical test demonstrating that the connection between variables could have transpired as a consequence of chance, at the designated level of significance.

Novel data New data collected as part of a research study.

Null hypothesis A prediction or educated guess that no relationship exists between the designated variables.

Objectivity The degree to which two researchers working independently would reach comparable findings or conclusions.

Observation Inconspicuous surveillance of people as they engage in everyday activities.

Observed score The actual score seen and/or printed by the instrument or tool.

Obstacle Something that resists, hampers the forward progress of, or reroutes movement in a certain way or path.

Open-ended questions Questions that permit the respondent to answer without any restrictions or barriers.

Operational definition The characterization of a concept or variable in terms of the operations or procedures by which it is to be measured for a specific research endeavor.

Opinions Attitudes and viewpoints that do not rest on adequate foundations to be viewed as completely without biases, and represent a person's beliefs, judgments, and/or values concerning a designated subject.

Ordinal scale A rank-order level of measurement.

Outcomes Results that proceed from an accomplishment or achievement; effects; consequences.

Outputs The work or practice of delivering a result.

Patient-oriented research Studies carried out with human subjects where a researcher openly interrelates with the participants.

Phenomenology A type of qualitative research in which the researcher endeavors to comprehend how individuals experience a phenomenon.

PICOT The five components of an evidence-based question: patient population of interest, intervention of interest, comparison of interest, outcome of interest, and time.

Population The complete group of individuals (or objects) possessing various characteristics to which a researcher wants to generalize the sample results; sometimes referred to as the universe population or target population.

Population-based research Studies incorporating epidemiology, social and behavioral sciences, public health, quality evaluation, and cost-effectiveness.

Predictive validity A characteristic based on the time between the collection of the alternative method tests to be validated and the criterion measured. It does not limit the researcher to using the Pearson Product Moment (PPM) to develop a validity coefficient, as a linear or logistic regression can also be used.

Primary data Information and/or data collected and/or observed directly from the project.

Primary sources First-hand testimony to facts, findings, or events; reporting of the research results structured by the individual who conducted the study.

Probability sampling Use of a specific sampling strategy using some form of random selection of elements.

Problem statement A declaration of the research problem, occasionally verbalized in the form of a research question.

Purposeful sampling Selecting of sample participants in a meaningful and direct way to ensure the representation within the sample members.

Purposive sampling A nonprobability sampling process in which the researcher chooses study participants based on personal decisions about which individuals would be most representative of the general population; also identified as judgmental sampling.

Qualitative analysis Examination and investigation using subjective reasoning established on nonquantifiable data.

Qualitative research The analysis of phenomena, characteristically in a comprehensive and holistic manner, through the compilation of abundant narrative notes based on an adaptable research model.

Qualitative research question An inquisitive sentence that poses a query about a selected practice, concern, or phenomenon to be investigated.

Quality assurance An orderly practice of examining a product or service to determine if it meets precise requirements.

Quality improvement A process utilized to investigate a policy, procedure, or protocol to determine if it addresses an aspect identified through an evidence-based practice process, and works to validate current practice.

Quality improvement (QI) project A project that is conducted to increase the effectiveness of the activities and processes used within a setting.

Quantitative analysis The numeric representation and manipulation of observations using statistical techniques for the express purpose of describing and explaining the outcomes of research as they pertain to the hypothesis.

Quantitative design The scrutinizing of a phenomenon that contributes to the collection of meticulous measurement and quantification, while using a painstaking and manipulative strategy.

Quantitative research Systematic, empirical investigation of observable activities using statistical measures to reach a conclusion.

Quasi-experimental design An experimental research design in which individuals are not randomly assigned to groups, but rather the researcher manipulates the independent variable and implements specific controls to augment the internal validity of the outcome.

Questionnaire A self-report data collection tool completed by research participants.

Quota sampling A nonrandom selection of participants by which the researcher identifies specific properties and/or characteristics that are used to establish the sample and determines sample size for the groups to increase their representativeness.

Random sampling Selection of a sample such that every member of a population has an equal possibility of being included in the sample.

Random selection Picking a group of individuals from a population where every member of the population has an equal chance of being included in the sample.

Randomization A selection system that creates assignments in a manner that augments the probability that the comparison groups will be equivalent on all extraneous variables.

Range The variation between the uppermost and lowest numbers in a data set.

Ranking The arranging of responses into ascending or descending sequence.

Ratio scale A level of measurement that has a true zero position, while also having the characteristics of the nominal (labeling), ordinal (rank ordering), and interval (equal distance) scales.

Receiver operand characteristics (ROC) A graphical chart illustrating the functioning of data points.

Reference librarian An information professional educated and qualified in library and information science, particularly in the area of collection of specialized or technical information or materials.

Reliability The extent to which a tool measures the attribute it is intended to evaluate; a measure of consistency.

Representative sample A sample that bears a resemblance to the target population.

Research A methodical examination that uses regimented techniques to resolve questions or decipher dilemmas.

Research articles Published manuscripts describing the results of research projects.

Research design The inclusive design for addressing a research question that incorporates the outline, plan, or strategy used to enhance the integrity of the study.

Research hypothesis A testable statement that predicts the relationship between two or more variables in a population of interest.

Research process Methodical process of conducting exploration and examination of an identified question.

Research question A statement of the particular inquiry the researcher desires to resolve through a research endeavor.

Research utilization The application of selected facets of a scientific analysis through a process unconnected to the fundamental research.

Researcher bias An intentional or unintentional manipulation of a study so that it achieves results consistent with what the researcher intends to uncover.

Respect The process of showing honor or appreciation; motivation to demonstrate thoughtfulness or gratitude.

Response rate The proportion of individuals in a sample who participate in a research project.

Retrospective research The analysis of existing data to address the question to be answered.

Rigor Firmness or precision.

Root cause analysis An approach for recognizing aspects involved in understanding what impacted the development of a harmful outcome in order to detect behaviors and/or actions useful in preventing recurrence of similar harmful outcomes.

Sample A division of a population chosen to participate in a study.

Sample size The number of individuals included in a sample; denoted by n.

Sampling The practice of extracting a designated group from a population.

Sampling bias Misrepresentations that occur when a sample is not representative of the target population from which the group was extracted.

Sampling error   The variation between a sample statistic and a population parameter.

Sampling interval   The total number within the target population divided by the preferred sample size; denoted by k.

Sampling plan   The plan for selection of the study participants proposed prior to the beginning of the study; it specifies the eligibility criteria, the sample selection process, and, in the case of quantitative studies, the number of subjects to be used.

Saturation   In qualitative research, the point at which sufficient data have been accumulated for all new data to produce redundant information.

Search engine   A web-based tool providing access to needed data. It takes a person to the information and helps to retrieve the information in a format that is accessible visually on screen at an on-site library or in downloadable written/readable format.

Secondary analysis   Data initially accumulated by various persons for a purpose other than the present research.

Secondary data   Data initially accumulated by various persons for a purpose other than the present research.

Secondary source   Second-hand explanation of proceedings or facts; explanation of a study or studies organized by someone other than the primary researcher.

Sensitivity   Frequency that a test will measure a "true" positive results when calculated.

Sentinel events   Unanticipated episodes resulting in a death or grave physical or psychological injury, or the risk thereof.

Simple hypothesis   A statement that specifies the relationship between two variables.

Simple random sampling   A population group extracted by a formula in which each member of the population has an equivalent possibility of being chosen.

Snowball sampling   A type of sampling in which every research contributor is asked to recommend additional prospective research participants; also referred to as network sampling.

Specificity   Determination of the capability of a test to establish a "true" negative result.

Stability   The determination of the results from trials and/or tests over a set time period that extends greater than 48 hours.

Standard error of measurement (SEM)   A statistic that reflects the fluctuation of the observed score due to the error score.

Statistical Package for the Social Sciences (SPSS)   A computer program used for statistical analysis; the initial program was made available in 1968.

Statistical significance   An idiom demonstrating that it is improbable that the results achieved in an examination of sample data would have been produced by luck at a particular level of probability.

Stratified random sampling A random selection of study participants from two or more levels of the population.

Subject A person who supplies information in a study. This term is predominantly used in quantitative research studies.

Systematic random sampling The selection of research study participants such that each kth individual (or facet) in a sampling frame is selected.

Systematic review A literature review directed by a research question that strives to recognize, evaluate, and integrate relevant research evidence.

t-test Statistical method used to determine the differences between the means of two groups.

Target population The total population to whom the research outcomes are to be generalized.

Teleology The use of final intention or design as a method of explaining phenomena within an ethical situation.

Tests Devices used to determine the selected intelligence, talents, behaviors, health status, or cognitive endeavor that is under investigation.

Theoretical sampling The qualitative research process of selecting new study participants based on emerging findings from previous data collection and analysis; followed until the point of data saturation.

Theory A rationalization that challenges how a phenomenon functions and why it functions as it does; a generalization or series of generalizations employed methodically to clarify certain phenomena.

Time-dimensional analysis A research tactic employing the investigation into the implications of patterns of change, growth, or trends across time.

Translational research Using both basic and applied research findings to ensure that best practices are incorporated within a population.

Trustworthiness An expression used in the appraisal of qualitative data; it is measured based on the decisive factors of credibility, transferability, dependability, and confirmability.

Validity The extent to which a research tool measures what it is proposed to measure.

Variable A characteristic of a person or entity that fluctuates.

Veracity Accuracy, truthfulness.

Vulnerable subjects Distinct groups of individuals whose rights require particular protection because of their inability to grant informed consent or because their state of affairs consigns them to higher-than-average risk of adverse effects from a proposed treatment or intervention.

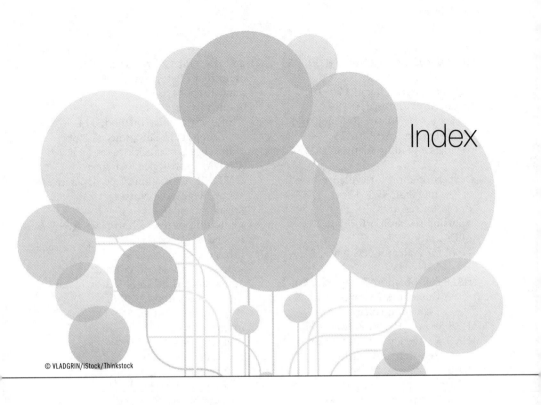

Index

Note: Page numbers followed by b, f, and t indicate material in boxes, figures, and tables respectively.